ESSENTIALS OF ANESTHESIA

Edited by:

Stefan Novevski

ALLIED HEALTH PRESS

Essentials of Anesthesia

Editor: **Stefan Novevski**

Allied Health Press
4164 Lakeshore Road
Burlington ON L7L 1A4
Canada
www.alliedhealthpress.com
Email: orders@arclereducation.com

ISBN: 978-1-77956-222-7

ABOUT THE EDITOR

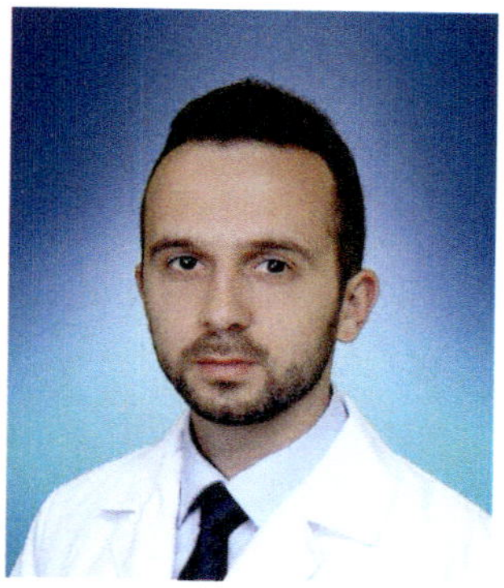

Stefan Novevski is a licensed veterinarian with 4 years of experience as a practitioner, currently working in a new up-to-date veterinary clinic that specializes in working with companion animals. His professional interests and continued education are aimed at working with small animals and he has a passion for reading, writing and researching different topics regarding veterinary medicine. His areas of interests include: internal medicine, obstetrics, pet nutrition, dermatology and animal welfare and behavior. He is dedicated to always staying up-to-date with newest research and is committed to practicing evidence-based veterinary medicine. During his studies and after obtaining his license, he gains first-hand experience in various fields of the veterinary industry through practical work, attending seminars and workshops, and international travel to other universities and private veterinary clinics. From 2023 he is a member of MSAVA (Macedonian Small Animal Veterinary Association).

Word Roots, Prefixes, and Suffixes by Chapter

Chapter 1 Introduction to Anesthesia

bacteri- bacteria
anti- against
Brady- slow
-esthesia sensation
-scopy visual examination

Chapter 2 Basic Pharmacologic Principles

Hypo- under, below
cavir - carbocyclic nucleosides
fenacin - muscarinic receptor antagonists
-ane Inhaled anesthetics
-tomy cutting

Chapter 3 Inhaled Anesthetics

pharyng/o pharynx
capn/o carbon dioxide
arteri(o)- of or pertaining to an artery
atri- an atrium (esp. heart atrium)
-asthenia weakness

Chapter 4 Intravenous Anesthetics

plasm/o plasma
pneum/o,pneumon/o lung, air
epi- on, upon, over
juxta- near, beside

Chapter 5 Local Anesthetics

aort/o Aorta
ather/o Yellowish, fatty plaque
echo- reflected sound
-esthesia nervous sensation

Chapter 6 Anesthetic Neurotoxicity

Myelo spinal cord
Dendr tree, branching, referring to dendrites
Hyper- over, excessive
Inter- between
-opathy disease or disorder

Chapter 7 Anesthesia Delivery Systems

gastr Stomach
enceph Brain
general- whole, entire
narco- numbness, stupor
-ine Amino acid

Chapter 8 Spinal, Epidural, and Caudal Anesthesia

Myel spinal cord
Caud tail
Lumb loin, lower back
Intra- within
-otomy cutting into

Chapter 9 Outpatient Anesthesia

Pre- Before
Post- After
Epidural- Upon the dura mater
Surg- Surgical repair
Analges- Pain relief

Chapter 10 Anesthesia for Trauma

Traum- Injury, wound
Lacer- Tear, rip
-oma Tumor, swelling
Osteo- Bone
Contus- Bruise
Pneumo- Lung, air

Table of Contents

LIST OF FIGURES

LIST OF TABLES

PREFACE

General anesthesia is a crucial component of modern medical practice, allowing for complex surgeries and procedures to be performed with patient comfort and safety.

This text "Essentials of Anesthesia" provides a comprehensive approach to the principles and practice of anesthesia for medical students, residents, and practicing anesthesiologists. This book aims to offer a thorough understanding of the basic concepts, techniques, and challenges involved in administering anesthesia, ensuring safe and effective patient care.

The book begins with an overview of the history and evolution of anesthesia, setting the stage for a detailed exploration of the pharmacology of anesthetic agents and their mechanisms of action. It covers the physiological and pharmacological principles underlying anesthesia, including anesthesia delivery systems, monitoring techniques, and perioperative care.

It also addresses the management of specific patient populations, such as pediatric, geriatric, and obstetric patients, highlighting the unique considerations and challenges involved in providing anesthesia to these groups. It emphasizes the importance of a multidisciplinary approach to anesthesia care, involving collaboration with surgeons, nurses, and other healthcare professionals to ensure optimal patient outcomes.

Throughout the book, key concepts are reinforced with clinical scenarios, case studies, and review questions to help readers apply their knowledge in real-world situations. The goal is to equip readers with the knowledge and skills necessary to provide safe, compassionate, and effective anesthesia care across a wide range of clinical settings. Integrating theoretical knowledge with practical insights, "Essentials of Anesthesia" aims to be a valuable resource for anyone involved in the field of anesthesia, from students and residents to experienced practitioners seeking to enhance their understanding and skills.

Chapter

INTRODUCTION TO ANESTHESIA

1

Contents

Introduction

A fundamental component of contemporary medicine, anesthesia produces a reversible state of unconsciousness, analgesia (pain relief), amnesia (memory loss), and muscle relaxation, all of which are necessary for surgical interventions and other medical procedures. Since its inception, this vital medical specialty has undergone significant evolution, completely changing the way that surgery and patient care are provided. Throughout ancient times, herbal remedies, alcohol, and even violent blows to the head were used as crude means of putting surgical patients to sleep. However, the development of ether and chloroform in the 19th century marked the beginning of the modern anesthesia era, allowing for painless surgeries and a dramatic decrease in patient suffering and death.

A set of fundamental principles that are intended to ensure patient safety, comfort, and ideal surgical conditions guide the practice of anesthesia. Anesthesiologists carefully assess patients before surgery, taking into account their health history, present condition, and the needs of the particular procedure in order to create customized anesthetic regimens. In the operating room, anesthesiologists use a variety of methods to induce and sustain anesthesia, such as intravenous drugs, nerve blocks, and epidurals, as well as inhalational agents. They keep a close eye on the patient's vital signs, the depth of anesthesia, and their responses throughout the process, adjusting as needed to maximize results and reduce risks.

Anesthesia encompasses perioperative care from preoperative assessment to postoperative recovery, and it doesn't stop in the operating room. Anesthesiologists are essential in controlling pain, avoiding complications, and guaranteeing a seamless transition between surgical stages. In addition, practicing anesthesia requires a thorough understanding of pharmacology, physiology, and patient management in addition to expert abilities in resuscitation, airway management, and crisis intervention. To provide comprehensive, patient-centered care, anesthesiologists work closely with surgical teams, nurses, and other medical specialists. Summing up, anesthesia is fundamental to contemporary medicine because it allows safe and efficient surgical procedures while putting the comfort, health, and success of the patient first.

Orientation and Directional Terms

Term	Definition	Illustration
Anesthesiologists	Anesthesiologists are medical doctors just like your primary care physician and surgeon. They specialize in anesthesia care, pain management, and critical care medicine, and have the necessary knowledge to understand and treat the entire human body.	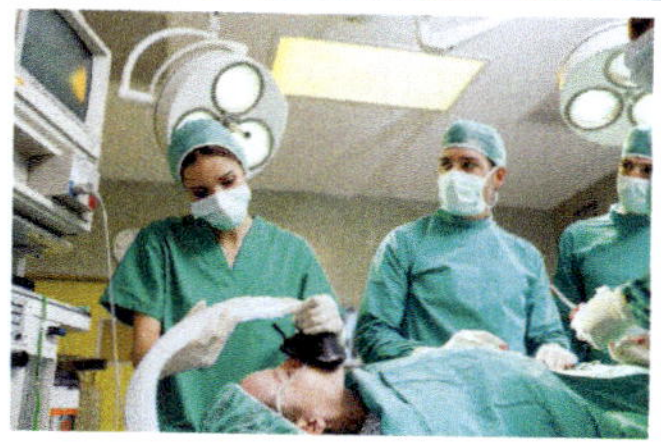
Halothane	Halothane is a general inhalation anesthetic used for induction and maintenance of general anesthesia. It reduces blood pressure and frequently decreases the pulse rate and depresses respiration. It induces muscle relaxation and reduces pain sensitivity by altering tissue excitability.	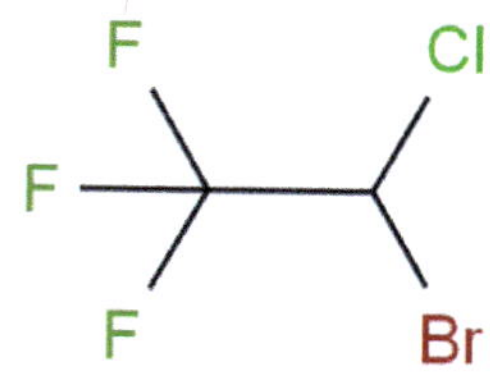
Laryngoscopy	A laryngoscopy is a procedure healthcare providers use to examine your larynx (voice box). This is performed with a laryngoscope, a thin tube with a light, lens and a video camera that helps providers look closely at your larynx.	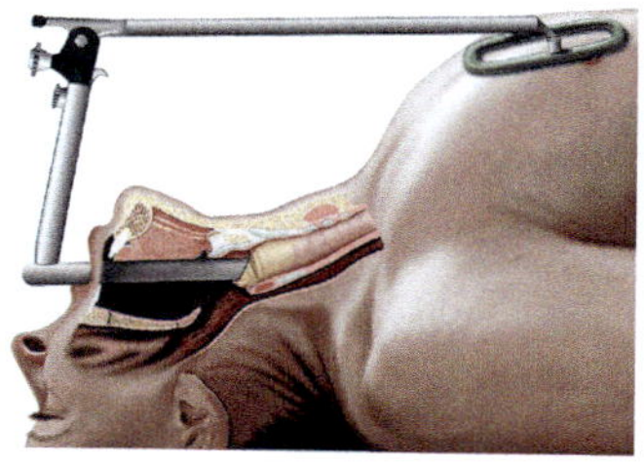
Obstetric anesthesia	Obstetric anesthesia also known as ob-gyn anesthesia or ob-gyn anesthesiology, is a sub-specialty of anesthesiology that provides peripartum pain relief (analgesia) for labor and anesthesia for cesarean deliveries	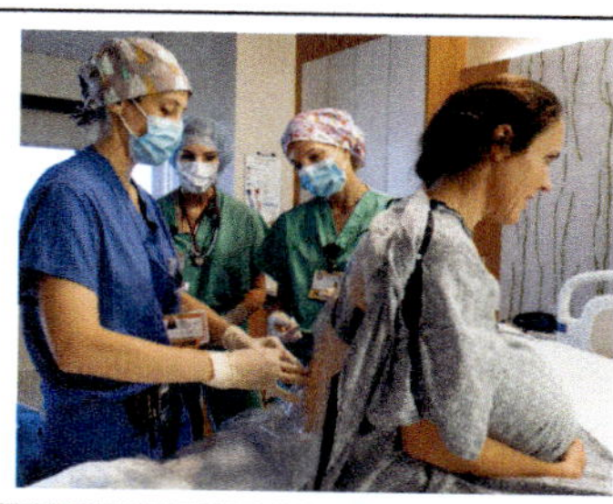
Anesthesia Information Management System (AIMS)	Anesthesia Information Management System (AIMS) is a software product that generates the medical record for an anesthesia encounter, including the pre-operative, intra-operative, and post-operative documentation.	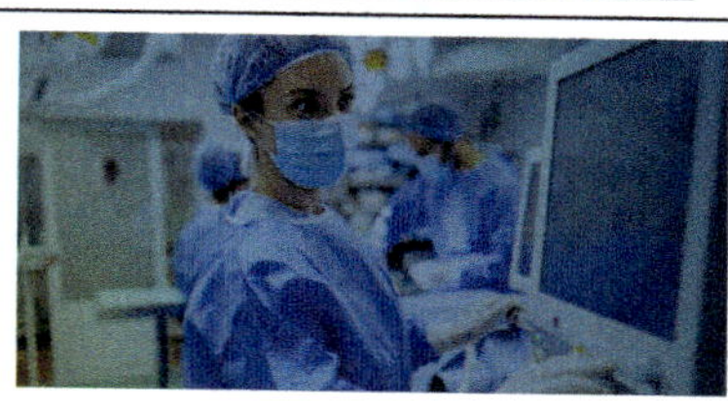

1.1. Anesthesia

Anesthesia is a medically induced state of controlled, transient loss of sensation or awareness. It may involve some or all of the following: amnesia (loss of memory), paralysis (relaxation of the muscles), analgesia (relief from or prevention of pain), and unconsciousness. An anesthetist is a person who administers anesthesia; the person under the influence of drugs is referred to as an anesthetized person.

1.1.1. Anesthetist

Physician specialists known as anesthetists are in charge of giving patients anesthesia during surgeries and other treatments. Anesthetists also provide pain management and critical care in addition to a variety of other practices that go beyond anesthesia for surgery. In NHS hospitals, anesthetists make up the majority of the specialty medical group. Following their qualification, these physicians made the decision to pursue at least seven years of postgraduate specialty training in pain management, intensive care medicine, and anesthesia.

An anesthetist cares for you during your operation and will:

- Discuss types of anesthesia with you and help you to make choices
- Discuss the risks of anesthesia with you
- Agree on a plan with you for your anesthetic and pain control
- Be responsible for giving you your anesthetic and for your wellbeing and safety throughout your procedure
- Manage any blood transfusions you may need
- Plan your care, if needed, in the Intensive Care Unit or High Dependency Unit
- Make your experience as calm and pain free as possible

In an attempt to reduce surgical pain, nitrous oxide, ether, chloroform, and ethyl chloride were tested in the 19th century. By today's standards, the technique used to administer these anesthetics was deemed extremely archaic. A significant advancement occurred when a device was developed that could regulate the amount of oxygen and nitrous oxide that flowed.

Prolonged administration of anesthetic agents, especially chloroform, resulted in significant physiological harm to the patients due to their toxicity. The use of chloroform became considerably less common after the discovery of trichlorethylene, also known as trilene. Despite being significantly safer, it still had a significant drawback in that it could not be utilized with a "closed circuit" anesthetic technique. When trilene passes through the chemical soda lime, which absorbs CO_2, it produces phosgene, a highly hazardous gas. Since 1945, a vastly different technique for putting patients to sleep has been extensively used. This technique is based on the finding that an intravenous injection of a refined extract of a naturally occurring poison called "curare" can be administered safely. It acts on the patient's neuromuscular system, causing a relaxation of the muscles. This means that different levels of physiological paralysis can be reached to perform more intricate surgery. When this technique is used for deep anesthesia, the patient's lungs become paralyzed, and the anesthetist must maintain the patient's life through carefully regulated artificial lung ventilation.

Sometimes, the extreme anesthesia used in modern surgery techniques necessitates many hours of anesthesia for the patient. In the past, the anesthetist found this to be an extremely difficult task that posed a significant risk to the patients' bodily integrity. Today's anesthetist has access to a wide range of advanced, dependable, patient, and gas monitoring devices. Thanks to the widely available compact gas analyzers, there is now even more control over the administration of anesthetic agents. These are able to track both the patient's inhaled gases and their exhaled gases. Surgical anesthesia is a drug-induced, reversible state of unconsciousness that suppresses enough reflexes to enable an operation to be carried out. The aforementioned statement makes clear that two prerequisites must be met to reach the state of surgical anesthesia. First and foremost, the patient should be unconscious, as this is all that matters to them! Next, there should be a slight reduction in muscular reflex activity, which the surgeon requires in order to perform delicate work. When an anesthetic is used in large enough doses for extended periods of time, overdose levels are reached, which can be fatal. Four stages can be distinguished in the progressive reflex depression of the central nervous system, starting from the moment the first discernible effect is produced and ending with a fatal overdose.

1.1.1.1 Stages of Anesthesia Based on Guedel's Classification

- ***Stage 1 - Analgesia or Disorientation*:** In a preoperative anesthesiology holding area, this stage can be started when the patient receives medication and may start to feel its effects, but they have not yet fallen unconscious. Typically, this phase is referred to as the induction stage. Despite being sedated, patients can converse. Breathing occurs steadily and slowly. At this point, the patient moves from analgesia without amnesia to analgesia and amnesia at the same time. The loss of consciousness marks the end of this phase.
- ***Stage 2 - Excitement or Delirium*:** Disinhibition, delirium, uncontrollable movements, loss of eyelash reflex, hypertension, and tachycardia are characteristics of this stage. During this stage, airway reflexes are still functional but frequently oversensitive to stimulation. It is best to refrain from performing any airway manipulation while under this level of anesthesia, including deep suctioning techniques and the insertion and removal of endotracheal tubes. At this point, laryngospasm—the involuntary tonic closure of the vocal cords—is more likely to occur, and any airway manipulation may make it worse. Consequently, the patient's airway may be compromised by the confluence of vomiting, spastic movements, and rapid, irregular breathing. Fast-acting agents make it easier to enter stage 3 and help minimize the amount of time spent in stage 2.
- ***Stage 3 – Surgical Anesthesia*:** When performing procedures that call for general anesthesia, this is the targeted anesthetic level. This stage is characterized by reduced respiratory depression and relaxed eye movements. At this point, airway manipulation is safe. For this stage, four planes are described. Constricted pupils, central gaze, and regular spontaneous breathing are all present during plane 1. Nonetheless, in this plane, the swallow, conjunctival, and eyelid reflexes typically vanish. In plane

2, there are sporadic respiratory arrests and a loss of laryngeal and corneal reflexes. There may also be an increase in lacrimation and halted ocular movements. The loss of the pupillary light reflex and total relaxation of the abdominal and intercostal muscles characterize plane 3. Because it works well for the majority of surgeries, this plane is known as true surgical anesthesia. Lastly, Plane 4 is characterized by complete diaphragm paralysis leading to apnea, paradoxical rib cage movement, and irregular breathing.

- ***Stage 4 - Overdose*:** This stage happens when an already severe brain or medullary depression gets worse due to the administration of an excessive amount of anesthetic agent in comparison to the amount of surgical stimulation. This phase lasts from the cessation of breathing to the possibility of death. At this point, the pupils are fixed and dilated, and the skeletal muscles are flaccid. The suppression of the cardiac pump and peripheral bloodstream vasodilation cause blood pressure to be significantly lower than normal and pulses to be weak and thready. This stage is fatal without cardiovascular and respiratory support. Because of this, the anesthetist's objective is to get the patient into stage 3 anesthesia as quickly as possible and maintain them there throughout the procedure.

1.1.2. General Anaesthetic Agents

1.1.2.1. Nitrous Oxide

Gas that is compressible and turns into liquid. Not flammable or explosive. A weak anesthetic agent with low toxicity. It served as the only anesthetic used during outpatient or dental procedures. When combined with other anesthetics, it can be used to maintain anesthesia during major surgery; however, it is not used by itself to achieve a deep level of anesthesia. Used on patients typically in a ratio of two-thirds nitrous oxide to one-third oxygen. In dentistry and obstetrics, nitrous oxide is used as an analgesic agent in an equal mixture with oxygen.

1.1.2.2. Halothane

Not flammable or explosive. Strong, organic compound with a heavy vapor costly; typically utilized in closed-circuit systems. It is vaporized using specialized equipment that can produce a known, calibrated concentration even at low anesthesia levels, and lowers blood pressure.

1.1.2.3. Non Anesthetic Gases

- Oxygen

  A concentration of roughly 21% is found in the atmosphere. While it cannot catch fire, its existence will facilitate burning. Exploding when exposed to oil or grease and under pressure. Patients shouldn't receive dosages greater than 40% of this medication.

- Carbon Dioxide

  It will deepen breathing by stimulating it, but not speed up the process. Used occasionally following surgery when spontaneous respiration fails to occur. When added in small amounts to the overall gas mixture being given, it can also help ensure a smooth induction of anesthetic agents. (i.e., decreases the patient's resistance to breathing in the anesthetic agent when used briefly before using nitrous oxide and oxygen.

1.1.3. Anaesthetic Equipment

1917 saw the development of the Boyles apparatus (on the left) explain more precisely where this boyles apparatus is. It was among the most often utilized anesthetic equipment kinds in the operating room. It works on the principle of continuous flow, in which gas flows continuously during the patient's inspiratory and expiratory phases of breathing, temporarily accumulating in a reservoir bag during expiration. The Boyles apparatus, though antiquated, remains in use in numerous hospitals and forms the basis for the majority of gas apparatus used today.

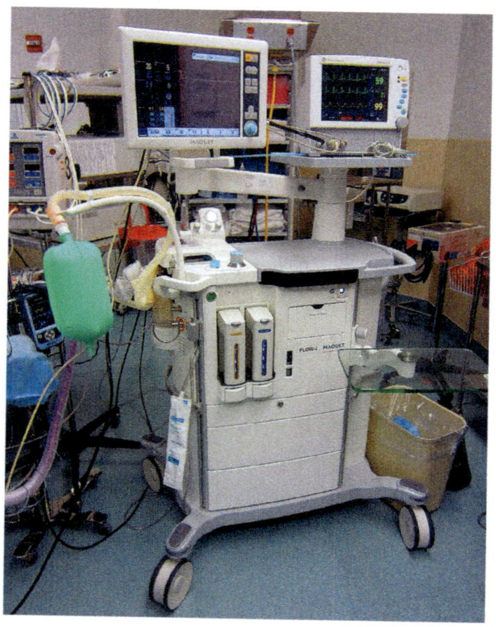

Figure 1.1. *Anesthetic equipment.*

Source: By DiverDave - Own work, CC BY-SA 3.0, https://commons.wikimedia.org/w/index.php?curid=19899416.

Gas anesthesia has been understood for more than a century and continues to be utilized today. The patient receives an anaesthetizing agent through flow controllers and mix controllers. Typically, a combination of nitrous oxide and oxygen is used to transport the primary agent, such as Halothane (Figure 1.1).

1.1.4. Systemic Effects of General Anesthesia

Physiological changes occur in multiple systems when under general anesthesia. Different anesthetic agents are preferred in different clinical contexts due to the varying systemic effects of the drugs used. Because of vasodilation, negative inotropy and chronotropy, and intravenous (propofol and thiopentone) and volatile agents all lower blood pressure in general. By obstructing the venous return to the heart, positive pressure ventilation (i.e., ventilating someone) can lower cardiac output and preload. Surgery's sympathetic stimulation is in opposition to these modifications. All respiratory depressants, including propofol, thiopentone, and etomidate, as well as volatile agents, weaken airway reflexes to varying degrees.

Propofol is especially good at causing brief apnea and lowering airway reflexes, which makes it easier to place supraglottic devices after induction. Sevoflurane is the least irritating to the respiratory system among volatile agents, which makes it ideal for gaseous induction and pediatric patients. Since desflurane irritates the airway, it is frequently used after anesthesia has been established.

Being bronchodilators, sevoflurane and isoflurane may even be used to treat brittle asthma. Ketamine is a unique intravenous medication because, in addition to its analgesic effects, it also preserves muscular tone, airway patency, and bronchodilates. Known as a "dissociative anesthetic," it allows the patient to be partially unconscious but with some degree of awareness and detachment from their environment. Due to its qualities, it can be helpful in field anesthesia, the developing world, and patients with hemodynamic instability.

1.1.5. Emergence and Recovery

After the anesthesia is no longer needed, the maintenance agents can be turned off. It is important to ensure adequate analgesia and anti-emesis before the patient emerges, and to restore neuromuscular junction function if a muscle relaxant is used. Emergence can be a time of physiological disturbances, as patients may experience agitation, laryngospasm, and breath-holding as they wake from anesthesia. Extubation is typically carried out after oropharyngeal suction, when the patient is breathing well, awake, and has regained airway reflexes. In some cases, extubation may be done while the patient is still under anesthesia to reduce the risk of complications such as coughing, laryngospasm, and hypertension. However, this leaves the airway unprotected against aspiration until the patient wakes up. The recovery room serves as a transitional space between the operating room and the ward, where immediate issues can be addressed, and vital signs, pain levels, and potential complications can be monitored (American Board of Anesthesiology; Adler-Milstein et al., 2015; Galvez et al., 2015)

1.2. Definition of Anesthesiology as a Specialty

A more formal definition of the specialty of anesthesiology is provided by The American Board of Anesthesiology (ABA). The ABA defines anesthesiology as a discipline within the practice of medicine dealing with but not limited to:

- Assessment of, consultation for, and preparation of patients for anesthesia.
- Relief and prevention of pain during and following surgical, obstetric, therapeutic, and diagnostic procedures.
- Monitoring and maintenance of normal physiology during the perioperative period.
- Management of critically ill patients including those receiving their care in an intensive care unit.
- Diagnosis and treatment of acute, chronic, and cancer-related pain.
- Management of hospice and palliative care.
- Clinical management and teaching of cardiac, pulmonary, and neurologic resuscitation.
- Evaluation of respiratory function and application of respiratory therapy.
- Conduct of clinical, translational, and basic science research.
- Supervision, instruction, and evaluation of performance of both medical and allied health personnel involved in perioperative or periprocedural care, hospice and palliative care, critical care, and pain management.
- Administrative involvement in health care facilities and organizations, and medical schools as appropriate to the ABA's mission.

The medical specialty board, the American Board of Anesthesiology (ABA), sets the requirements for becoming a certified specialist in anesthesiology. Like other medical specialties, anesthesiology is represented by professional societies such as the American Society of Anesthesiologists and the International Anesthesia Research Society, as well as scientific journals such as Anesthesia and Analgesia, Anesthesia, and Anesthesia Review Committee. The ACGME has delegated authority to this committee to establish and ensure that anesthesia residency training programs adhere to published standards. The ABA and other specialty boards have also created requirements for certification maintenance that include periodic evaluations of professional standing, cognitive proficiency in practice performance, and improvement, in addition to an ongoing program of self-evaluation and lifetime learning. That's how the American system is. There are certification programs for anesthesiologists in other nations and cultures. Some countries work collectively to educate and certify specialists in anesthesiology (e.g., the European Society of Anesthesia) (American Board of Anesthesiology; Adler-Milstein et al., 2015; Galvez et al., 2015)

1.3. Evolution of Anesthesia as a Multidisciplinary Medical Specialty

Over the past half-century, the field of anesthesiology has gradually expanded its reach beyond operating rooms. Pain management and adult critical care medicine were initially the two non-operating room patient care skills that anesthesia providers developed the most. Rotation experiences in these areas were mandatory for anesthesia residents starting in the 1980s. The first recognized subspecialty of anesthesiology was established in 1985 when the American Board of Subspecialty Physicians (ABA) started awarding subspecialty certificates in critical care medicine to candidates who had finished at least a year of specialty training. Beginning in 1991, when the ABA started to issue certificates, pain medicine was the second subspecialty to receive official recognition. At this point, fellowship programs were being developed across a wide range of specializations, and residency programs mandated rotations in multiple areas. This was a reflection of both the increasing specialization in all areas of medicine and the growing complexity of health care.

1.3.1. Pain Management

Both chronic pain conditions and the perioperative period require pain management. The more closely the relationship between postoperative pain control and functional outcomes (such as mobility following joint replacement surgery), the more complicated the management of perioperative pain has become. In addition, more specialized acute pain management services, typically overseen by anesthesiology, are being provided as a result of the growing usage of neuraxial and regional anesthesia techniques for postoperative pain management. Patients with chronic pain are usually treated by an outpatient-based pain management center, with sporadic consultations held in the hospital (e.g., for patients with chronic pain who require surgery that leads to acute and chronic pain). Chronic pain management is a multidisciplinary field that encompasses neurology, neurosurgery, medicine, psychiatry, physical medicine, and physical therapy.

1.3.2. Critical Care Medicine

Since critical care medicine was acknowledged as a separate subspecialty of anesthesiology thirty years ago, its complexity has grown dramatically. Patient care protocols are being developed with an increasing amount of data from large randomized clinical trials. Most often, one or more specialties (e.g., medical, surgical, neurosurgical, cardiac) are used to categorize ICU patients.

The critical care medicine specialist may complete their residency training in multiple specialties, such as anesthesiology, medicine, surgery, neurology, pulmonary medicine, nephrology, or emergency medicine, due to the wide range of specialties that may be involved. Anesthesiologists play prominent local leadership roles in critical care medicine in many institutions.

1.3.3. Pediatric Anesthesia

Pediatric anesthesia has been a part of anesthesia residency training since the 1980s, and there have long been distinct pediatric anesthesia fellowships available. However, the ABA has only been awarding subspecialty certification since 2013. In place of the customary six years, a five-year combined integrated training program in pediatrics and anesthesiology was introduced in 2009 by the American Board of Pediatrics and the American Association of Boards of Pediatrics. Pediatric anesthesiologists have a very defined role in pediatric hospitals. However, when pediatric and adult surgeries are carried out in the same hospital, the procedure (as well as the staffing issues that arise) becomes more complicated. Common inquiries include: what is the minimum age requirement for patients to receive anesthesia from a pediatric anesthesiologist (rather than from anesthesiologists who treat adult patients)? How should anesthesia be provided in the event that pediatric anesthesiologists are unavailable? In certain hospitals, pediatric anesthesiologists also oversee patients in the pediatric intensive care units.

1.3.4. Cardiac Anesthesia

Residency programs have long mandated cardiac anesthesia rotations, and at least as long, elective cardiac anesthesia fellowships have been offered. Since the adult cardiothoracic anesthesia fellowships were first accredited by the ACGME in 2006, they have become more structured and standardized, with the addition of an echocardiography training requirement. Adult and perioperative transesophageal echocardiography certifications are available from the National Board of Echocardiography to anesthesiologists. A common certification for cardiac anesthesiologists is this one.

1.3.5. Obstetric Anesthesia

Obstetric anesthesia experiences have always been an important part of anesthesia training programs due to the unique physiology and patient care issues associated with childbirth. Fellowship training in obstetric anesthesia has been available for many years, with the ACGME accrediting obstetric anesthesiology fellowships starting in 2012. This accreditation has led to standardized and structured training programs to prepare future leaders in obstetric anesthesia, similar to other ACGME anesthesia fellowships. As of now, the ABA does not offer subspecialty certification in obstetric anesthesia.

1.3.6. Other Surgical Areas of Anesthesia

The remaining surgical specialties may offer non-ACGME fellowship training, but anesthesia is not linked to any additional certification procedures. Cardiothoracic, colon and rectal, general surgery, neurological, ophthalmic, oral and maxillofacial, urology, vascular, hospice and palliative care are some of these subspecialties. Without receiving any further training beyond what is offered by a typical anesthesiology residency, anesthesiologists typically provide anesthesia for the remaining surgical subspecialties. The number of patients in an institution frequently determines whether specialized anesthesia teams can provide anesthesia. Institutions that perform a lot of neurosurgical or outpatient surgery, for instance, might have different specialized teams (American Board of Anesthesiology; Adler-Milstein et al., 2015; Galvez et al., 2015).

1.4. Perioperative Patient Care

1.4.1. Preoperative Evaluation

Preoperative assessment, immediate preoperative care, intraoperative care, PACU, acute postoperative pain management, and potentially ICU care are all included in perioperative care. The majority of surgical patients were expected to show up the morning of the procedure rather than the night before starting in the late 1990s and early 2000s. This alteration often required that the preoperative assessment for anesthesia be completed on the morning of surgery. However, because surgical procedures and patient medical risks can be complicated, many institutions established preoperative clinics where patients could be assessed one or more days before the surgery date. These clinics are run by anesthesiologists and have grown to be highly advanced. Anesthesiologists may oversee the care given by nurses or nurse practitioners, or they may assess patients directly. A patient may occasionally require further assessment for particular patient care concerns from the primary care physician or other specialists.

1.4.2. Operating Room Theaters

The management of operating room theaters is becoming more and more difficult. It is a mental challenge in and of itself to match the operating room available time with anticipated surgical complexity and duration. "Throughput" refers to how well each patient's experience was executed. Surgical teams have been permitted to perform simultaneous operations in two or three operating rooms for decades. The risks associated with multiple surgeries are being questioned for the first time in many years. In some cases, the PACU's bed shortage causes throughput delays rather than operating room availability. A patient's scheduled progress may be delayed by some steps in the perioperative pathway, such as preoperative evaluation, the precision of estimating the duration and complexity of surgical care, and patient flow in and out of PACUs. For example, after surgery, patients might have to wait in the operating room for a PACU bed. More and more hospitals are hiring perioperative or operating room directors who oversee the operating rooms or plan the whole perioperative process from the preoperative clinic to the patient's departure from the PACU. These jobs demand a great deal of skill and clinical acumen and can be administratively demanding. Anesthesiologists typically hold these positions, though occasionally a surgeon, nurse, or hospital administrator may serve as the director.

1.4.3. Postanesthesia Care Unit

A tertiary care hospital's PACU plays a crucial role. In addition to recuperating from anesthesia and surgery, patients are also being instructed on how to receive proper care following their PACU stay, which lasts from the ICU to discharge. Even today, operating room theater throughput delays are frequently caused by a lack of PACU beds. Numerous scenarios serve as examples of this fundamental issue. There is nowhere in the PACU to move patients who are fully recovered if all of the regular hospital beds are taken. Patients who require anesthesia and recuperation from surgery performed in an operating room will not have any beds if those patients remain in the PACU. The start of surgery is postponed when this issue is predicted. Hospitals will need more PACU beds in the future as anesthesiologists treat patients with increasingly complicated medical risks. The effectiveness and quality of care during the perioperative phase depend heavily on patient logistical management in addition to the quality of care provided.

1.5. Training and Certification in Anesthesiology

1.5.1. Postgraduate (Residency) Training in Anesthesiology

After earning a degree as a doctor of medicine or doctor of osteopathic medicine, candidates for postgraduate training in anesthesiology in the United States must complete four years of supervised experience in an authorized program. During the first year of postgraduate training in anesthesiology, basic clinical skills in medicine are taught. All facets of clinical anesthesia are studied during the second, third, and fourth postgraduate years (clinical anesthesia years 1 through 3). This includes subspecialty experience in pain management, recovery room care, pediatric anesthesia, cardiothoracic anesthesia, neuro anesthesia, and anesthesia for outpatient surgery. Four months of training in critical care medicine are necessary in addition to these subspecialty experiences. There are differences in the length and format of anesthesiology education among nations. On what, however, qualifies as sufficient training in anesthesiology and its perioperative duties, there is broad international consensus.

The breadth of anesthesiology's application as a medical specialty is reflected in the curriculum of the clinical anesthesia years. In fact, in the operating room, the anesthesiologist should serve as both the internist or pediatrician and the clinical pharmacologist. Moreover, anesthesiology encompasses more than just the operating room; it also includes research, critical care medicine, cardiopulmonary resuscitation, and acute and chronic pain management. More flexibility has recently been added to anesthesia training programs. Programs may provide options for substantial research time as well as integrated residency and fellowship training. Leaders in subspecialty clinical fields and research may come from these more specialized training programs. Furthermore, the American Board of Anesthesia (ABA) has provided backing for the establishment of integrated residency programs in internal medicine, pediatrics, and, most recently, emergency medicine. It is obvious that the goal of anesthesia education programs is to produce anesthesiologists capable of taking on new challenges.

The American College of Geriatrics and Medicine (ACGME) has approved about 131 postgraduate training programs in anesthesiology. The Residency Review Committee (RRC) for Anesthesiology reviews approved programs once a year to make sure that they continue to adhere to the program's published requirements. The American Society of Anesthesiologists, the American Medical Association, and the American Board of Pain Management have all appointed members to the RRC for Anesthesiology (American Board of Anesthesiology; Adler-Milstein et al., 2015; Galvez et al., 2015).

1.5.2. American Board of Anesthesiology

In 1938, the American Board of Surgery affiliated with the ABA was formed. 87 doctors received certification as ABA diplomates following the first voluntary examination. In 1941, the American Board of Medical Specialties acknowledged the ABA as an independent board. Upon successful completion of an approved postgraduate training program, passing both an oral and written exam, and fulfilling licensure and credentialing requirements, over 30,000 anesthesiologists have been certified as diplomates of the American Board of Anesthesiologists (ABA) to date. "Board-certified anesthesiologists" is the term used to describe these diplomates, and the ABA certificate is considered the primary certificate. The ABA, like the majority of other specialty boards, started issuing time-limited certificates with a 10-year limit on January 1, 2000. All diplomates are required to take part in a program called Maintenance of Certification in Anesthesiology (MOCA) to become certified again. This program underwent a redesign in 2016 and became MOCA 2.0. Diplomates who have not had their certificates revoked (those who obtained their certificates before January 1, 2000) are eligible to actively participate in MOCA.

The MOCA program places a strong emphasis on public accountability, ongoing self-improvement—the cornerstone of professional excellence—and the assessment of clinical skills and practice performance. The constituents comprise of four elements: (1) unrestricted state license and professionalism; (2) lifelong learning and self-assessment through formal and informal continuing medical education [CME], encompassing patient safety; (3) assessment of knowledge, judgment, and skills through the completion of thirty MOCA minute pilot questions every calendar quarter); and (4) optimization of medical practice. This last element could be any number of self-directed tasks, such as developing clinical pathways, improving quality, or simulating situations. The American Board of Pain Management (ABA) certifies diplomates in pain medicine, critical care medicine, hospice and palliative medicine, sleep medicine, and pediatric anesthesiology in addition to many other specialties. The requirements for each certificate include completing a year of additional postgraduate training in the relevant subspecialty, meeting licensure and credentialing requirements, and passing a written exam. A ten-year period is likewise attached to these certificates. The ABA shift to the Maintenance of Certification in Anesthesiology for Subspecialties Program (MOCA-SUBS) is causing ongoing changes to the requirements for recertification.

1.5.3. Credentialing and Privileging

Anesthesiologists who have completed their residency and joined a hospital's medical staff are required to go through the credentialing and privileging process. This allows the relevant institutions to gather, confirm, and assess all information related to a clinician's professional performance. The American Board of Medical Specialties and the ACGME collaborated to create three new ideas recently. The medical staff evaluates clinicians based on general competencies, which include patient care, medical/clinical knowledge, practiced-based learning and improvement, interpersonal and communication skills, professionalism, and systems-based practice. Further information about a specific clinician can be obtained through targeted professional practice evaluation. Ongoing professional practice evaluation is the final new idea. Essentially, procedures must be created to locate an issue as quickly as feasible.

1.6. Other Anesthetic Providers

1.6.1. Certified Registered Nurse Anesthetists

Most anesthetics administered in the United States are likely administered by certified registered nurse anesthetists (CRNAs), most of whom work under a physician's supervision. After receiving a registered nurse degree and working as a critical care nurse for a year, candidates must enroll in an approved nurse anesthesia training program and spend two to three years learning the didactic and clinical skills necessary to administer anesthesia. Curriculum development for nurse anesthesia training programs and the creation of requirements for CRNA certification are under the purview of the American Association of Nurse Anesthetists. Under the guidance (medical direction) of an anesthesiologist, CRNAs' duties often involve providing intraoperative care for patients during anesthesia. It is congruent with the idea that administering anesthesia constitutes the practice of medicine for a physician-nurse anesthetist team (anesthesia care team). CRNAs sometimes provide anesthesia without the medical guidance or oversight of an anesthesiologist.

1.6.2. Anesthesiologist Assistants

A master of medical science in anesthesia is awarded to anesthesiologist assistants upon completion of a graduate-level program, which takes about 27 months, from an approved training program (currently Case Western Reserve University, Emory University School of Medicine, Nova Southeastern University, South University, and University of Missouri). As members of the anesthesia care team, anesthesiologist assistants collaborate with the anesthesiologist to carry out the anesthesia care plan (American Board of Anesthesiology; Adler-Milstein et al., 2015; Galvez et al., 2015)

1.7. Quality of Care and Safety in Anesthesia

1.7.1. Continuous Quality Improvement

In the practice of medicine, quality is a hard term to define. However, it is widely acknowledged that focusing on quality enhances patient safety and satisfaction with anesthetic care. The National Academies of Sciences, Engineering, and Medicine (formerly the Institute of Medicine) brought attention to these problems in medicine generally in 2000 with their report "To Err Is Human," although the specialty of anesthesiology has long placed such a premium on these matters. New terms that we used often started to appear regularly in our vocabulary (e.g., competency metrics, continuous evaluation, standardization, time limits, system approaches, checklists, and practice guidelines). The requirements of The Joint Commission, formerly known as the Joint Commission on Accreditation of Healthcare Organizations [JCAHO], frequently serve as the basis for quality improvement programs in the anesthesia industry. Three factors are taken into consideration when evaluating the quality of care: (1) structure (the people and resources used to deliver it), (2) process (the order and coordination of patient care tasks like administering and documenting a preanesthetic evaluation, and continuously attending to and monitoring the patient during anesthesia), and (3) outcome. These three fundamental elements of care are the focus of a quality improvement program, which measures and enhances them. Continuous quality improvement (CQI) programs use a "systems" approach, acknowledging that random errors are hard to prevent from the start, as opposed to quality assurance programs that look for "outliers." On the other hand, system errors ought to be under control and strategies for reducing them ought to be achievable. A CQI program might concentrate on unfavorable results to find areas where the organization and delivery of care could be improved.

Reductions in the frequency of unfavorable outcomes are frequently used to gauge improvements in the quality of care. Measuring improvement is challenging, though, because unfavorable outcomes in anesthesia are relatively uncommon. CQI programs may concentrate on sentinel events and critical incidents in addition to outcome measurement. Critical incidents, such as the disconnecting of a ventilator, are situations that injure people or have the potential to do so if they are not identified and addressed quickly. Patient safety may be enhanced by measuring the frequency of significant critical events, which could take the place of uncommon anesthesia outcomes. Sentinel events are singular occurrences that may point to a systemic issue (e.g., a syringe exchange due to inadequate labeling, a drug administration error resulting from the patient leaving unnecessary medications on the anesthetic cart).

Adequate monitoring, current knowledge, and vigilance are critical components in preventing anesthesia-related patient harm. It goes without saying that adherence to the guidelines recommended by the American Society of Anesthesiologists is crucial. In this sense, formal, published standards of practice have been developed and implemented by

American anesthesiology, which has led the way in organized medicine. The way anesthesia is administered in the US has been greatly impacted by these standards (e.g., practice parameters). Quality and safety have received a lot of attention and focus over the past few years, but occasionally the standards are not applied as quickly and thoroughly as intended. Lately, proposals have been put forth to include credentials requirements as well as sanctions for noncompliance (American Board of Anesthesiology; Adler-Milstein et al., 2015; Galvez et al., 2015)

1.8. Organizations with Emphasis on Anesthesia Quality and Safety

1.8.1. Anesthesia Patient Safety Foundation

Ellison C.'s administration saw the establishment of the Anesthesia Patient Safety Foundation (APSF). Pierce Jr, MD, in his year as the American Society of Anesthesiologists' president. The American Society of Anesthesiologists initially contributed funds for the establishment of the APSF, and they still do. Moreover, businesses, specialized societies, and private donors provide financial support to APSF. Ensuring that no patient is harmed by anesthesia is the goal of the APSF. To carry out this goal, the APSF offers research grants to fund studies intended to improve our knowledge of avoidable anesthetic injuries and encourages national and international exchange of knowledge and concepts regarding the origins and mitigation of anesthesia-related harm. The APSF newsletter, which is published quarterly and is the most widely distributed anesthesia publication worldwide, focuses on patient safety issues related to anesthesia. In medicine, anesthesiology is the only specialty with a foundation devoted exclusively to patient safety concerns. Modeled after the APSF, the National Patient Safety Foundation was established by the American Medical Association in 1997.

1.8.2. Anesthesia Quality Institute

To serve as the main information source for anesthesiology practices looking to improve their quality, the Anesthesia Quality Institute (AQI) was established in 2008. It keeps track of information that's useful for "evaluating and enhancing patient care." Quality and safety information that could be utilized to satisfy legal requirements will eventually be available from the AQI. Aiming to improve the quality of care, societies, research, and clinical care already use the AQI as a source of data. The National Anesthesia Clinical Outcomes Registry (NACOR) is organized according to the AQI website, which also explains how data enters and leaves the NACOR.

1.8.3. American Society of Anesthesiologists Closed Claims Project and Its Registries

A database of past evaluations of court cases that had unfavorable results is maintained by the ASA Closed Claims Project and its Registries. This continuous study has made it easier to pinpoint patient and practice risk areas that frequently encounter issues and need more care from the specialty in terms of quality and safety.

1.8.4. Foundation for Anesthesia Education and Research

The Foundation for Anesthesia Education and Research (FAER) is a very significant vehicle for supporting anesthesiology-related research, even though it is not directly related to quality and safety. The American Society of Anesthesiologists provided financial support for FAER's establishment in 1986. Furthermore, corporations, specialty societies, and individual donors provide financial support to FAER. FAER's mission is to promote anesthesiology, perioperative medicine, and pain management research, teaching, and scientific innovation. FAER has supported the training of academic anesthesiologists and funded several research grants over the years.

1.9. Professional Liability

Malpractice claims have decreased in number and severity as a result of a strong commitment to quality and safety. Consequently, over the previous 20 years, malpractice premiums have dropped significantly. However, it is necessary to comprehend the underlying ideas. First, legal disputes still arise. For instance, between 1995 and 2007, 93 claims were made in the United Kingdom. The majority of the sixty-two claims concerned drug administration errors involving muscle relaxants. Additionally, 19 claims mentioned paralyzed patients who were awake. Such errors can be reduced by labeling properly and double-checking. It is obvious that the anesthesiologist is in charge of anesthesia management and recovery. Compared to other anesthesiologists, doctors who administer anesthesia are expected to use ordinary and reasonable care or skill, but they are not expected to guarantee a positive outcome for the patient. It is not negligence (below the standard of care) if the expected outcome does not materialize or if problems arise. Furthermore, unless the mistake is judged to be outside the scope of the anesthesiologist's expertise, they cannot be held accountable for it. Nonetheless, an anesthesiologist's duty as a specialist is to make medical decisions that adhere to national, not local, standards. In the event of a court ruling against them, anesthesiologists are financially protected by professional liability (malpractice) insurance. Furthermore, CRNAs may be legally accountable for the technical facets of anesthesia administration. However, it is likely that the doctor in charge of overseeing the anesthesia administration will share legal liability for the CRNA's actions (American Board of Anesthesiology; Adler-Milstein et al., 2015; Galvez et al., 2015).

Anesthesiologists are best protected against medicolegal actions by practicing anesthesia with thoroughness and up-to-dateness; they also show interest in their patients by keeping meticulous records of their anesthesia course, as well as by attending preoperative and postoperative visits (automated information systems provide the resources to collect and record real-time actual data). Additionally, all anesthesia providers need to be ready for the switch to automated information systems for anesthesia record keeping. In particular, the information technology system of a medical center should completely integrate the use of automated anesthetic records. Regretfully, putting electronic health records (EHRs) into practice is challenging, expensive, time-consuming, and full of unforeseen consequences—including failing to meet safety regulations. Nonetheless, a study of national data from 2008 to 2014 shows significant advancements in the use of EHRs, with 75% of hospitals now having at least a basic EHR system, up from 59% in 2013. The Office of the National Coordinator (ONC) for Health Information Technology is leading the way in the United States when it comes to the adoption and application of health IT.

1.9.1. Adverse Events

The anesthesiologist should promptly record the details of any accident or anesthesia-related complication in the patient's medical record and notify the relevant agencies right away. This notification should start at the department level and continue with the quality improvement administration and risk management office of the medical center. When necessary, seek advice from other doctors and record the patient's treatment. A thorough report of the incident should be given by the anesthesiologist to the hospital and the organization that handles the physician's professional liability insurance. In conjunction with the doctors, nurses, and other healthcare professionals involved in the patient's care, a root cause analysis (RCA) may be conducted as part of the investigation and discussion of adverse events and complications.

1.10. Risks of Anesthesia

Even though many patients express fear of dying while under anesthesia, the number of deaths associated with anesthesia has dropped significantly over the past 20 years. Anesthesiologists' professional liability insurance premiums have dropped since fewer adverse events are being linked to anesthesia. It is assumed that improved anesthesia medications and monitoring (capnography, pulse oximetry) along with more anesthesiologists in training are to blame for the improved safety of anesthesia, particularly for patients undergoing elective surgery and without significant coexisting diseases. Although anesthesia is thought to be safe, side effects can still happen, and opinions on how much the death rate from anesthesia has decreased vary. The 244,000 surviving patients who had surgery and anesthesia serve as the basis for improvement. The 1 in 250,000 death rate from anesthesia is estimated using this series. Persuading patients to give up smoking, reduce their body weight, abstain from excessive alcohol consumption, and attain optimal medical control of their essential hypertension, diabetes mellitus, and asthma before undergoing elective surgeries is probably a good way to increase the safety of anesthesia and surgery.

Determining the cause and effect mechanism of perioperative adverse events is frequently challenging. In many cases, it is impossible to distinguish between an unavoidable mishap (error, coincidental event) that happened despite the best of care and an adverse event brought on by an inappropriate action on the part of the anesthesiologist (a "lapse of vigilance" or a breach in the standard of care). Peripheral nerve damage, brain damage, aspiration, intraoperative awareness, eye injury, fetal/newborn injury, airway trauma (usually from difficult tracheal intubation), and other negative outcomes are examples of unfavorable outcomes other than death. Anesthesiologists have historically believed that the biggest risk to patient safety during anesthesia is difficult airway management. A survey conducted among sizable anesthesia groups has brought to light additional patient safety issues.

With better patient monitoring, hopefully, anesthesiologists will be even more vigilant and human error will play a smaller part in anesthetic morbidity and death rates. A significant amount of adverse anesthesia events are, in fact, the consequence of human error, which can arise from attentional or vigilant failings. The anesthesiologist's capacity to exercise vigilance is weakened by a variety of factors present in the operating room. Among these, sleep deprivation and exhaustion rank highly, as they have been shown to negatively impact productivity at work and on cognitive tasks (such as clinical decision-making and monitoring). The day following a 24-hour in-hospital call, anesthesia residents are not permitted to be given clinical responsibilities, according to the RRC for Anesthesiology. The National Academies' Health and Medicine Division (HMD) has issued very specific recommendations about resident work hours, and it is likely that it will issue recommendations for physicians generally as well, some of which may eventually become mandates. The focus on productivity in the operating room, known as "production pressures," may take precedence over patient safety and lead to mistakes that compromise patient safety. However, not every untoward incident that occurs during anesthesia can be avoided because it was caused by a mistake made by a person (American Board of Anesthesiology; Adler-Milstein et al., 2015; Galvez et al., 2015)

1.11. Hazards of Working in the Operating Room

A long day in the operating room exposes anesthesiologists to vapors from chemicals (volatile anesthetics), ionizing radiation, and infectious agents (human immunodeficiency virus, hepatitis viruses). The need for constant attention to detail when caring for patients under anesthesia causes psychological stress. Interactions with the surgical team (nurses, surgeons) can also cause varied degrees of interpersonal stress.

Although there isn't enough proof to suggest that scavenging, or the removal of waste anesthetic gases, has improved the health of anesthesia staff, it has reduced exposure to trace amounts of these gases. Universal precautions are recommended in the care of every patient in an attempt to prevent the transmission of blood-borne infections, particularly by accidental needlestick injuries. Substance abuse, mental illness (depression), and suicide seem to occur with increased frequency among anesthesiologists, perhaps reflecting the impact of occupational stress. Lastly, infection control for both patients and clinical personnel in the operating rooms requires increasingly strict rules regarding specific procedures in the operating room such as washing hands.

1.12. Structured Approach to Anesthesia Care

Preoperative, intraoperative, and postoperative care are provided by anesthesia providers to the surgical patient. Critical choices regarding patient care involve evaluating the preoperative assessment, developing the anesthesia plan, setting up the operating room, and overseeing the intraoperative anesthetic, postoperative care, and results. The learning process will be aided by comprehension of this framework.

1.12.1. Preoperative Evaluation

Preoperative evaluation aims to address patients' concerns, modify risks, assess the likelihood of coexisting diseases, and talk about options for anesthesia care. The novice trainee ought to become familiar with the questions that are most crucial to comprehending the patient and the suggested procedure. The following are some particular queries and their possible significance.

Table 1.1. *American Society of Anesthesiologists Physical Status Patient Classification System*

ASA class I	A normal healthy patient
ASA class II	A patient with mild systemic disease
ASA class III	A patient with severe systemic disease
ASA class IV	A patient with severe systemic disease that is a constant threat to life
ASA class V	A moribund patient who is not expected to survive without an operation
ASA class VI	A declared brain-dead patient whose organs are being removed for donor purposes

Source: Elo, J. A., & Sun, H.-H. (2016). Anesthesia and Sedation. InTech. doi: 10.5772/63539.

What is the indication for the proposed surgery? Is it elective or an emergency? The indication for surgery may have particular anesthetic implications. For example, a patient requiring esophageal fundoplication will likely have severe gastroesophageal reflux disease, which may require modification of the anesthesia plan (e.g., preoperative nonparticulate antacid, intraoperative rapid sequence induction of anesthesia) (Table 1.1).

The choice of anesthetic may also be impacted by a particular procedure. For example, general anesthesia, peripheral nerve blockade, local anesthesia, or occasionally a combination of methods can be used to achieve anesthesia for hand surgery. Without raising the risk of complications, the urgency of a particular procedure (such as acute appendicitis) may prevent a long surgical delay for further testing. (e.g., appendiceal rupture, peritonitis). What are the inherent risks associated with this surgical procedure? Various surgical procedures carry inherent risks. A patient receiving a coronary artery bypass graft, for instance, is at a high risk of complications like myocardial infarction, stroke, or death. There is a rare chance that a patient receiving cataract extraction will sustain serious organ damage.

To anticipate the effects of a particular medical problem, the anesthesia provider must understand the physiologic effects of the surgery and anesthetic and the potential interaction with the medical problem. Does the patient have coexisting medical problems? Does the surgery or anesthesia care plan need to be modified because of them? To help with tracheal intubation, a patient with poorly managed systemic hypertension, for instance, is more likely to react to direct laryngoscopy with an exaggerated hypertensive response. To raise the induction dose of an intravenously given anesthetic, the anesthesia provider may alter the anesthetic plan (e.g., propofol) and use a β-adrenergic blocker with a short half-life (e.g., esmolol) before airway instrumentation. At any point during the procedure, the anesthesia plan may need to be modified based on the medical issue. Has the patient had anesthesia before? Were there complications such as difficult airway management? Does the patient have risk factors for difficult airway management? Anesthesia records from previous surgery can yield much useful information. The most important fact is the ease of airway management techniques such as direct laryngoscopy. If physical examination reveals some risk factors for difficult tracheal intubation, but the patient had a clearly documented uncomplicated direct laryngoscopy for recent surgery, the anesthesia provider may choose to proceed with routine laryngoscopy. Other useful historical information includes intraoperative hemodynamic and respiratory instability and the occurrence of postoperative nausea.

1.12.2. Creating the Anesthesia Plan

The completion of the anesthesia plan can come after the preoperative evaluation. A comprehensive list of drug selections, dosages, and potential issues should be included in the plan. Numerous modifications to a given plan might be appropriate, but the specifics should be agreed upon beforehand by the trainee and the supervising anesthesia provider.

1.12.3. Preparing the Operating Room

The trainee has to set up the operating room after deciding on the anesthetic protocol. Regular preparation for the operating room involves things like inspecting the anesthesia machine. Preparing extra equipment may depend on the details of the anesthesia plan. For instance, special tools needed for fiberoptic tracheal intubation may be stored in a cart specifically intended for managing difficult airways.

1.12.4. Managing the Intraoperative Anesthetic

The anesthesia plan is usually followed for intraoperative anesthesia management, although it should be modified following the patient's reactions to anesthesia and surgery. In order to decide whether to alter the patient's care, the anesthesia provider must assess a variety of information sources. The trainee needs to develop the ability to handle several tasks at once and process information from various sources. The general mental activity cycle consists of observation, judgment, action, and subsequent assessment. Being vigilante, or being aware and watchful, is essential for providing safe patient care, but it is insufficient on its own. The anesthesia provider may feel overburdened by the volume of information or by information that is changing quickly as they consider the importance of each observation. Clinical events that occur during surgery can encourage critical thinking and interactive dialogue between the supervisor and trainee.

1.12.5. Patient Follow-up

After emerging from anesthesia, the patient needs to be evaluated again. In addition to reviewing for complications like dental injury, nausea, nerve injury, and intraoperative recall, this follow-up entails gauging general satisfaction with the anesthetic. The effects of anesthesia, particularly the long-term effects of hypotension, inhaled anesthetic dosage, and "deep" levels of anesthesia, are receiving more and more attention.

1.13. Learning Strategies

The cornerstone of clinical training is acquired through supervised direct patient care. Direct patient care cannot be the only element of the teaching program due to the broad scope of anesthesia practice and the variety of competencies that trainees must master. Additional teaching methods consist of lectures, debates in groups, role-playing, and individual reading. Giving lectures can be an effective way to convey a lot of information. However, there isn't much opportunity for audience participation during a lecture. Smaller, more interactive groups with fewer than 12 participants are the most productive. This format works well for journal clubs, quality assurance conferences, and problem-based case discussions. A teaching strategy known as the "flipped classroom" can incorporate elements of both group discussions and lectures. A well-liked method for implementing the flipped classroom is to use an online video lecture that needs to be watched before class. Discussions and other active learning techniques are used in class, but they work best when the student has already seen the material. There are various types of simulations available: task-based simulators for practicing specific procedures like laryngoscopy or intravenous catheter placement; mannequin-based simulators for simulating intraoperative crises like cardiac arrest or malignant hyperthermia; and computer-based simulators for repeatedly managing sophisticated cardiac life support algorithms (Tables 1.2 and 1.3).

Table 1.2. *American Society of Anesthesiologists Fasting Guidelines*

Ingested Material	Minimum Fasting Period
Clear liquids	2 h
Breast milk	4 h
Infant formula	6 h
Nonhuman milk	6 h
Light meal	6 h
Fatty meal	8 h

Source: Elo, J. A., & Sun, H.-H. (2016). Anesthesia and Sedation. InTech. doi: 10.5772/63539.

Table 1.3. *Tracking Staff Behavior-an Example: From Left to right: (1) Intervention ID Number, (2) OR Location, (3) Surgery Type (Orthopedic or Cardiac), (4) Duration of the Intervention, (5) Number of Detected Objects, (6) Number of Doors, (7) Number of Objects Discarded Because of an Insufficient Detection Rate (Undetermined (u) >50%), (8) Mean/std Value of the Percentage of Undetermined Status of the Different Objects*

ID	Site	Surgery	Duration h:mm	Nb Detected Objects	Nb Doors	Nb Discarded Objects	% Undet. Mean ± std
1	16	ort	2:33	9	1	1	6.4 ± 7.7
2	16	ort	2:33	7	1	0	14.4 ± 9
3	16	ort	2:32	11	1	2	14.6 ± 6.6
4	16	ort	3:17	8	1	3	10 ± 6.2
5	07	ort	4:02	11	2	3	12.9 ± 6.6
6	07	ort	3:19	13	2	7	23.8 ± 18.3
7	15	ort	2:30	10	2	0	9.9 ± 11.1
8	15	ort	2:50	10	2	1	11.5 ± 8.7
9	15	ort	2:55	10	2	1	12.9 ± 8.3
10	15	ort	2:25	13	2	0	8 ± 4.9
11	15	ort	2:12	14	2	0	8.1 ± 5.9
12	06	ort	1:58	9	1	0	11.3 ± 7.6
13	06	ort	1:56	12	1	0	15.4 ± 4.7
14	06	ort	2:06	11	1	1	8.8 ± 7.7
15	06	ort	2:31	11	1	0	10.5 ± 6.7
16	06	ort	2:35	10	1	0	8.6 ± 7.2
17	13	car	4:39	9	1	0	7.1 ± 2.4
18	13	car	6:22	10	1	0	10 ± 9.5
19	13	car	6:52	8	1	0	9.5 ± 6.1
20	17	car	5:06	14	3	1	11.1 ± 6
21	17	car	6:51	13	3	0	9.5 ± 6.7
22	17	car	4:42	12	3	1	8.2 ± 6.1
23	17	car	4:11	11	3	0	9.2 ± 6.7
24	03	car	4:50	12	1	1	14.8 ± 6.2
25	03	car	4:52	11	1	2	11 ± 8.3
26	03	car	6:51	13	1	1	9.8 ± 6.2
27	03	car	5:53	10	1	0	14.3 ± 9.3
28	03	car	5:30	15	1	1	11.3 ± 7.7
29	01	car	4:04	12	4	1	6.1 ± 2.7
30	01	car	6:14	15	4	1	14 ± 5.4

Source: Azevedo-Coste C, Pissard-Gibollet R, Toupet G, Fleury É, Lucet J-C, Birgand G. Tracking Clinical Staff Behaviors in an Operating Room. Sensors. 2019; 19(10):2287. https://doi.org/10.3390/s19102287.

1.13.1. Learning Orientation versus Performance Orientation

It is possible to characterize the trainee's approach to a learning challenge as either "learning orientation" or "performance orientation." The objective of learners with a learning orientation is to increase situational mastery, whereas learners with a performance orientation seek to validate their abilities. Training participants who have a learning orientation are more likely to see feedback as helpful, whereas those who have a performance orientation are more likely to see it as just a tool to point out areas of weakness. Strong learners have a higher chance of succeeding in a demanding and challenging training environment (American Board of Anesthesiology; Adler-Milstein et al., 2015; Galvez et al., 2015)

1.14. Anesthesia and Health Information Technology

Anesthesia professionals generate and document a staggering volume of physiologic, pharmaceutical, and care management data. An exponential increase has occurred in the use of computerized anesthesia information management systems (AIMS), both as stand-alone systems and as components of an electronic health record (EHR) for patient care, since the publication of the previous edition of this text in 2011. Few academic anesthesia practices and even fewer private practice settings had AIMS installations in the late 1990s. On the other hand, by 2007, about 44% of academic medical centers had either finished or were in the process of implementing AIMS. According to a 2014 follow-up survey, 84% of U. S. By the end of that year, academic medical centers would have an AIMS in place. It was predicted that in a few years, very few residents in anesthesia programs would have completed their residency with a paper anesthetic record. The increasing number of auxiliary electronic devices and other software will probably be incorporated into EHRs as well, bringing all of this together under the umbrella of health information technology, or health IT. Anesthesia providers need to be aware of the potential advantages and risks of these technologies due to the significant influence that health information technology has on patient care. Medical informatics, the branch of information science that deals with health care and biomedicine, which includes medical computer science, health informatics, and computers in medicine, is the scientific field that forms the basis of health IT.

Anesthesia providers should play a major role in the creation, evaluation, selection, and implementation of perioperative health IT due to their unique set of abilities and knowledge. These days, anesthesia teams must be conversant in the relevant theory and application of medical informatics.

1.14.1. History of Anesthesia Documentation and Aims

The paper record that neurosurgeon and physiologist Harvey Cushing and his medical school classmate E created in 1895 is where the current AIMS got its start. An. Cody. Codman and Cushing had pushed one another to advance their anesthetic practices as pioneers of anesthesia quality improvement. Just 50 years after the discovery of anesthesia, they were the first to gather and analyze physiologic data using written anesthesia records to achieve this aim. Approximately concurrently, Cushing and associates initiated the utilization of recently developed automated hemodynamic monitors featuring paper-based documentation, encompassing noninvasive arterial blood pressure assessments. The anesthetic record kept the same fundamental structure for displaying hemodynamics over the next fifty years, even though the quantity and kinds of data recorded increased gradually. These two innovations served as the cornerstone for the development of the modern AIMS: the automated real-time recording of hemodynamic vital signs and the documentation of noteworthy events that occurred during actual anesthesia and surgery.

In the late 1970s and early 1980s, the computerized anesthesia automated record keeper (AARK) was introduced and evaluated, but its commercialization and widespread use were hindered by the limited availability of affordable and reliable computer hardware and software. Despite these challenges, the benefits of AARKs were evident, even with the emerging technology. AARKs addressed issues with paper records such as recall bias, illegible writing, missing or incomplete data (impacting regulations and billing), and the lack of a proper audit trail for legal and medical purposes. Clinical studies showed that AARKs provided a more accurate recording of hemodynamic variables compared to handwritten charts. Notably, handwritten anesthetic records tended to have more "data smoothing," where data points were often approximated, leading to less variability between individual recordings, unlike AARKs.

The 1990s and early 2000s heralded a proliferation of advanced computer hardware and software, such as local area networks, the Internet, digital hemodynamic monitors, medical communication protocols such as Health Level Seven International (HL7), and a significant reduction in the cost of computer processing power. Coupled with the voracious demand for more data that paper records could not satisfy, the relatively simple AARKs evolved into full fledged AIMS, with numerous additional capabilities.

1.14.2. The Demand for Data

To enhance patient safety, the Anesthesia Patient Safety Foundation (APSF) supported and promoted "the use of automated record keeping in the perioperative period and the subsequent retrieval and analysis of the data in 2001." Additionally, requests for anesthesia and perioperative data were made for quality assurance, research, compliance documentation, and the expediting of billing and administrative tasks. The fast adoption of EHRs in the U.S. in the twenty-first century may have been primarily sped up by federal government action. Enacted as a component of the American Recovery and Reinvestment Act of 2009, the Health Information Technology for Economic and Clinical Health (HITECH) Act included provisions for financial incentives and penalties to promote the adoption and appropriate use of health IT.

In 2011, the U.S. Department of Health and Human Services (HHS) Centers for Medicare & Medicaid Services (CMS) initiated the Medicare and Medicaid EHR Incentive Programs. Their Meaningful Use (MU) criteria encourage U.S. health care providers and organizations to adopt health IT through a staged process, via variable payments or penalties. For ongoing MU compliance, organizations must—by 2017—satisfy Stage 3 rules, which consolidate and update many of the Stage 1 and 2 requirements, as well as add requirements for privacy and security practices and the electronic submission of clinical quality measure (CQM) data for all providers. Reporting compliance within the MU system is complex. For instance, there are specific reporting, incentive, and hardship exemption rules that may apply to anesthesia providers. Advice from the American Society of Anesthesiologists, HHS, Office of the National Coordinator for Health Information Technology (ONC), and health IT professionals may help navigate these requirements. The requirements are dynamic, and in early 2016, in response to stakeholder feedback, the federal government was developing the Advancing Care Information program. This new program intends to simplify or replace the MU program, focusing on improving interoperability (see later) and creating user-friendly technology designed to support physician workflows. Up-to-date information about federal guidelines and requirements for health IT is available online.

One of the main justifications given for implementing health IT is the ability to collect and report data discretely within a healthcare organization. Reporting facilitates workflow analysis, directs efforts to improve scheduling, utilization, and resource management, allows for the measurement of costs, quality, and clinical outcomes, complies with regulations regarding compliance, supports research studies, and may be mandated by outside public and private agencies. Since crucial data frequently exists in several systems, the Data Warehouse—a centralized location for integrated data gathered from one or more disparate sources—has grown in popularity. Despite the enormous potential of local reporting, these local data are contributing to the establishment of large national and international databases known as data registries. The fields of anesthesia and perioperative care are the focus of several observational data registries, including the Pediatric Regional Anesthesia Network, the Anesthesia Quality Institute (AQI), the National Anesthesia Clinical Outcomes Registry (NACOR), the Multicenter Perioperative Outcomes Group (MPOG) data registry, the Society for Ambulatory Anesthesia (SAMBA) database (SAMBA Outcomes Registry, SCOR), and the Society for Cardiovascular Anesthesiologists Adult Cardiac Anesthesia Module. Health IT can send data directly to these data registries, but there are a few obstacles that make data sharing from local health IT challenging. First, mapping local clinical concepts to the registry data schema requires a major time and resource commitment. The lack of a widely accepted "data dictionary" for anesthesia is another obstacle to fully harvesting the information present in these datasets due to the inconsistent types of clinical taxonomies. The incomplete or erroneous data in health IT anesthesia documentation is a third problem. It is unrealistic to expect clinicians to be proficient data entry workers while also providing anesthesia and patient care, so this issue may remain unsolvable in the absence of large resource or technological investments. Lastly, a large portion of health IT data is expressed in plain text, or natural or human language, rather than being discrete, structured, or categorized. Much of this data cannot be used extensively until natural language processing (NLP), an area of artificial intelligence where computer software understands human languages, develops.

Local and national registries have a lot of potential for quality improvement and health care research, despite these obstacles. These data enable the sharing of lessons learned, process and outcome measure benchmarking across organizations, and an explanation of the current status of clinical care. Additionally, when clinical outcomes are uncommon, pooled data can be used to investigate the relationships between particular patient care factors and these outcomes. However, there are worries that these large, observational cohort studies have significant limitations when compared to conventional prospective randomized controlled trials. However, huge datasets, sometimes referred to as "big data," have assisted big businesses in other industries in visualizing unique customer-product relationships and formulating fresh tactics. Big data approaches may prove to be a time- and money-efficient means of enhancing future interventional studies and fundamental science research in anesthesia. Big data is expected to be used in a variety of ways, such as simulating perioperative patient complications and feeding that data back to EHR systems to inform clinical decision support

(CDS) rules, potentially averting issues before they arise. Big data may allow new computer methods like machine learning and cognitive inference computing to use data to make conclusions that humans are unable to.

1.14.3. Professional Performance Data Reporting With Health It

A specific use of health IT data, professional quality electronic reporting is the driving force behind many reporting initiatives. Individual qualified practitioners and group practices provide quality data to the Physician Quality Reporting System (PQRS) on behalf of CMS. The purpose of PQRS quality measures is to assist qualified practitioners and groups in evaluating their performance in various quality areas. CMS intends to combine a number of existing value- and quality-based assessment systems (such as PQRS and MU) in 2019 into advanced Alternative Payment Models (APMs) or Merit-based Incentive Payment Systems (MIPS) that are a result of the most recent Medicare Access and CHIP Reauthorization Act of 2015 (MACRA).

It is acknowledged that reporting on quality metrics is an essential component of an EHR. There are systems that allow you to record high-quality documentation directly within the EHR. On the other hand, to lower the possibility of unintended legal discovery, perhaps this reporting should be done outside of the EHR. Joining a qualified clinical data registry that has been approved by CMS as an alternative to direct documentation gives you the ability to gather and submit PQRS quality measure data on behalf of individual providers. According to the HHS's Patient Safety Rule, the AQI is presently recognized as a qualified clinical data registry in addition to being a Patient Safety Organization. To promote accurate reporting, patient safety organizations and qualified clinical data registries are highly protected from medicolegal discovery. Participants in NACOR and MPOG can use their participation in these data registries to meet federal reporting requirements because MPOG is also a 2015-qualified clinical data registry through its Anesthesiology Performance Improvement and Reporting Exchange registry (ASPIRE).

1.14.4. Features of the Electronic Health Record in Anesthesia and Perioperative Care

An electronic health record (EHR) is a longitudinal database containing patient health information gathered from one or more visits in any type of healthcare setting. Using EHRs has many potential benefits for patients, providers, and the health care organization, both realized and potential. However, there are also many potential drawbacks. A successful EHR could be the difference between a project that fails and one that succeeds. Since supporting necessary clinical and administrative tasks is the EHR's primary goal, it must be user-friendly, and intuitive, and provide users access to the appropriate information at the appropriate moment to meet the demands of contemporary healthcare.

The AARK core functions (permanent recording of device data/device integration from hemodynamic monitors, anesthesia machines, and other clinical devices), the management of perioperative orders, the documentation of preoperative evaluation (including the use of structured data to support reporting and CDS), and the integration with the patient's electronic health record and other records in various health IT systems are among the system feature requirements specific to AIMS.

Key targets for integration include the following:

- Medication data (requiring integration with pharmacy systems, which encompasses patient allergies, medication orders, administrations, interactions, formulary, and costs)

- Laboratory and radiology systems (study orders and results, ability to record point-of-care test results)
- Provider orders, notes, and consults
- Nursing assessments including "ins and outs"
- Billing functions (create charges to patients and their insurance plan)
- Patient tracking (integration with admission/discharge/ transfer application)
- Perioperative management systems (e.g., case ordering, scheduling, utilization management)

This integration may be operationalized through shared databases and procedures for modular AIMS (parts of a larger EHR) (e.g., the AIMS module records medication orders and administrations in the enterprise database shared with the pharmacy and other clinical applications). To prevent a perioperative information "black hole," standalone AIMS may need multiple interfaces (hardware and software) to exchange data with the other health IT systems (previously discussed). The most crucial aspect of an EHR may be its dependability. Fault tolerance refers to the ability of the EHR to withstand a variety of problems, including network errors, hardware malfunctions, hacking, software "bugs," and even natural disasters. Creating a fail-safe workflow (such as scanning paper records) and redundant data storage are important steps in ensuring business continuity following a failure. Two popular data protection models are (1) data mirroring, where a local workstation application uses locally stored data that is automatically copied to remote storage (or the cloud), and (2) client-server, where data is stored on a remote computer (the server) and accessed from a local workstation (the client). Data mirroring has the potential to withstand momentary network outages, which is advantageous. Client-server architectures, which centralize data and software to facilitate backup and maintenance procedures, can streamline system administration. (Xie, 2015)

1.14.5. Health Care Information Privacy and Security

Healthcare professionals have a moral and legal duty to safeguard patient privacy and the security of the electronic health record. The U.S. has regulations for privacy, security, and breach notification under the Health Insurance Portability and Accountability Act (HIPAA) rules that make this duty legally binding. The Privacy Rule establishes guidelines for the use and disclosure of protected health information (PHI) in any format, including written, spoken, and electronic. Any information that could be used to identify a patient is considered PHI. When information is kept digitally, it is referred to as electronic PHI (ePHI). The Security Rule mandates some safety measures to ensure that only authorized individuals have access to health IT systems. Health care organizations and providers are required by the Breach Notification Rule to notify HHS, patients, and, in certain situations, the media of any breach involving patient privacy or a breakdown in health IT security.

The HIPAA Security Rule is managed and enforced by the Office for Civil Rights at HHS. The HHS website provides a detailed description of the intricate details. The protection of ePHI may also be governed by applicable federal, state, and local laws, in addition to HIPAA, as well as the policies of health care organizations. One of the most important HIPAA regulations is requiring all patients to receive an official notice of their privacy rights, usually at "check-in" or admission. Thus, further consent is usually not needed for routine use of clinical data for anesthesia care. However, sharing PHI with other organizations might need the patient's consent. Patients are entitled to control access to their PHI and to view their own medical records. Laws also prohibit tampering with electronic records to obtain fraudulent information. Comprehensive audit trails and integrity checks should be included in modern EHRs in order to spot changes.

Since data security is a constantly changing field, new vulnerabilities appear along with enhanced features offered by new system capabilities. HHS has issued a warning regarding a rise in recent ePHI privacy breaches, which are described in an ONC document on ePHI security and privacy. In order to prevent breaches, both individual providers and institutions are accountable. Health IT security is a major worry; for instance, unidentified hackers have held EHR data hostage on hospital systems. At the health care organizational level, the security officer must perform a risk analysis, develop a risk mitigation plan, and approve electronic systems, such as an EHR. Purchasers of health IT must conduct security risk analyses upon installation or upgrade. The health care organization may also benefit from the work of the Health Information Trust Alliance (HITRUST), a U.S. organization that, in collaboration with health care, technology, and information security leaders, has established a Common Security Framework. This includes a prescriptive set of controls that seek to harmonize the requirements of multiple regulations and standards and can be employed by organizations that create, access, store, or exchange sensitive and regulated data. MU Stage 3 includes provisions that the Food and Drug Administration will deliver new tools to help mobile health product developers manage health care data security.

1.14.6. Selected Key Topics for Health IT

1.14.6.1. Interoperability

A core application (computer program) and additional modular applications or data sources (both inside and outside the organization) that increase functionality are typically found in health care data collection and management systems. Certain organizations adopt a primarily modular strategy, utilizing numerous distinct applications from various vendors to fulfill their comprehensive health IT requirements (e.g., the orders system, the laboratory system). A company is said to have an enterprise system if most of its operations are centralized within the same general application. Interoperability is the capacity of the various modules to communicate with one another as well as with external applications and data sources. Organizations utilizing various kinds or versions of health IT can still share data thanks to high-level interoperability. There are several ways to operationalize interoperability in software applications: (1) through built-in functionality; (2) through application programming interfaces (APIs) or standardized formats (e.g., HL7) for data sharing between applications; or (3) through remote interfaces through health information exchanges (HIEs), which are sizable data repositories that compile information from multiple health care providers. Medication errors and redundant testing are decreased when ineffective paper workflows are replaced with interoperability. Along with enhancing provider communication, interoperability also promotes improved chronic illness management and preventive care.

Applications that are modular in nature must be able to exchange and use electronic health information without requiring the user to take extra steps to comply with MU regulations. To direct the present and future development of a learning health system, the ONC has created an "interoperability road map.." For the EHR to automatically collect data from physiologic monitors, anesthesia machines, ventilators, intravenous pumps, medication dispensers, and other electronic devices, multiple device integration is another aspect of interoperability. The term "Internet of Things" (IOT) refers to the broader trend in interoperability whereby a wide range of electronic devices, including cars, home appliances, and personal health devices, are becoming connected to each other. This rapid expansion of functionality comes with a corresponding rise in security risks. Even though it requires a lot of work and resources, interoperability is a crucial and promising aspect of future health IT.

1.14.6.2. System Design, User Interface, and Usability

Laboratory test and imaging results, demographic data, billing and compliance data, scheduling, materials management, pharmacy data, physiologic data, and provider clinical documentation are just a few of the countless pieces of medical data that can be found in an EHR. Users may need to locate information across multiple screens, at different levels within the same application, or across multiple applications to conduct a clinical assessment of a patient. A "hunt and peck" strategy, or the display of data on screens in a way that hinders global comprehension, places a heavy cognitive and memory load on users and ignores human factors. Inadequate user interface and data visualization design can hinder accurate documentation, clinical evaluation, and effective pattern recognition in addition to decreasing efficiency. More generally, bad system and user interface design can hinder clinicians' ability to integrate information, anticipate future events, and plan ahead—a skill known as situational awareness—in addition to making it difficult for them to comprehend what is happening to a patient. Although it was first introduced in the aviation industry, situational awareness has also been used in the anesthesia industry. It pertains to complex systems involving teams of clinicians and computer systems in perioperative care and is defined as the collective functioning of teams.

The term "user interface" in computer science and informatics refers to all aspects of an information device that a user can interact with, such as the system's invitation and response mechanisms. A well-designed health IT user interface makes it possible for medical professionals to safely and effectively process vast amounts of data with speed and understanding. The overall layout of the health IT system may place restrictions on the user interface. Therefore, the principles of computer-human interaction must inform the overall design of the system. The practice of human factors engineering takes into account the needs and capabilities of the user of technology in the real world, assuming that people will act like humans and make mistakes when interacting with technology as well as have limited memory and cognitive capacity. User-centered design, an iterative technology development workflow, is one method for enhancing the performance of human-computer systems. It involves designing and developing prototypes based on early user-based evaluation, such as simulation and user interface evaluation during development. The adoption of more user-acceptable technologies and the avoidance of costly "redos" could result in significant savings even though such iterative engineering techniques might have higher upfront costs.

Design concepts from sectors other than aviation and computer science can also be effectively applied to health IT. Health care and anesthesia IT have used the industrial safety concept of a hierarchy of controls, which describes levels of intervention to defeat a hazard in order of most to least effective. The best controls are those that just take away a risk—that is, they make it impossible for the undesirable result to happen. A hard-stop rule that forbids ordering a medication with a lethal dose is one example. The next stage of intervention is substitution, where a less risky procedure is used in place of the riskier one. Examples of this include switching from anesthesia-drawn medications to prefilled syringes with standardized concentrations or, in the case of health IT, switching from free text to designated check boxes or buttons. Engineering the controls is the process of using system design to make it simpler to prevent a hazard. For instance, by requiring the bar code scanning of identification bracelets for vital activities like blood product transfusion, or by including patient identification photographs on various important screens in the EHR, the risk of a COWPIE (charting on the wrong patient in the EHR) can be decreased. The foundation of the next level of risk avoidance is administrative or organizational procedures and training, like checklists before procedures (which can be incorporated into AIMS workflows). Individual control measures, like instructing staff members to constantly click on a link to verify allergies before taking on a case, are the least successful. AIMS engineers and governance members should make every effort to avoid risks (e.g., patient safety, billing concerns, and compliance issues) at higher control levels, and collaborate with clinical and institutional leadership to remove, swap out, or engineer them out.

The degree to which technology enables users to accomplish their objectives in a fulfilling, successful, and efficient way while working within the limitations and complexity of their workplace is known as its usability. Usability guidelines are advised by the American Medical Informatics Association (AMIA) when developing electronic health records. Reversibility (the ability to reverse simple user errors), minimalism (the ability to quickly access core functions), and memory (memory load reduction, to lessen the cognitive burden of operating the system, preserving memory capacity for core tasks) are some of these principles that are especially applicable to technology implemented in the perioperative environment.

The value of system customization is highlighted by the AMIA's recommendation for flexibility. It is evident that tailoring the interface to the roles and preferences of users can improve usability. The advantages of standardizing user interfaces and system behaviors in accordance with regional and national standards do, however, also exist, so health IT developers must carefully weigh the advantages of customization against standardization. Standardized questionnaires, simulation, and screen and video recording have been used to assess user satisfaction, charting accuracy, situational awareness (effectiveness), and the number of "clicks" required to complete a task (efficiency) in an old versus a new AIMS, despite the fact that there is no one recognized evaluation tool for evaluating health IT usability. The purpose of such testing should be to evaluate and guide improvements in human interaction with the hardware, software, and human workflows that make up the entire system, both before and after rollout.

The resilience of the users is a crucial corollary of usability. Health care workers will typically find a way to achieve their objectives despite the limitations of health IT systems, even if they are difficult to use. In these situations, even though the health IT system seems to be functioning properly, the demands placed on the user's memory and focus (like having their "face buried in the computer screen" or relying on system "work-arounds") may cause the system to operate less effectively overall as well as negatively impact situational awareness, clinical performance, and user satisfaction.

1.14.6.3. Clinical Decision Support

CDS is an important feature of effective modern health IT and one of the most touted reasons for organizations to purchase health IT:

> To improve health and health care, clinical decision support gives clinicians, employees, patients, and other people person-specific knowledge and information that is intelligently filtered or presented at the right times. A range of tools are included in CDS to improve decision-making in the clinical workflow. Among other things, these tools include clinical guidelines, focused patient data reports and summaries, focused order sets for specific conditions, computerized alerts and reminders for patients and healthcare providers, documentation templates, diagnostic support, and contextually relevant reference material.

CDS can be passive, in which case the system helps the clinician make decisions by giving them the appropriate information at the appropriate moment. Passive CDS, which is closely related to user interface design, includes the display of pertinent laboratory results or vital signs as well as quick access to the proper checklists, protocols, standards, or policies. A patient's basic situational awareness, or understanding of what is happening to them right now, is supported by passive CDS. In Active CDS, logic (i.e., rules) identifies specific clinical situations and subsequently carry out operations, like producing an automated action, warning, or alert. An electronic health record (EHR) has the capability to autonomously track a patient's vital signs and laboratory results. In the event that a significant anomaly is identified, like symptoms of systemic inflammatory response syndrome, the EHR can initiate various alerts, such as a pop-up message, a smartphone alert, a pager alert, a dashboard alert, or recommendations for lab or medication orders. Higher level situational awareness deficiencies, such as the inability to combine and evaluate data from multiple sources in order to understand a clinical scenario, can be addressed by active CDS. CDS can be operated at the multi patient level, at the user level, in real time, or over an extended duration (e.g., an efficiency dashboard for the operating room).

In terms of managerial workflows, the care process, and ultimately the results of the care, CDS offers a great deal of potential and achieved benefits. With regard to anesthesia, CDS has enhanced adherence to the cardiac workup protocol, alerted patients about their anticoagulation status before a regional block, provided near-real-time alerts and reminders for intraoperative and critical care, and decreased certain unfavorable outcomes like postoperative nausea and vomiting. A major drawback of CDS is that it cannot use data that are not readily available, like medical history records from unintegrated health systems or data that are not yet entered into the EHR. Automation-induced complacency describes the situation in which clinicians become overly dependent on alerts or other CDS and then fail to recognize and act on that same situation when CDS fails to warn them. What good is a drug-drug interaction alert that fails to appear because it does not know the patient's home medications or signals after the concerning medication has already been given? These errors may be decreased by ensuring sufficient EHR data and structure so that CDS is not a black box—that is so that the provider knows how the CDS operates and what data it depends on.

A National Patient Safety Goal from 2016 aims to decrease unnecessary alerts and alarms. This goal tackles the opposite scenario, where an excessive number of ineffective CDS warnings lead to confusion and a decline in clinician performance due to alert fatigue. In light of the potential consequences of misdirected or inadequately signaled alerts, CDS—especially active CDS—should be assessed in a manner akin to that of hemodynamic alarms or laboratory tests. In addition to their quantifiable sensitivity and specificity, they also have positive and negative predictive values, which indicate the likelihood that the existence or nonexistence of a true significant situation is reflected in the presence or absence of a CDS alert. Health IT management should test an active CDS intervention "in the background" to identify the warning characteristics and, once it is implemented, measure the impact the tool has on health care providers' behavior, such as when they order a new test or medication. It is generally advised to avoid hard stops as much as possible because they can unintentionally completely prevent a user from performing productive work. This situation is made much worse when faulty design makes it impossible to comply with the rule that caused the hard stop, which is a major disadvantage for user satisfaction and efficacy. If the use of hard stops is necessary for vital patient safety, it might be best to test the rule as a caution or soft stop at first, watch for appropriate behavior, and activate the hard stop functionality only after it has been validated.

1.14.7. Transitioning to Health IT: From Paper Records to an AIMS, and Beyond

Decisions regarding the migration of a new health IT system or the transition from a traditional paper workflow should be made with consideration for factors like risk mitigation, clinical work enhancement, CDS and reporting support, and usability in mind. It is important to recognize these risks, and any evaluation of an IT system should involve a thorough analysis and continuous watch for any negative effects.

The purchase of new perioperative information management systems, or AIMS, is largely the responsibility of anesthesia and perioperative leaders. They should collaborate closely with possible vendors and application developers and take the lead in considering new anesthesia and perioperative health IT. They still have a crucial responsibility to share their assessment of the AIMS and perioperative modules and determine which elements are appropriate (or not), even if their healthcare organization is investing in an enterprise-wide EHR. Take note of the project communication, implementation plan, role of change management, and how the new technology interacts with the organization's culture. Important "people factors" for a successful rollout include a project champion with strong political and social skills, early and frequent engagement of end users in the project from the start of design to the end of evaluation, and deeply committed leadership. Users' impressions of a new system's usefulness—what it can accomplish?—may pique their interest more in it than its apparent simplicity of use. Since both are crucial, project education should cover both system operations as well as how the new tool can enhance clinical care or the efficacy and efficiency of the user. When launching a new AIMS or related health IT system, keep in mind that the main objective of these systems is to enhance each patient's quality of health. Its support for the organizational "health" in terms of quality, management, and finances is essential. Provider satisfaction and system usability will probably suffer, though, if excessive data entry is required to support these secondary goals. "As value-based care and accountable care models grow, the primary purpose of the EHR should remain the facilitation of seamless patient care to improve outcomes while contributing to data collection that supports necessary analyses," states a recent position paper from the American College of Physicians, highlighting these tensions. Despite the fact that many stakeholders might want more information to be entered into the medical record, clinical leaders and health IT governance should rank these tasks based on institutional priorities. In order to ensure that the use of new technology enhances rather than worsens patient care, they must also promote its general usability.

1.14.8. Legal Issues and Responsibilities of the AIMS User

Numerous instances in the literature have discussed the dangers of utilizing AIMS with defects in design, insufficient training, or improper user practices, including potential legal ramifications. When switching from paper records to an AIMS, one of the most frequent concerns about AIMS is device integration. The providers have expressed concerns regarding the potential medicolegal risks associated with the now apparent increased variation in auto documented vital signs and the inevitable data artifacts. There is historical evidence that the appropriate use of an AIMS does not result in significant medicolegal negative consequences for providers generally, despite the risks associated with artifacts, unnoticed data dropouts, and inaccurate auto documentation. Actually, the field of anesthesia may benefit from the automatic recording of physiological data since it eliminates the known issues associated with human data filtering and increases the record's credibility. However, EHR users need to be aware of the fundamentals of device data acquisition workflow and be able to identify and fix data capture errors. EHRs should also make it simple to note mistakes in data collection or artifacts.

These concerns are demonstrated by a case report of a patient undergoing a craniotomy. Legal documents state that the responsible anesthesia provider discovered, upon returning from a break, that the vital sign/device data stream had failed. The interim anesthesia provider, who had taken care of the patient during the break, was not aware of this. 93 minutes of data were therefore not included in the chart. The absence of anesthetic documentation may have played a role in resolving the patient's postoperative quadriplegia. Because the "active" window covered up the data's graphic display, the anesthesiologist was unable to understand how the data was transmitted. This case highlights the need for the anesthesia provider to exercise caution and the fact that monitoring devices can malfunction occasionally.

The use of CDS to display an alert when data flow is interrupted is one example of how AIMS design has improved since this case, but in the end, it is the health IT user's responsibility to adhere to institutional, local, and national standards in order to create an accurate and comprehensive anesthetic and medical record. Depending on the institutional policy, users might even need to manually enter missing data on a regular basis or mark data gaps and artifacts. These procedures are also applicable in the event of a network or system outage. When there are problems with the data, it is best to fully and transparently record the events and to make the necessary corrections as soon as possible. Discoverable audit trails document the data's source and the time of modification. It goes without saying that extremely late alterations to an anesthetic record may appear improper. Evidence suggests that health IT does have genuine benefits, and its ubiquity and inevitable nature make it inevitable. However, the design and specifics are critical. Health IT should support the organization's financial and management needs in addition to the clinical needs of patients and providers. Every anesthesiologist needs to be aware of how health IT affects patient care. To guarantee that present and future IT systems meet the unique requirements of perioperative care, anesthesia providers must be involved in IT decision-making and development. As they understand that IT systems can be helpful for teaching and learning, anesthesia trainees do, in fact, have a role to play in the advancement of health IT. Health IT is still developing quickly, so it's important to keep an eye on and research how it's used in critical and perioperative care. Perioperative Surgical Home (PSH) is a concept that requires the use of health information technology.

Every organization's future changes will be influenced by the collection and use of data. It is stated that something you cannot measure, you cannot manage. Health IT has the potential to significantly transform and improve patient care beyond what has been accomplished thus far, once a large number of organizations contribute their patient data into aggregated data pools. (Vigoda et al., 2011; Xie, 2015)

A Closer Look

Anesthesia for Oculoplastic Surgery

Anesthesia for oculoplastic surgery involves careful consideration of the patient's medical history, the specific procedure being performed, and the preferences of both the patient and the surgical team. Oculoplastic surgery encompasses a range of procedures involving the eyelids, tear ducts, orbit, and surrounding structures, and anesthesia choices may vary depending on factors such as the complexity of the surgery and the patient's overall health.

Local anesthesia with sedation is commonly used for many oculoplastic procedures, providing adequate pain control and patient comfort while allowing them to remain awake and responsive during surgery. Local anesthetic agents are injected around the surgical site to numb the area, and sedative medications may be administered intravenously to help relax the patient and alleviate anxiety.

In some cases, general anesthesia may be preferred or necessary, particularly for more extensive or invasive oculoplastic surgeries. General anesthesia induces a state of unconsciousness, allowing the patient to remain asleep and pain-free throughout the procedure. This approach may be chosen for complex reconstructive surgeries, orbital surgeries, or procedures requiring prolonged operative times.

Regional anesthesia techniques, such as peribulbar or retrobulbar blocks, may be used to provide anesthesia and akinesia (muscle paralysis) for certain oculoplastic procedures involving the globe or orbit. These techniques involve injecting local anesthetic agents around the eye to block sensory and motor function while maintaining patient comfort and minimizing systemic effects.

The choice of anesthesia for oculoplastic surgery is carefully tailored to each patient's individual needs, taking into account factors such as the patient's medical history, allergies, preferences, and the surgeon's expertise. Anesthesia providers work closely with the surgical team to ensure optimal patient safety, comfort, and outcomes throughout the perioperative period. Preoperative assessment, intraoperative monitoring, and postoperative care are essential components of anesthesia management for oculoplastic surgery, aimed at minimizing risks and optimizing patient recovery.

Summary

- Anesthesia represents a cornerstone of modern medicine, facilitating surgical interventions and medical procedures by inducing a reversible state of unconsciousness, analgesia (pain relief), amnesia (memory loss), and muscle relaxation.
- Anesthetists are specialist doctors who are responsible for providing anesthesia to patients for operations and procedures. In addition, anesthetists have a range of practices that extends beyond anesthesia for surgery to include pain management and intensive care.
- General anesthesia leads to multi-system physiological changes. The systemic effects of anesthesia vary with the drugs used so different agents are favored in different clinical contexts. In general, intravenous (propofol and thiopentone) and volatile agents all reduce blood pressure as a result of vasodilation, and negative inotropy and chronotropy.
- Pain management is required in the perioperative setting as well as for chronic pain conditions. The management of perioperative pain has become more complex as the relationship between postoperative pain control and functional outcomes (e.g., mobility after joint replacement surgery) has become more tightly linked.
- Anesthesiologists can obtain certification from the National Board of Echocardiography for perioperative transesophageal echocardiography as well as adult echocardiography.
- The role of the PACU is pivotal. Not only are patients recovering from anesthesia and surgery, they also are receiving direction for appropriate care after their PACU time which spans from ICU to discharge.
- Postgraduate training in anesthesiology in the United States consists of 4 years of supervised experience in an approved program after the degree of doctor of medicine or doctor of osteopathy has been obtained.
- Anesthesiologists spend long hours in an environment (operating room) associated with exposure to vapors from chemicals (volatile anesthetics), ionizing radiation, and infectious agents (hepatitis viruses, human immunodeficiency virus).
- Anesthesia providers care for the surgical patient in the preoperative, intraoperative, and postoperative periods. Important patient care decisions reflect on assessing the preoperative evaluation, creating the anesthesia plan, preparing the operating room, and managing the intraoperative anesthetic, postoperative care, and outcome.
- The EHR is a longitudinal electronic record of patient health information generated by one or more encounters in any care delivery setting. Although there are significant realized and potential advantages of using EHRs for patients, providers, and the health care organization, there are also many potential pitfalls.
- Health care providers are morally and legally obligated to protect the privacy of their patients as well as the security of the EHR. The Health Insurance Portability and Accountability Act (HIPAA) Privacy, Security, and Breach Notification Rules are U.S. regulations that codify this obligation into law.
- Clinical decision support provides clinicians, staff, patients, or other individuals with knowledge and person-specific information, intelligently filtered or presented at appropriate times, to enhance health and health care.

References

1. Adler-Milstein, J., DesRoches, C., Kralovec, P., et al. (2015). Electronic health record adoption in US hospitals: Progress continues, but challenges persist. *Health Affairs, 34*(12), 2174–2180.
2. Apfelbaum, J. L., Aveyard, C., Cooper, L., et al. (2009). Outsourcing anesthesia preparation. *Anesthesiology News*, 1–6.
3. Berlinger, N. T. (2006). Robotic surgery: Squeezing into tight places. *New England Journal of Medicine, 354*, 2099–2101.
4. Braun, B. R. A., Donofrio, K., Hafiz, H., & Loeb, J. (2012). The Joint Commission—Improving patient and worker safety: Opportunities for synergy, collaboration, and innovation. *The Joint Commission*. Retrieved from: http://www.jointcommission.org/improving_patient_worker_safety/ (accessed on 29 July 2024).
5. Centers for Medicare & Medicaid Services (CMS). (2016). *EHR Incentive Programs*. Retrieved from: https://www.cms.gov/Regulations-and-Guidance/Legislation/EHRIncentivePrograms/index.html (accessed on 29 July 2024).
6. Centers for Medicare & Medicaid Services (CMS). (2016). *HIPAA Basics for Providers: Privacy, Security, and Breach Notification Rules*. Retrieved from: http://www.hhs.gov/hipaa/for-professionals/index.html (accessed on 29 July 2024).
7. Centers for Medicare & Medicaid Services (CMS). (2016). *PQRS Measures*. Retrieved from: https://www.cms.gov/medicare/quality-initiatives-patient-assessment-instruments/pqrs/measurescodes.html (accessed on 29 July 2024).
8. Committee on Quality of Health Care in America, Institute of Medicine. (2000). *To Err Is Human*. Washington, DC: National Academy Press.
9. Cooper, J. B., & Gaba, D. G. (2002). No myth: Anesthesia is a model for addressing patient safety. *Anesthesiology, 97*, 1335–1337.
10. Cranshaw, J., Gupta, K. J., & Cook, T. M. (2009). Litigation related to drug errors in anesthesia: An analysis of claims against the NHS in England 1995–2007. *Anaesthesia, 64*, 1317–1323.
11. Dexter, F. (2012). A brief history of evidence-based operating room management: Then and now. *Anesthesia & Analgesia, 115*, 10–11.
12. Dexter, F. (2014). High-quality operating room management research. *Journal of Clinical Anesthesia, 26*, 341–342.
13. Directors ABO. (2001). APSF endorses use of automated record keepers. *Anesthesia Patient Safety Foundation Newsletter, 16*(4).
14. Dutton, R. P. (2015). Making a difference: The Anesthesia Quality Institute. *Anesthesia & Analgesia, 120*(3), 507–509.
15. Ehrenfeld, J. M., McEvoy, M. D., Furman, W. R., et al. (2014). Automated near-real-time clinical performance feedback for anesthesiology residents: One piece of the milestones puzzle. *Anesthesiology, 120*(1), 172–184.
16. Epstein, R. H., Dexter, F., & Patel, N. (2015). Influencing anesthesia provider behavior using anesthesia information management system data for near real-time alerts and post hoc reports. *Anesthesia & Analgesia, 12*(3), 678–692.
17. Furukawa, M. F., Eldridge, N., Wang, Y., et al. (2016). Electronic health record adoption and

rates of in-hospital adverse events. *Journal of Patient Safety, 16(2), 137–142*. https://doi.org/10.1097/PTS.0000000000000257.

18. Galvez, J. A., Rothman, B. S., Doyle, C. A., et al. (2015). A narrative review of meaningful use and anesthesia information management systems. *Anesthesia & Analgesia, 121*(3), 693–706.
19. Hallinan, J. T. (2005). Once seen as risky, one group of doctors changes its ways. *The Wall Street Journal*.
20. Healthcare Information and Management Systems Society (HIMSS). (2016). *What is interoperability?* Retrieved from: http://www.himss.org/library/interoperability-standards/what-is-interoperability (accessed on 29 July 2024).
21. Karsh, B. T., Weinger, M. B., Abbott, P. A., & Wears, R. L. (2010). Health information technology: Fallacies and sober realities. *Journal of the American Medical Informatics Association, 17*(6), 617–623.
22. Kheterpal, S. (2014). In the land of the blind, the one-eyed man is king. *Anesthesiology, 120*(3), 523–525.
23. Kuhn, T., Basch, P., Barr, M., & Yackel, T. (2015). Clinical documentation in the 21st century: Executive summary of a policy position paper from the American College of Physicians. *Annals of Internal Medicine, 162*(4), 301–303.
24. Lagasse, R. S. (2002). Anesthesia safety: Model or myth? A review of the published literature and analysis of current original data. *Anesthesiology, 97*, 1609–1617.
25. Mangalmurti, S. S., Murtagh, L., & Mello, M. M. (2010). Medical malpractice liability in the age of electronic health records. *New England Journal of Medicine, 363*(21), 2060–2067.
26. Matthay, M. A., & Liu, K. D. (2016). New strategies for effective therapeutics in critically ill patients. *JAMA, 315*(8), 747–748.
27. Mello, M. M., & Livingston, E. H. (2016). Managing the risks of concurrent surgeries. *JAMA, 315*, 1563–1564.
28. Miller, R. D. (2005). Report from the Task Force on Future Paradigms of Anesthesia Practice. *ASA Newsletter, 69*, 2–6.
29. Miller, R. D. (2008). The pursuit of excellence. The 47th Annual Rovenstine Lecture. *Anesthesiology, 110*, 714–720.
30. Molnar, C., Nemes, C., Szabo, S., & Fulesdi, B. (2008). Harvey Cushing, a pioneer of neuroanesthesia. *Journal of Anesthesia, 22*(4), 483–486.
31. Nair, B. G., Horibe, M., Newman, S. F., et al. (2014). Anesthesia information management system-based near real-time decision support to manage intraoperative hypotension and hypertension. *Anesthesia & Analgesia, 118*(1), 206–214.
32. Nolan, T. (2000). System changes to improve patient safety. *BMJ, 320*, 771–773.
33. Office of the National Coordinator for Health Information Technology. (2015). *Health IT.gov*. Retrieved from: http://www.healthit.gov/ (accessed on 29 July 2024).
34. Office of the National Coordinator for Health Information Technology (ONC). (2015). *Connecting Health and Care for the Nation: A Shared Nationwide Interoperability Roadmap*. Retrieved from: https://www.healthit.gov/sites/default/files/hie-interoperability/nationwide-interoperability-roadmap-final-version-1.0.pdf (accessed on 29 July 2024).

35. Pierce, E. C. (1996). The 34th Rovenstine Lecture: 40 years behind the mask: Safety revisited. *Anesthesiology, 84*, 965–997.

36. Schulz, C. M., Endsley, M. R., Kochs, E. F., et al. (2013). Situation awareness in anesthesia: Concept and research. *Anesthesiology, 118*(3), 729–742.

37. Shah, N. J., Tremper, K. K., & Kheterpal, S. (2011). Anatomy of an anesthesia information management system. *Anesthesiology Clinics, 29*(3), 355–365.

38. Sittig, D. F., & Wright, A. (2015). What makes an EHR "open" or interoperable? *Journal of the American Medical Informatics Association, 22*(5), 1099–1101.

39. Spiess, B. D., Wahr, J. A., & Nussmeier, N. A. (2010). Bring your life into FOCUS. *Anesthesia & Analgesia, 110*, 283–287.

40. Stabile, M., & Cooper, L. (2013). Review article: The evolving role of information technology in perioperative patient safety. *Canadian Journal of Anesthesia, 60*(2), 119–126.

41. Stoelting, R. K. (1999). APSF survey results identify safety issues priorities. *Spring APSF Newsletter*, 6–7. Retrieved from: http://www.apsf.org (accessed on 29 July 2024).

42. Stol, I. S., Ehrenfeld, J. M., & Epstein, R. H. (2014). Technology diffusion of anesthesia information management systems into academic anesthesia departments in the United States. *Anesthesia & Analgesia, 118*(3), 644–650.

43. U.S. Department of Health & Human Services (HHS). (2016). *Health Information Privacy*. Retrieved from: https://www.hhs.gov/hipaa/for-professionals/security/laws-regulations/ (accessed on 29 July 2024).

44. Vetter, T. R., & Redden, D. T. (2015). The power and perils of big data: It all depends on how you slice, dice, and digest it. *Anesthesia & Analgesia, 121*(3), 582–585.

45. Vigoda, M. M., & Lubarsky, D. A. (2006). Failure to recognize loss of incoming data in an anesthesia record-keeping system may have increased medical liability. *Anesthesia & Analgesia, 102*(6), 1798–1802.

46. Vigoda, M. M., & Rembold, S. D. (2011). Implications of electronic discovery. *ASA Monitor, 75*, 20–21.

47. Vigoda, M. M., Rothman, B., & Green, J. A. (2011). Shortcomings and challenges of information system adoption. *Anesthesia Clinics, 29*(3), 397–412.

48. Xie, J. (2015). Up to speed: A role for trainees in advancing health information technology. *Pediatrics, 136*(3), 412–414.

Chapter

BASIC PHARMACOLOGIC PRINCIPLES

2

Contents

Introduction

An anesthesia provider's knowledge base must include the fundamentals of pharmacology. The behavior of anesthetic drugs is described in this chapter with reference to important clinical pharmacology concepts. Drug clearance, drug volumes of distribution, drug transfer from plasma to tissues, and drug binding to circulating plasma proteins are examples of pharmacokinetic concepts. The physiological mechanisms governing pharmacokinetics and the mathematical models utilized to connect dose to concentration are both introduced in the section on pharmacokinetics. Seldom do anesthesiologists use just one medication. Specializing in analgesia, sedation, and muscle relaxation, most anesthetics are blends of multiple medications. Therefore, the anesthetic effect can be significantly influenced by pharmacodynamic interactions. While determining the appropriate dosage of anesthetic, a number of patient characteristics must be taken into account, including age, body habit, sex, history of long-term use of opioids, benzodiazepines, or alcohol, presence of heart, lung, kidney, or liver disease, and degree of dehydration or blood loss. These patient factors that affect the pharmacology of anesthetic drugs will be discussed, with two of them being body habitus and age.

Orientation and Directional Terms

Term	Definition	Illustration
Pharmacokinetic	Pharmacokinetics, sometimes described as what the body does to a drug, refers to the movement of drug into, through, and out of the body—the time course of its absorption, bioavailability, distribution, metabolism, and excretion.	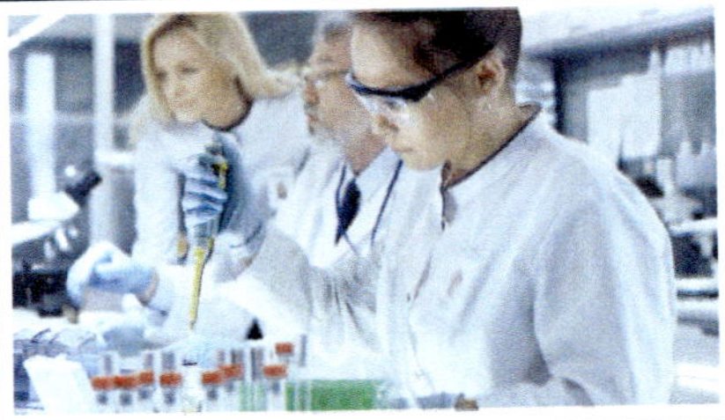
Plasma volume	Plasma volume can be measured by using Evans blue dye, which binds to plasma proteins, or by injecting serum albumin labeled with radioactive iodine. The average PV in a normal 70 kg adult is approximately 3.5. L (50–55 mL/kg).	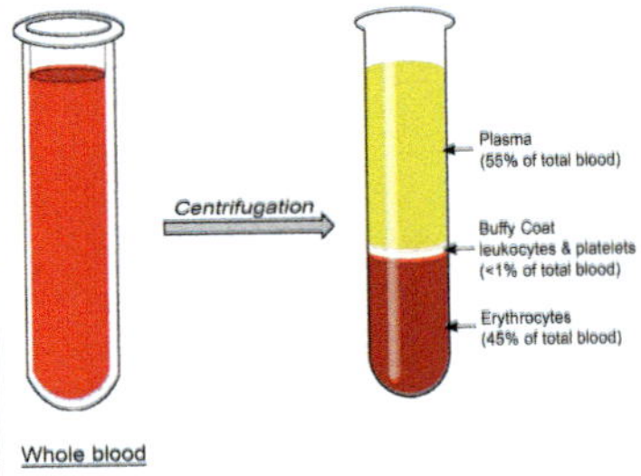
Peripheral artery disease	Peripheral artery disease is similar to coronary artery disease. Peripheral artery disease, or PAD, is a narrowing of the peripheral arteries that carry blood away from the heart to other parts of the body. The most common type is lower-extremity PAD, in which blood flow is reduced to the legs and feet.	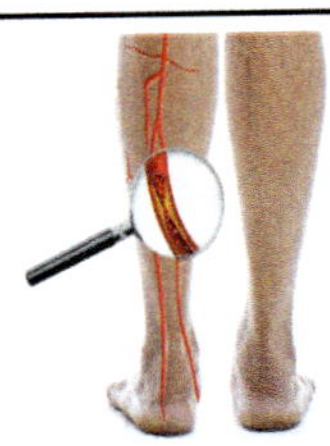
Bispectral index (BIS)	Bispectral index (BIS) is one of several technologies used to monitor depth of anesthesia. BIS monitors are used to supplement Guedel's classification system for determining depth of anesthesia. Titrating anesthetic agents to a specific bispectral index during general anesthesia in adults (and children over 1 year old) allows the anesthetist to adjust the amount of anesthetic agent to the needs of the patient, possibly resulting in a more rapid emergence from anesthesia.	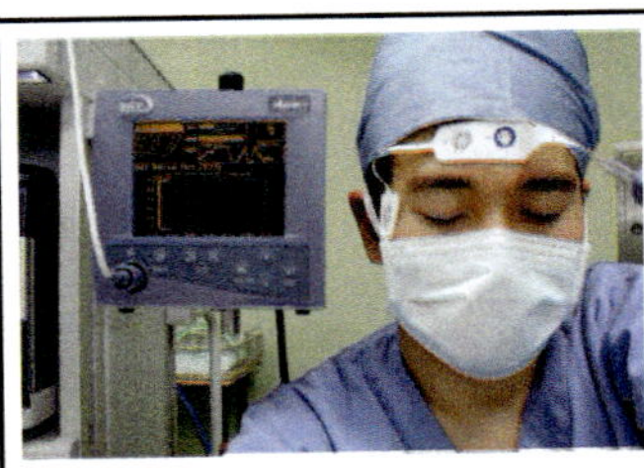
Fat-free mass (FFM)	Fat-free mass (FFM) or lean body mass is the primary determinant of TEE in all age groups. FFM is the metabolically active tissue in the body. Hence, most of the variation in REE between people can be accounted for by the variation in their FFM.	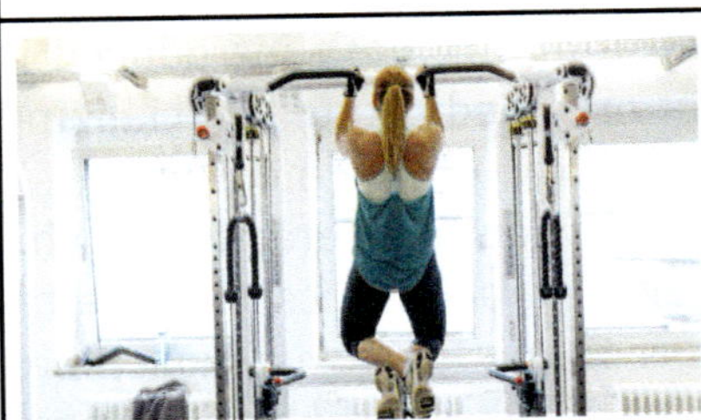

2.1. Pharmacokinetic Principles

The relationship between drug dose and drug concentration in plasma or at the site of drug effect over time is referred to as pharmacokinetics. This relationship is controlled by the processes of absorption, distribution, and elimination (metabolism and excretion). While absorption is relevant to all other drug delivery routes, it does not apply to drugs administered intravenously. Drugs administered intravenously have a time course that depends on both distribution volume and clearance. Pharmacokinetic parameters describe estimates of clearances and distribution volumes. Mathematical formulas fitted to measured blood or plasma concentrations over time after a known drug dose are used to derive pharmacokinetic parameters.

2.1.1. Fundamental Pharmacokinetic Concepts

2.1.1.1. Volume of Distribution

The dilution of a drug dose into a water tank represents an oversimplified model of drug distribution throughout plasma and tissues. Once the drug has had enough time to fully mix within the tank, the volume of distribution (Vd) is the apparent size of the tank needed to explain a measured drug concentration from the tank water. The distribution volume is estimated using the simple relationship between dose (e.g., mg) and measured concentration (e.g., mg/L) as presented in Eq. 1.

$$\text{Volume of distribution} = \frac{\text{Amount of dose (mg)}}{\text{Concentration (mg/L)}} \quad (1)$$

Once the tank volume is estimated, the drug concentration following a bolus dosage can be computed. Similarly to how a tank has a fixed volume regardless of the presence of drug within it, distribution volumes in individuals are inherent characteristics regardless of the administration of any medication. Human bodies do not function like water tanks. As soon as a drug is administered, it starts to be eliminated from the body (Figure 2.1).

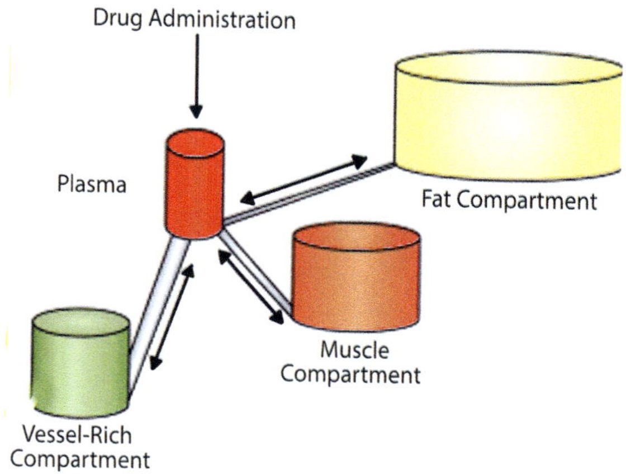

Figure 2.1. *Drug distribution.*

Source: Elo, J. A., & Sun, H.-H. (2016). Anesthesia and Sedation. InTech. doi: 10.5772/63539.

Using Equation 1, estimating the volume of distribution without accounting for elimination leads to the volume of distribution estimates that become larger than the initial volume. To refine the definition of distribution volume, the amount of drug that is present at a given time t is divided by the concentrations at the same time.

$$\text{Vd} = \frac{\text{Amount } (t)}{\text{Concentration } (t)} \quad (2)$$

The volume of distribution determined by Equation 2 will remain constant if elimination proceeds as a first-order process, meaning that it is proportionate to the concentration at that particular moment. A drug given intravenously distributes to peripheral tissues primarily, with some remaining in the vascular volume. Often, this distribution is shown as more distribution volumes (tanks) attached to a central tank (blood or plasma volume). The volume of distribution as a whole is increased by peripheral distribution volumes. Peripheral tissue drug distribution is represented by the peripheral tank. To accurately depict the entire drug disposition in the body, more than one peripheral tank (volume) may exist. The peripheral volume size indicates the solubility of a drug in tissue in comparison to blood or plasma. The peripheral volumes of distribution of a drug increase with its solubility in peripheral tissue as compared to blood or plasma. (Figures 2.2 and 2.3).

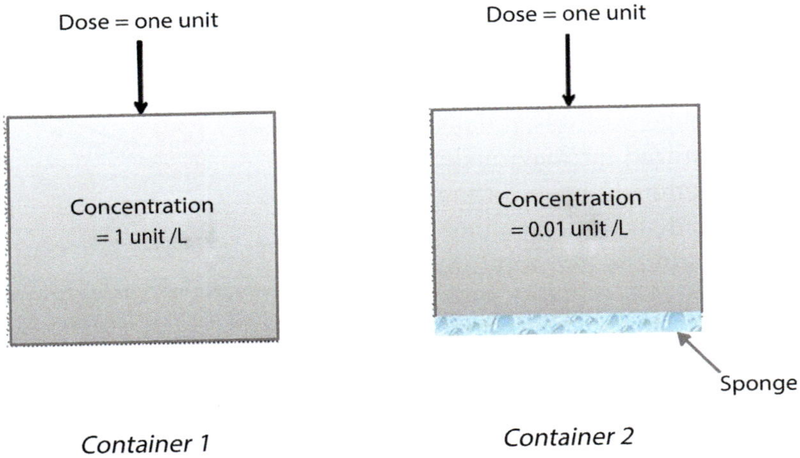

Figure 2.2. *A clarification of the concept of VD of a drug dissolved in two containers containing water. The Vd is an apparent volume term that is determined from the amount of drug added and the resulting concentration. Given the same dose amount and the 100-fold reduction in drug concentration in Container 2, the VD of the drug in Container 2 is 100 times larger than that of the same drug present in Container 1.*

Source: Kok-Yong, S., & Lawrence, L. (2015). Drug Distribution and Drug Elimination. InTech. doi: 10.5772/59929.

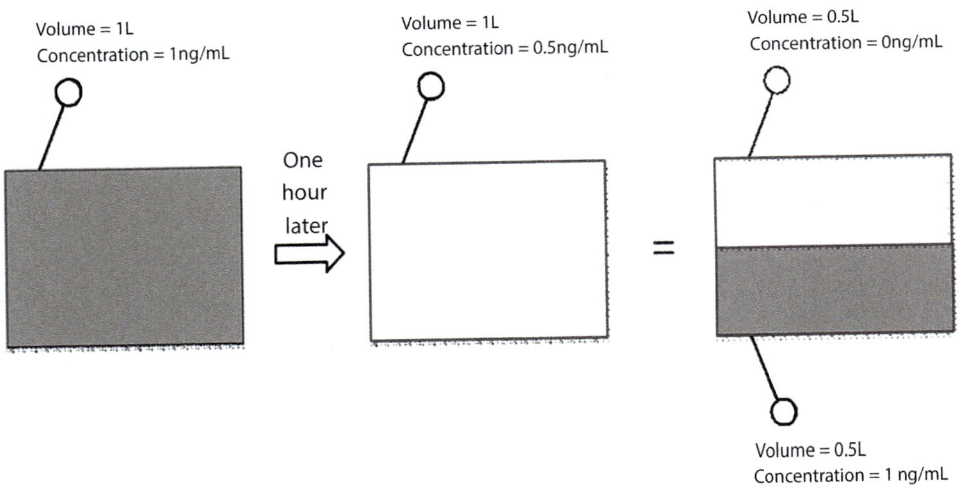

Figure 2.3. *Clearance.*

Source: Kok-Yong, S., & Lawrence, L. (2015). Drug Distribution and Drug Elimination. InTech. doi: 10.5772/59929.

The fact that the drug binds to the tissue in the peripheral tank in addition to distributing to it and increasing its volume of distribution is a crucial point. The central tank's measurable concentration is further reduced by this process. As a result, the distribution's overall volume might even exceed the sum of the two tanks. Certain anesthetics actually have enormous distribution volumes; for example, fentanyl appears to have an 8 L/kg distribution volume, which is much greater than the extracellular (0.02 L/kg) or vascular (0.07 L/kg) volumes of an individual.

The distribution volume is no longer constant over time with an extra tank. At time = 0, the estimated volume of distribution is 4.3. L, which is also the value of the single-tank model. Over the course of the following ten minutes, the distribution volume rises to 48 L. The drug's distribution to the peripheral volume and subsequent elimination from the body are the causes of the increase. A common occurrence is that during the first few minutes following drug administration, more drug enters peripheral tissue than is removed. Take a look at a simulation of a propofol bolus, for instance, which shows how much propofol accumulates in peripheral tissues and how much is eventually eliminated. The amount that is transferred to peripheral tissue during the first four minutes is greater than the amount that is expelled from the body. After four minutes, the amounts are the opposite.

2.1.1.2. Clearance

The term "clearance" refers to the pace at which drugs leave plasma or blood. Systemic (out of the tank) and intercompartmental (between the tanks) clearance are the two processes that lead to drug clearance. Drugs are eliminated from the body permanently through systemic clearance, which can also involve the conversion of the drug into metabolites. Drugs are moved between peripheral tissue tanks and plasma tanks through intercompartmental clearance. To be clear, the terms "tank" and "compartment" are used interchangeably.

The volume of drug entirely cleared per unit of time, or L/min, is the unit of flow used to define clearance. Elimination rate (e.g., mg/min) and clearance are not the same thing. (Figures 2.4 and 2.5).

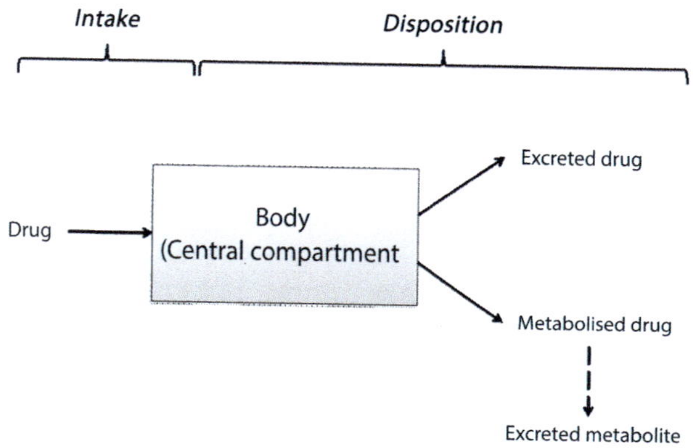

Figure 2.4. *A one-compartment model with first-order input for describing the drug plasma concentration versus time profile. The arrows indicate the movement of the drug with respect to the body. Further, the diagram depicts that part of the drug may be excreted unchanged and some part may be metabolised by enzymes in the body.*

Source: Kok-Yong, S., & Lawrence, L. (2015). Drug Distribution and Drug Elimination. InTech. doi: 10.5772/59929.

The total amount of drug can be computed at each measured drug concentration using the volume of distribution. Despite having the same duration of one minute, time window A's concentration change is greater than time window B's. For time windows A and B, the elimination rates are 12 mg/min and 27, respectively. They are distinct from one another, and neither can be utilized as a predictor of drug concentrations when a different drug dosage is given. Owing to this restriction on elimination rate, clearance was created in order to give a single figure that would represent the decline in drug concentration.

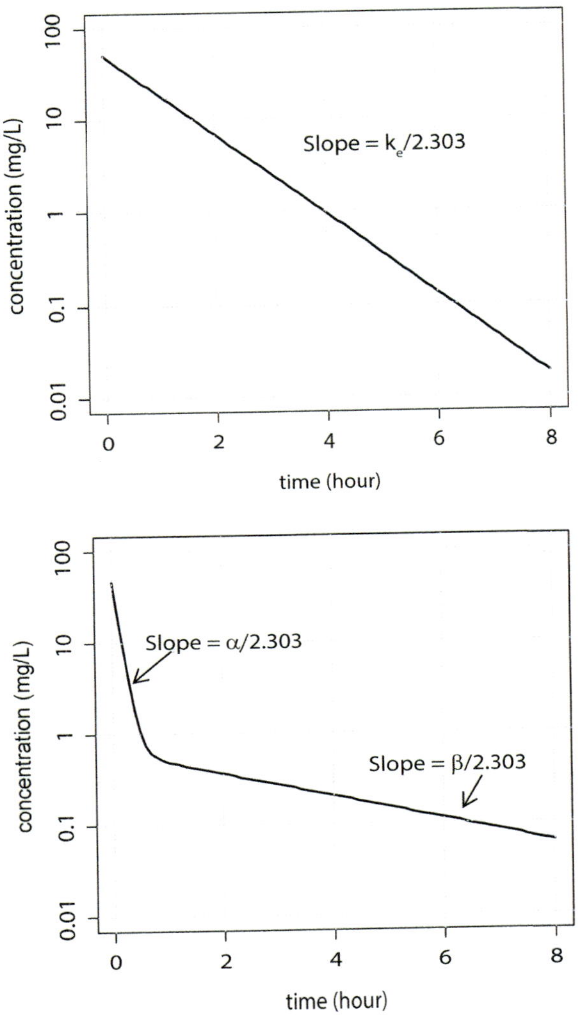

Figure 2.5. *Plasma concentration versus time profiles following I.V. bolus administration on a semi-logarithmic graph for a drug exhibiting a one-compartment model (upper panel) and a two-compartment model (lower panel). For the two-compartment model, the slopes α and β denote the rates of combined distribution plus elimination, and elimination, respectively, of the drug from the central compartment.*

Source: Kok-Yong, S., & Lawrence, L. (2015). Drug Distribution and Drug Elimination. InTech. doi: 10.5772/59929.

Assume for the sake of discussion that the force required to force the drug out of the water tank is concentration.

The more drug that is eliminated, the higher the concentration. The amount of drug eliminated is scaled to concentration to standardize the elimination rate. For instance, the elimination rate in time window A (27 mg/min) is 0.001807 mg/min/mg/L when scaled to the mean concentration (15 µg/mL) during that time window. Unit reduction results in 0.002 L/min. The same outcome as in A is obtained by normalizing the elimination rate in time window B to concentration. If the time interval is narrowed so that the time window approaches zero, the definition of clearance becomes:

$$\text{Clearance} = \frac{dA/dt}{C\ (t)} \tag{3}$$

where dA/dt is the rate of drug elimination at a given time t, and C (t) is the corresponding concentration at time t.

Rearranging Equation 3, clearance can be expressed as follows:

$$\text{Clearance} = \frac{Q(C_{in} - C_{out})}{C_{in}} \tag{4}$$

where Q is the blood flow to metabolic organs, C_{in} is the concentration of drug delivered to metabolic organs, and C_{out} is the concentration of drug leaving metabolic organs. The fraction of inflowing drug extracted by the organ is $(Cin - C_{out})/C_{in}$ and is called the extraction ratio (ER). Clearance can be estimated as organ blood flow multiplied by the ER. Equation 4 can be simplified as shown here:

$$\text{Clearance} = Q \times ER \tag{5}$$

The total clearance is the sum of each clearance by metabolic organs such as the liver, kidney, and other tissues.

The hepatic clearance has been extensively studied. For instance, the connection between liver blood flow, clearance, and the extraction ratio. A change in liver blood flow results in a nearly proportionate change in clearance for medications with an extraction ratio of almost 1 (such as propofol). The rate of liver blood flow has little effect on the clearance of medications with low extraction ratios, such as alfentanil. If the liver extracts almost all of the drug, this suggests that the liver has a large amount of drug metabolism capacity. Here, the drug's passage to the liver is the rate-limiting step in metabolism; as a result, these medications are referred to as "flow limited." It is normal for anesthesia to cause a reduction in liver blood flow, which will also likely cause a decrease in clearance. However, because the hepatic metabolic capacity is far greater than the demand, slight modifications in the hepatic metabolic function per se will not significantly affect clearance.

The extraction ratio for many medications, such as alfentanil, is significantly less than 1. The liver's ability to absorb and metabolize the drug limits the amount of these medications that can be cleared. These medications are referred to as "capacity limited." "Any alteration in the liver's ability to metabolize such drugs, whether due to enzymatic induction or liver disease, will alter clearance." However, because the liver only processes a small portion of the drug that it sees, changes in liver blood flow—which may be brought on by the anesthetic state itself—typically have little effect on clearance.

2.1.1.3. Front-End Kinetics

The term "front-end kinetics" describes the behavior of an intravenous drug right after it is administered. The peak plasma drug concentration is directly influenced by how quickly a drug enters peripheral tissues from the blood. One key premise of compartmental models is that an intravenous bolus immediately mixes in the central volume, reaching its peak concentration at injection time and not being eliminated or distributed to the periphery. The initial concentration and distribution volume at time = 0 are extrapolated as though the circulation had been infinitely fast for simulation purposes.

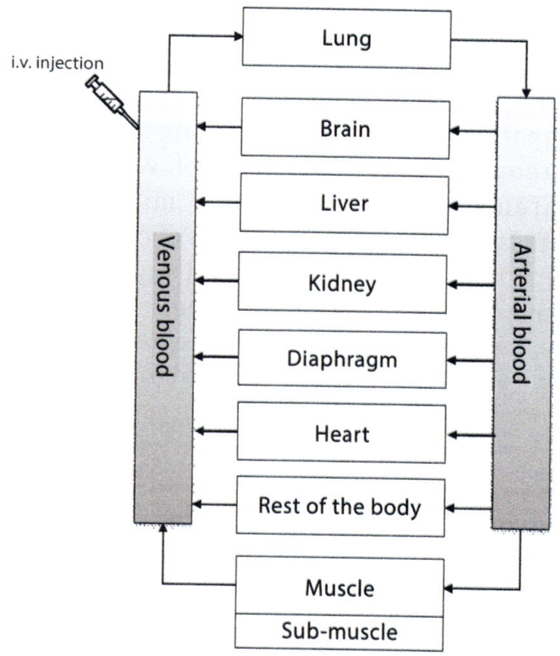

Figure 2.6. *A physiologically based pharmacokinetic (PBPK) model for the description of drug pharmacokinetics in anatomically relevant tissues and organs. Here, the drug is administered as a bolus dose into the venous blood compartment.*

Source: Kok-Yong, S., & Lawrence, L. (2015). Drug Distribution and Drug Elimination. InTech. doi: 10.5772/59929.

Naturally, this isn't true. The drug enters the arterial circulation 30 to 40 seconds after injection if it is injected into an arm vein and the initial concentration is measured in a radial artery. The delay most likely indicates the amount of time the medication needs to travel through the heart's venous volume, the great vessels, the peripheral arterial circulation, and the upper arm. More complex models (such as a recirculatory model) take this delay into account and are helpful in describing the behavior of a drug right after a bolus is administered, as in the case of induction agents, where the duration and speed of action are important parameters (Figure 2.6).

2.1.1.4. Compartmental Pharmacokinetic Models

There is no physiological equivalent for compartmental models. They are constructed by reparametrizing in terms of volumes and clearances after employing mathematical expressions fit to concentration over time data. There is only one volume and one clearance in the one-compartment model. This model may be oversimplified for anesthetic drugs, despite being used for several other drugs. Clinical pharmacologists have created two or three-compartment models with multiple tanks connected by pipes to more accurately simulate anesthetic medications. The volume of distribution at steady state, or Vdss, is the total of all volumes. The central or metabolic clearance is the process by which the central compartment is released for the exterior. The intercompartmental clearances are those that exist between the central and peripheral compartments.

2.1.1.5. Multicompartment Models

The curve above represents the plasma concentrations over time following an intravenous bolus. When administered as an intravenous bolus, this curve shares the properties of the majority of medications. Initially, the concentrations gradually drop over time. Secondly, the initial decline rate is steep but keeps getting flatter until it reaches a log-linear portion. Many drugs can be divided into three distinct phases. As soon as the bolus is injected, a rapid-distribution phase (blue line) starts. This phase is characterized by a very fast drug transfer from plasma to the quickly equilibrating tissues. The drug then moves into tissues that equilibrate more slowly and returns to plasma from tissues that equilibrate most quickly, indicating a second slow distribution phase (red line). (Figures 2.7 and 2.8).

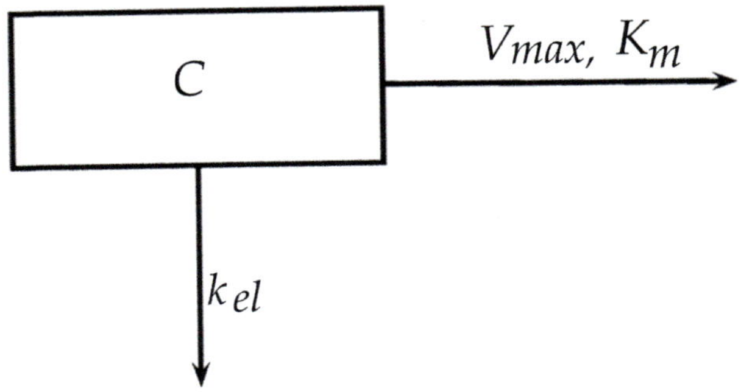

Figure 2.7. *Schematic representation of I.V. bolus injection with mixed drug elimination.*

Source: Egbelowo O. Nonlinear Elimination of Drugs in One-Compartment Pharmacokinetic Models: Nonstandard Finite Difference Approach for Various Routes of Administration. Mathematical and Computational Applications. 2018; 23(2):27. https://doi.org/10.3390/mca23020027.

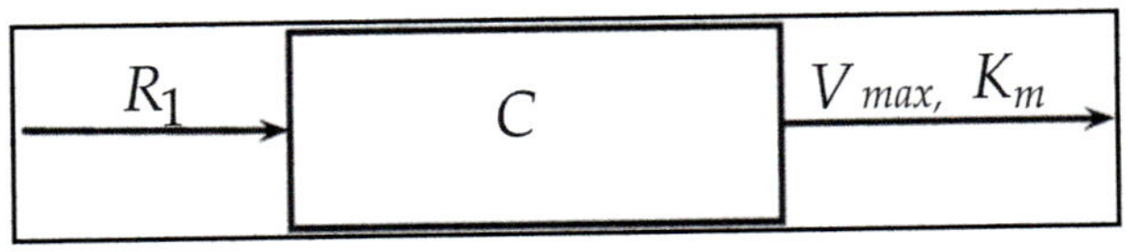

Figure 2.8. *Schematic representation of IV infusion with Michaelis-Menten elimination.*

Source: Egbelowo O. Nonlinear Elimination of Drugs in One-Compartment Pharmacokinetic Models: Nonstandard Finite Difference Approach for Various Routes of Administration. Mathematical and Computational Applications. 2018; 23(2):27. https://doi.org/10.3390/mca23020027.

Third, when plotted on a semilogarithmic graph, the terminal phase (green line) is almost exactly a straight line. Because drug elimination from the body is the main mechanism for lowering drug concentration during the terminal phase, the phase is frequently referred to as the "elimination phase.." The drug's relative proportion in plasma and peripheral volumes of distribution stays constant, and the plasma concentration is lower than tissue concentrations, which is what characterizes the terminal elimination phase. The drug returns to plasma during this terminal phase from the rapid- and slow-distribution volumes, where it is eventually eliminated by excretion or metabolism.

A characteristic that distinguishes a mammillary model with three compartments is the existence of three separate phases following bolus injection. Three tanks are depicted in this model, which correspond to the slowly equilibrating peripheral compartment, the central compartment (the plasma into which the drug is injected), and the rapidly equilibrating peripheral compartment, from left to right. The horizontal pipes stand for metabolic clearance (for the pipe that drains onto the page) or intercompartmental clearance. The fentanyl compartment volumes and the volumes of each tank match. The intercompartmental and systemic clearance of fentanyl are correlated with the pipe cross-sectional areas. Each tank's water level reflects the amount of drug present. We can track the mechanisms that lead to a gradual drop in drug concentration following bolus injection by utilizing this hydraulic model. Initially, the drug travels via intercompartmental clearance from the central compartment to both peripheral compartments and then exits the model entirely through metabolic clearance. Because the drug can go in three different directions, the concentration in the central compartment drops off quickly. The most rapidly equilibrating compartment plays a different role at the intersection of the blue and red lines. The concentration in the rapidly equilibrating compartment rises above the concentration in the central compartment at this transition, and the flow direction between them is switched. Drugs in plasma can only exit the drain pipe or enter the slowly equilibrating compartment after this transition (red line). The drug's return to plasma from the compartment that is rapidly equilibrating partially offsets these processes. In summary, the concentration in the central compartment decreases much more slowly than it did initially after the rapidly equilibrating compartment reaches equilibration.

The only way to lower the plasma concentration is through metabolic clearance, which occurs through the drain pipe, once the concentration in the central compartment falls below the levels in the compartments that equilibrate both quickly and slowly (green line). The rate at which the drug concentration in plasma decreases is significantly slowed down when the drug returns from both peripheral compartments to the central compartment.

Curves that continuously decrease over time, with a continuously increasing slope, can be described by a sum of negative exponentials. In pharmacokinetics, one way of denoting this sum of exponentials is to say that the plasma concentration over time is as follows:

$$C\ (t) = Ae^{-\alpha t} + Be^{-\beta t} + Ce^{-\gamma t} \qquad (6)$$

where t is the time since the bolus injection, C (t) is the drug concentration after a bolus dose, and A, α, B, β, C, and γ are parameters of a pharmacokinetic model. A, B, and C are coefficients, whereas α, β, and γ are exponents.

After a bolus injection, all six of the parameters in Equation 6 will be greater than 0. Poly exponential equations are used mainly because they describe the plasma concentrations observed after bolus injection, except for the misspecification in the first few minutes, mentioned previously. Models of compartmental pharmacokinetics are exclusively empirical. These models don't have an anatomical equivalent. They are based only on equations that fit measured plasma concentrations after a dose that is known. Models that describe concentration changes over time in terms of volumes and clearances are derived from kinetic models. Despite being more logical, they lack a physiological counterpart. The smallest exponent is frequently assigned special significance. The slope of the last log-linear segment of the curve is determined by this exponent. Unless specified otherwise, the half-life of a medication is the terminal half-life when it comes to references to it in medical literature. For medications with multiple exponential terms, the terminal half-life is nearly impossible to interpret. The time needed for concentrations to drop by 50% following drug administration is limited by the terminal half-life. The time required for a 50% decrease will typically be substantially less than that maximum.

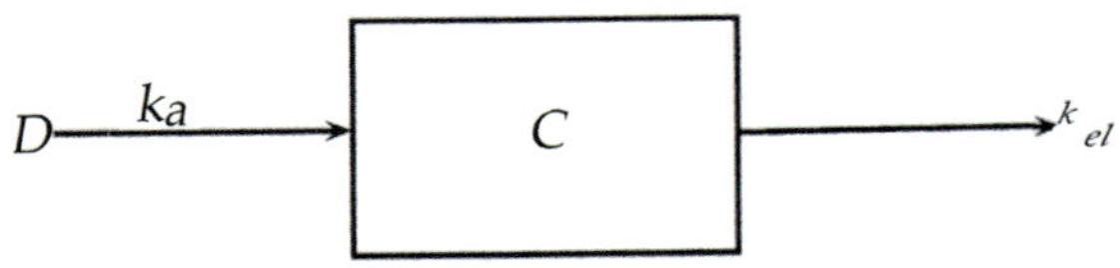

Figure 2.9. *One-compartment pharmacokinetic model for first-order drug absorption and first-order elimination.*

Source: Egbelowo O. Nonlinear Elimination of Drugs in One-Compartment Pharmacokinetic Models: Nonstandard Finite Difference Approach for Various Routes of Administration. Mathematical and Computational Applications. 2018; 23(2):27. https://doi.org/10.3390/mca23020027.

Pharmacokinetic compartmental models are still popular because they can be converted from an incomprehensible exponential form to a more understandable compartmental form. The rate at which drugs move from compartment i to compartment j is determined by microrate constants, or k_{ij}. The microrate constant for processes acting through metabolism or elimination that remove drugs irreversibly from the central compartment is k10 (analogous to k for a one-compartment model), where compartment 0 is the compartment outside the model. The microrate constants (k_{12}, k_{21}, etc.) between compartments.] explain the flow of medication between the peripheral and central compartments. At least two microrate constants—one for drug entry and one for drug exit—are present in each peripheral compartment (Figure 2.9).

2.1.1.6. Back-End Kinetics

Back-end kinetics is a helpful tool that characterizes the behavior of intravenous drugs when given as continuous infusions, using estimates of distribution volume and clearance. Descriptors of how plasma drug concentrations fall when a continuous infusion is stopped are provided by back-end kinetics. Decrement time is one illustration. It forecasts how long it will take, after an infusion stops, to attain a specific plasma concentration. The length of the infusion determines the degradation times. Examine the following example: decrement times for a series of ongoing infusions that are target-controlled. Propofol target-controlled infusion (TCI) is simulated with a concentration of 4 μg/mL maintained for 30, 60, and 120 minutes. The time to reach 0.5 μg/mL is estimated after the infusion is stopped. As demonstrated, the amount of time needed to reach 0.5 μg/mL increases with the length of the infusion. This illustration shows how medications build up in peripheral tissues after extended infusions. The decrement time is extended by this accumulation.

Decrement times can also be used to compare medications within a class of drugs (such as opioids). Plots of decrement times as a function of infusion duration are shown as a comparator. When applied in this manner, decrement times are calculated as the amount of time needed to attain a desired concentration percentage right after a continuous infusion is stopped. Figure 2.10 shows examples of 50 percent and 80 percent decrement times for specific opioids and sedatives. Notably, both classes of anesthetic drug degradation times are comparable for shorter infusions. Significant variations in decrement times occur once the infusion duration surpasses two hours. The context-sensitive halftime, or 50% decrement time, is a widely used decrement time. Context-sensitive describes how long an infusion takes. The 50% decrement time is referred to as half-time.

2.1.1.7. BioPhase

The biophase is the interval of time between alterations in plasma concentration and the therapeutic effect. The biophase takes into consideration the time needed for the drug to diffuse from the plasma to the site of action as well as the time needed for the drug to produce an effect once it has arrived at the site of action. Figure 2.11 shows a simulation of different propofol bolus doses and their expected impact on the bispectral index scale (BIS) of the electroencephalogram (EEG). Every dose has the same time-to-peak effect (roughly 1.5 hours after the peak plasma concentration). The strength and duration of the effect vary with each dose. A key principle is that when drug concentrations are in flux (i.e. Changes in drug effect will occur later than changes in drug concentration, particularly during the induction of anesthesia and the emergence from it. The phenomenon known as hysteresis, in which two different plasma concentrations correspond to one drug effect or one plasma concentration corresponds to two drug effects, is typically caused by this lag between the plasma concentration and effect. As an illustration, Figure 2.11 demonstrates how the various concentrations at C and c match the same BIS score. An "effect site" compartment is frequently added to the central compartment to model this lag, collapse the hysteresis between plasma concentration and effect, and match one plasma concentration to one drug effect. Biophase is described by the kinetic microrate constants k_{e0} and k_{1e}. K_{e0} describes the drug's removal from the effect site compartment, while K_{1e} describes the drug's movement from the central compartment to the effect site. With regard to the effect-site compartment, two key presumptions exist: (1) there is no volume estimate to the effect-site compartment, and (2) the amount of drug that travels from the central compartment to the effect-site compartment is negligible.

Typically, the relationship between plasma and the site of drug effect is modeled with an effect-site model. The site of drug effect is connected to plasma by a first-order process. Eq. 7 relates effect-site concentration to plasma concentration:

$$dCe = \frac{k_{e0} \times (Cp - Ce)}{dt} \qquad (7)$$

where k_{e0} is the drug elimination rate constant, Ce is the effect-site concentration, and Cp is the plasma drug concentration. The rate at which the effects of drugs rise and fall is described by the constant ke0.

In conclusion, anesthesia professionals deal with medications whose clinical behavior is not well described by half-life, so they are not very familiar with the conventional pharmacokinetic term half-life.

The pharmacokinetic principles discussed in this section (such as volume of distribution, clearance, elimination, front-end kinetics, back-end kinetics, context-sensitive half-time, and biophase) better illustrate how an anesthetic will behave. (Youngs and Shafer, 1999)

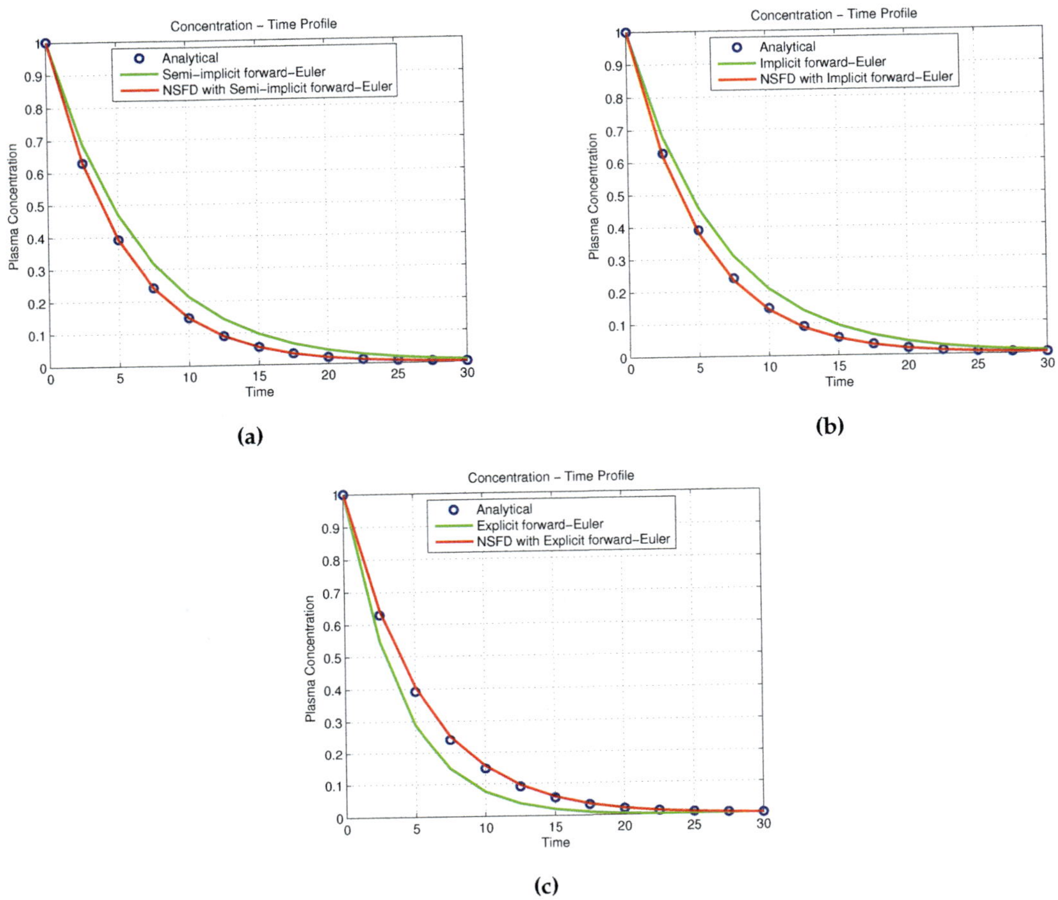

Figure 2.10. *(a) The nonstandard finite difference (NSFD) scheme (31) in case 1 plotted against the analytical solution (19) and the corresponding SFD scheme (25); (b) NSFD scheme (33) in case 2 plotted against the analytical solution (19) and the corresponding SFD scheme (32) and (c) NSFD scheme (36) in case 3 plotted against the analytical solution (19) and the corresponding SFD scheme.*

Source: Egbelowo O. Nonlinear Elimination of Drugs in One-Compartment Pharmacokinetic Models: Nonstandard Finite Difference Approach for Various Routes of Administration. Mathematical and Computational Applications. 2018; 23(2):27. https://doi.org/10.3390/mca23020027.

2.2. Pharmacodynamic Principles

Pharmacodynamics specifically explains the connection between drug concentration and pharmacologic effect. Similar to pharmacokinetic models, the models used to explain concentration-effect relationships are derived from observations and utilized to build a mathematical model. Drug effects and plasma drug levels are measured concurrently to build a pharmacodynamic model. Take into account, for instance, the recorded plasma concentrations of an intravenous anesthetic medication after a bolus dose and the corresponding variations in the EEG spectral edge frequency, which is a gauge of anesthetic depth, in a single person. The spectral edge begins to decrease shortly after the plasma concentration peaks, reaches a nadir, and then returns to baseline when the plasma concentrations approach zero. A hysteresis loop is produced by combining data from multiple individuals and graphing the measured concentrations against the observed effect (which is changed to represent a percentage of the maximal effect across all individuals). Rising drug concentrations are represented by the loop's ascending section (see arrow). The increase in drug effect rises, but it does so more slowly than the increase in drug concentration. The drug effect diminishes more slowly in the descending loop than the drug concentration does.

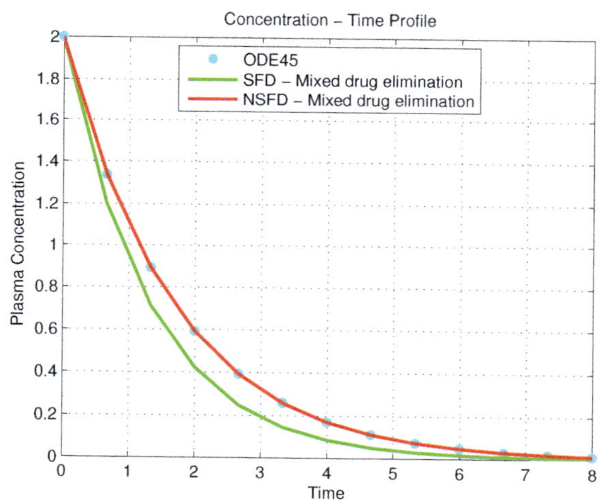

Figure 2.11. *Trajectory representation of the one-compartment I.V. bolus injection model that follows mixed drug elimination.*

Source: *Egbelowo O. Nonlinear Elimination of Drugs in One-Compartment Pharmacokinetic Models: Nonstandard Finite Difference Approach for Various Routes of Administration. Mathematical and Computational Applications. 2018; 23(2):27. https://doi.org/10.3390/mca23020027.*

The hysteresis loop is collapsed using modeling techniques that take into account the lag time between plasma concentrations and the observed effect in order to produce a pharmacodynamic model.

These modeling techniques provide an estimate of the lag time, known as the $t_{½}k_{e0}$, and an estimate of the effect-site concentration (Ce) associated with a 50% probability of drug effect (C_{50}). Most concentration-effect relationships in anesthesia are described with a sigmoid curve. The standard equation for this relationship is the Hill equation, also known as the sigmoid E_{max} relationship (Equation 8):

$$\text{Effect} = E_0 + (E_{\max} - E_0)\ (C^{\gamma}/(C_{50}{}^{\gamma} + C^{\gamma})) \qquad (8)$$

where E_0 is the baseline effect, E_{max} is the maximal effect, C is the drug concentration, and γ represents the slope of the concentration-effect relationship; γ is also known as the Hill coefficient. For values of γ less than 1, the curve is hyperbolic, and for values greater than 1, the curve is sigmoid.

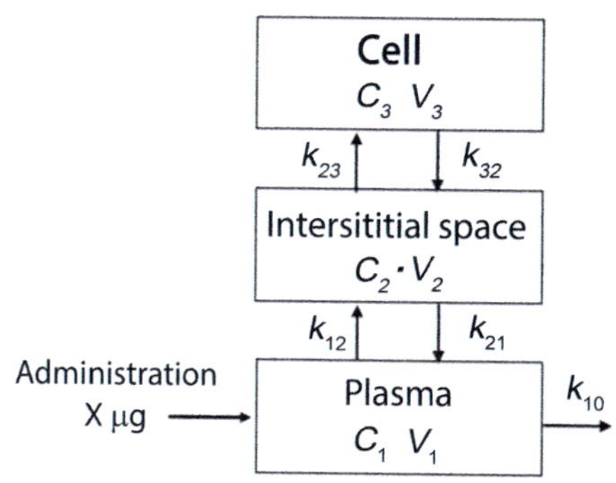

Figure 2.12. *Schematic of a proposed three-compartment pharmacokinetic model.*

Source: *Uno Y, Ogawa E, Aiyoshi E, Arai T. A Three-Compartment Pharmacokinetic Model to Predict the Interstitial Concentration of Talaporfin Sodium in the Myocardium for Photodynamic Therapy: A Method Combining Measured Fluorescence and Analysis of the Compartmental Origin of the Fluorescence. Bioengineering. 2019; 6(1):1. https://doi.org/10.3390/bioengineering6010001.*

An example of this relationship: a fentanyl effect-site concentration-effect curve for analgesia. This example illustrates how C_{50} and γ characterize the concentration-effect relationship. (Figures 2.12 and 2.13).

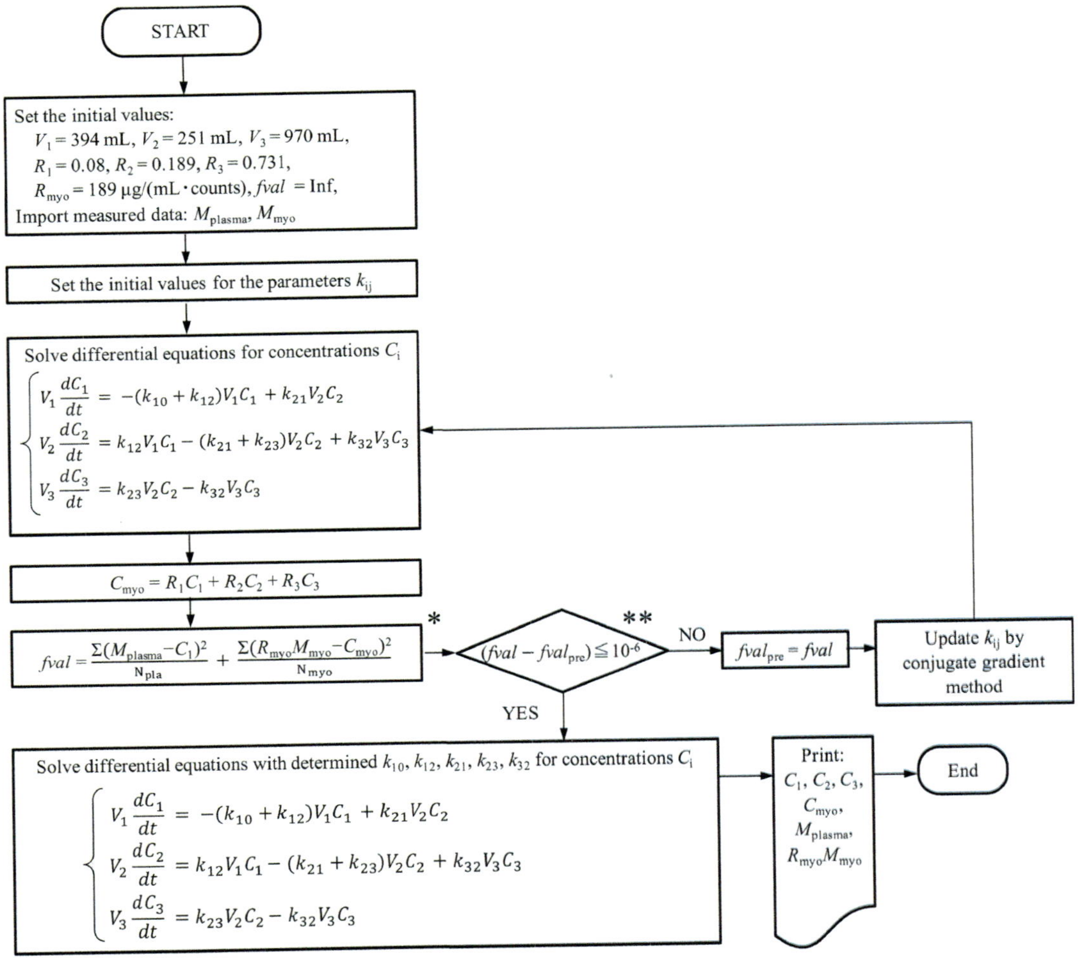

Figure 2.13. *An example of the optimization of a three compartment model:* Npla and Nmyo represent the number of data points for the plasma *concentration and myocardial fluorescence, respectively.* ** *fval pre represents the previously calculated value of fval.*

Source: Uno Y, Ogawa E, Aiyoshi E, Arai T. A Three-Compartment Pharmacokinetic Model to Predict the Interstitial Concentration of Talaporfin Sodium in the Myocardium for Photodynamic Therapy: A Method Combining Measured Fluorescence and Analysis of the Compartmental Origin of the Fluorescence. Bioengineering. 2019; 6(1):1. https://doi.org/10.3390/bioengineering6010001.

2.2.1. Potency and Efficacy

This relationship involves two key concepts: efficacy and potency. The term "potency" refers to the quantity of a drug needed to produce an effect. One often used metric to characterize potency is the C_{50}. Drugs are thought to be more potent if their concentration-versus-effect relationship is shifted to the left (small C_{50}), and the opposite is true for drugs whose concentration-versus-effect relationship is shifted to the right. The analgesia C_{50} for some fentanyl congeners, for instance, varies from small for sufentanil (0.04 ng/mL) too large for alfentanil (75 ng/mL). Sufentanil is therefore more effective than alfentanil (Tables 2.1 and 2.2).

Table 2.1. *An Example Study of a Pharmacokinetic Model for CLR1404, a Phospholipid Ether Analog that, Labeled with 124I/131I: First-Order Sensitivity Indexes Si, Which Account for the "Relative Importance" of the Parameters at First-Order Iterations. By Definition, Si Takes Values Between 0 and 1 and ΣΣSi≤1*[a]

$k_{i,j}$	Marrow	Heart wall	Kidneys	Liver	Lungs	Spleen	Tumor	Blood	Renal
Blood to heart fast	0.00	0.13	0.00	0.00	0.00	0.00	0.00	0.00	0.00
Heart fast to blood	0.00	0.25	0.00	0.00	0.00	0.00	0.00	0.00	0.00
Heart fast to slow	0.00	0.00	0.00	0.00	0.00	0.00	0.00	0.00	0.00
Blood to kidney fast	0.00	0.00	0.06	0.00	0.00	0.00	0.00	0.01	0.09
Kidney fast to blood	0.00	0.00	0.07	0.00	0.00	0.00	0.00	0.01	0.13
Kidney fast to slow	0.00	0.00	0.00	0.00	0.00	0.00	0.00	0.00	0.00
Blood to tumor fast	0.00	0.00	0.00	0.00	0.00	0.00	0.13	0.00	0.00
Tumor fast to blood	0.00	0.00	0.00	0.00	0.00	0.00	0.26	0.00	0.00
Tumor fast to slow	0.00	0.00	0.00	0.00	0.00	0.00	0.02	0.00	0.00
Tumor slow to fast	0.00	0.00	0.00	0.00	0.00	0.00	0.02	0.00	0.00
Blood to lung fast	0.00	0.00	0.00	0.00	0.07	0.00	0.00	0.00	0.00
Lung fast to blood	0.00	0.00	0.00	0.00	0.05	0.00	0.00	0.00	0.00
Lung fast to slow	0.00	0.00	0.00	0.00	0.01	0.00	0.00	0.00	0.00
Liver fast to blood	0.00	0.00	0.00	0.02	0.00	0.00	0.00	0.00	0.00
Blood to liver fast	0.00	0.00	0.00	0.01	0.00	0.00	0.00	0.00	0.00
Liver fast to slow	0.00	0.00	0.00	0.00	0.00	0.00	0.00	0.00	0.00
Blood to BM fast	0.05	0.00	0.00	0.00	0.00	0.00	0.00	0.00	0.00
BM fast to blood	0.05	0.00	0.00	0.00	0.00	0.00	0.00	0.00	0.00
BM fast to slow	0.00	0.00	0.00	0.00	0.00	0.00	0.00	0.00	0.00
Blood to RT fast	0.04	0.02	0.05	0.05	0.05	0.03	0.00	0.58	0.02
RT fast to blood	0.02	0.01	0.02	0.03	0.02	0.02	0.00	0.27	0.00
RT fast to RT slow	0.00	0.00	0.00	0.00	0.00	0.00	0.00	0.02	0.00
Kidney fast to urine	0.00	0.00	0.00	0.00	0.00	0.00	0.00	0.01	0.07
Spleen to blood	0.00	0.00	0.00	0.00	0.00	0.00	0.00	0.00	0.00
Blood to spleen	0.00	0.00	0.00	0.00	0.00	0.00	0.00	0.00	0.00
f_s									
f_{Blood}(BM)	0.18	0.00	0.00	0.00	0.00	0.00	0.00	0.00	0.00
f_{Blood}(Heart wall)	0.00	0.00	0.00	0.00	0.00	0.00	0.00	0.00	0.00
f_{Blood}(Kidneys)	0.00	0.00	0.06	0.00	0.00	0.00	0.00	0.00	0.00
f_{Blood}(Liver)	0.00	0.00	0.00	0.24	0.00	0.00	0.00	0.00	0.00
f_{Blood}(Lungs)	0.00	0.00	0.00	0.00	0.14	0.00	0.00	0.00	0.00
f_{Blood}(Spleen)	0.00	0.00	0.00	0.00	0.00	0.49	0.00	0.00	0.00

[a]The higher the Si value, the higher the relative importance of the parameter by first-order iterations. A Si = 0 does not necessarily imply null contribution to the model. Those indexes greater than zero were highlighted for a better visualization.

Source: *Neira S, Gago-Arias A, González-Crespo I, Guiu-Souto J, Pardo-Montero J. Development of a Compartmental Pharmacokinetic Model for Molecular Radiotherapy with 131I-CLR1404. Pharmaceutics. 2021; 13(9):1497. https://doi.org/10.3390/pharmaceutics13091497.*

A drug's efficacy is determined by how well it occupies a receptor. Even though they both have the same receptor occupancy, similar medications that act on the same receptor may differ in their efficacy. When it comes to G protein-coupled receptors, for instance, certain medications may bind to the receptor in a way that results in a more noticeable activation of second messengers, having a greater effect than others. Full agonists are defined as drugs that produce their maximum effect, while partial agonists are defined as drugs that produce their least amount of effect.

Table 2.2. *An Example Study of a Pharmacokinetic Model for CLR1404, a Phospholipid Ether Analog that, Labeled with 124I/131I: Total-Order Sensitivity Indexes ST,i, which Account for the "Relative Importance" of the Parameters to the Model by Higher Order Iterations*[a]

$k_{i,j}$	Marrow	Heart wall	Kidneys	Liver	Lungs	Spleen	Tumor	Blood	Renal
Blood to heart fast	0.00	0.54	0.00	0.00	0.00	0.00	0.00	0.00	0.00
Heart fast to blood	0.00	0.66	0.00	0.00	0.00	0.00	0.00	0.00	0.00
Heart fast to slow	0.00	0.02	0.00	0.00	0.00	0.00	0.00	0.00	0.00
Blood to kidney fast	0.00	0.00	0.45	0.00	0.00	0.00	0.00	0.01	0.48
Kidney fast to blood	0.00	0.00	0.42	0.00	0.00	0.00	0.00	0.01	0.53
Kidney fast to slow	0.00	0.00	0.05	0.00	0.00	0.00	0.00	0.00	0.00
Blood to tumor fast	0.00	0.00	0.00	0.00	0.00	0.00	0.52	0.00	0.00
Tumor fast to blood	0.00	0.00	0.00	0.00	0.00	0.00	0.66	0.00	0.00
Tumor fast to slow	0.00	0.00	0.00	0.00	0.00	0.00	0.21	0.00	0.00
Tumor slow to fast	0.00	0.00	0.00	0.00	0.00	0.00	0.12	0.00	0.00
Blood to lung fast	0.00	0.00	0.00	0.00	0.40	0.00	0.00	0.01	0.00
Lung fast to blood	0.00	0.00	0.00	0.00	0.32	0.00	0.00	0.00	0.00
Lung fast to slow	0.00	0.00	0.00	0.00	0.05	0.00	0.00	0.00	0.00
Liver fast to blood	0.00	0.00	0.00	0.20	0.00	0.00	0.00	0.00	0.00
Blood to liver fast	0.00	0.00	0.00	0.20	0.00	0.00	0.00	0.00	0.00
Liver fast to slow	0.00	0.00	0.00	0.04	0.00	0.00	0.00	0.00	0.00
Blood to red marrow fast	0.35	0.00	0.00	0.00	0.00	0.00	0.00	0.00	0.00
BM fast to blood	0.27	0.00	0.00	0.00	0.00	0.00	0.00	0.00	0.00
BM fast to slow	0.03	0.00	0.00	0.00	0.00	0.00	0.00	0.00	0.00
Blood to RT fast	0.34	0.20	0.34	0.35	0.34	0.30	0.08	0.64	0.15
RT fast to blood	0.22	0.12	0.23	0.23	0.22	0.18	0.04	0.32	0.09
RT fast to RT slow	0.01	0.01	0.01	0.01	0.01	0.01	0.00	0.03	0.00
Kidney fast to urine	0.00	0.00	0.01	0.00	0.00	0.00	0.00	0.01	0.45
Spleen to blood	0.00	0.00	0.00	0.00	0.00	0.00	0.00	0.00	0.00
Blood to spleen	0.00	0.00	0.00	0.00	0.00	0.05	0.00	0.00	0.00
f_s									
f_{Blood}(BM)	0.42	0.00	0.00	0.00	0.00	0.00	0.00	0.00	0.00
f_{Blood}(Heart wall)	0.00	0.06	0.00	0.00	0.00	0.00	0.00	0.00	0.00
f_{Blood}(Kidneys)	0.00	0.00	0.29	0.00	0.00	0.00	0.00	0.00	0.00
f_{Blood}(Liver)	0.00	0.00	0.00	0.60	0.00	0.00	0.00	0.00	0.00
f_{Blood}(Lungs)	0.00	0.00	0.00	0.00	0.34	0.00	0.00	0.00	0.00
f_{Blood}(Spleen)	0.00	0.00	0.00	0.00	0.00	0.85	0.00	0.00	0.00

[a]e.g., Iterations of Parameters with One Another. By Definition, ST,i ≥ Si. Figure SM1: Parallel coordinates Plot Representing the Relative Differences Between the Full Compartmental Model and Bioexponential Fits with Different Combinations of Four Time-Points.

Source: Neira S, Gago-Arias A, Gónzalez-Crespo I, Guiu-Souto J, Pardo-Montero J. Development of a Compartmental Pharmacokinetic Model for Molecular Radiotherapy with 131I-CLR1404. Pharmaceutics. 2021; 13(9):1497. https://doi.org/10.3390/pharmaceutics13091497.

2.2.2. Anesthetic Drug Interactions

A typical clinical anesthetic typically consists of a mix of medications to produce the desired effects of muscle relaxation, analgesia, and hypnosis. When used with other medications, hypnotics, analgesics, and muscle relaxants rarely act the same way as when taken alone due to their mutual interactions. When an analgesic is given with a hypnotic, for instance, the analgesia is stronger in combination with the hypnotic than it is on its own, and the hypnosis is stronger in combination with the analgesic than it is on its own. Consequently, the practice of applied drug interactions is anesthesia. This phenomenon is probably caused by the fact that different receptors are affected differently by each class of drug.

Numerous investigations have been conducted to examine the interactions between anesthetic medications. Interactions have been classified as antagonistic, additive, and synergistic. When two medications with additive interactions are taken together, the combined effect of both is what is known as the overall effect.

Table 2.3. *A Review Summarizing the Prevalence (%) of Potentially Inappropriate Medications (PIM) and Drug–Drug Interactions (DDI) (Total, Severe and Moderate) and Polymedication (Mean or Median) in Elderly Patients in Nursing Home Settings*[a]

	Author	Year	Country	Age (Mean, Median or Threshold)	Sample Size	Study Style P–R	Source of Data (Medical Chart–Database)	PIM Criteria	Prevalence of PIM (% Patients with at least 1 PIM)	DDI Checkers (Access Date or Version)	Prevalence of DDI (% of Patients)				Polymedication (Mean or Median Number of Medications)
											All Risk Rating	Severe and Moderate Risk Rating	Severe	Moderate	
1	Bitter K et al.,[15]	2019	Germany	84	103	R	Medical chart	PRISCUS	16	ABDA (2018)		40	ND	ND	13
2	Kolar J et al.,[16]	2018	Slovak Republic	79.9	70	R	Medical chart	Topinkova list (2012)	34.3	Lexicomp (2016)	88.4		8.2	100	7.87
3	Fog AF et al.,[17]	2017	Norway	85.9	2465	P	Medical chart	NORGEP, STOPP/ START	1.2	DRUID (2017)	4.4		ND	ND	9.8
4	Alves-Conceição V et al.,[18]	2017	Brazil	81.8	125	R	Medical chart	Beers Criteria (2012)	73.6	Micromedex (2014)	62.4		ND	ND	ND
5	Lao CK et al.,[19]	2013	Macao	86.6	114	R	Medical chart	STOPP/ START	46.5	Micromedex (2012), Lexicomp (2012)	37.8		ND	ND	6.9
6	Xavier-Pinto MC et al.,[20]	2013	Brazil	76.7	151	R	Medical chart	Beers Criteria (2012)	25.8	Micromedex (2012)	54.1		3.1	81.4	3.3
7	Bakken MS et al.,[21]	2012	Norway	84.7	157	P	Medical chart	NORGEP	25.5	DRUID (2011)	52.9		1.3	6.4	6.0
8	Varallo FR et al.,[22]	2012	Brazil	>60 (t)	120	R	Medical chart	Fick criteria (2003) (updated Beers Criteria), WHO criteria	29.2	Micromedex (2011)		8.3	1.7	6.7	ND
9	Haassum Y et al.,[23]	2012	Sweden	85.6	86721	R	Database (Swedish Prescribed Drug Register (SPDR))	Swedish National Board of Health and Welfare	30.2	Swedish Physicians' Desk Reference (2010)	ND	ND	3.3		7.2
10	Halvorsen KH et al.,[24]	2012	Norway	85.3	2986	R	Database (Norw-egian presc-ription database)	NORGEP	31.4	DRUID (2011)	48		1	6	5.7

11	Hosia-Randell HMV et al., [25]	2008	Finland	83.7	1987	R	Medical chart	Fick criteria 2003 (updated Beers Criteria)	34.9	Swedish, Finnish, Interaction X-refer-encing (SFINX) (2007)	ND	ND	4.8		7.9
12	Nygaard HA et al., [26]	2003	Norway	86.3	1042	R	Medical chart	Beers Criteria (1997)	12.8	Norwegian Pharm-aceutical Products Comp-endium (2000)	ND	10.4	3.0	10.1	5
13	Giron MST et al., [27]	2001	Sweden	>81 (t)	493	P	Medical chart	Swedish National Formulary	80.1	Swedish Physicians' Desk Reference (1998)	ND	24.5	ND	ND	4.5
					96,534				**29.7**		**31.1**	**15.9**	**3.3**	**10.9**	
14	Stuhec M et al., [28]	2019	Slovenia	80.6	24 Mental health disease	P	Medical chart	Beers criteria (2015), PRISCUS	70.8	Lexicomp (2019)	ND	ND	50	ND	12.2
15	Bazargan M et al., [29]	2019	USA	75.2	193 Hyper-tension	P	Medical chart (drug conta-iners)	Beers criteria (2015)	46	Beers criteria (2015)	NA	23	ND	ND	7,3
16	Allegri N et al., [30]	2017	Italy	80.4	860 Mental health disease	R	Medical chart	Beers criteria (2015)	44.4	Drugs.com (2016)	ND	30.9	ND	ND	5.9
17	Pasina L et al., [31]	2016	Italy	84.9	272 Mental health disease	P	Medical chart	(2012) Beers criteria, STOPP/ START	74.6 (psychotropic drugs)	INTERcheck (2013)	86.4	53.3	ND	ND	7

18	Hanlon JT et al., [32]	2015	USA	>65	1076 Mental health disease (mild to moderate)	R	Database (Medication dispensing information from the Pharmacy Benefits Management services (PBM))	Beers criteria (2012)	27.2	VA PBM and Medical Advisory Panel Cholinesterase inhibitor criteria for use (2003)		7.9			
					227 Mental health disease (severe)				25.1			5.3			
19	Hanlon JT et al., [33]	2011	USA	>65	877 Mental health disease	P	Database (Medication dispensing information from the Pharmacy Benefits Management services (PBM))	AMDA Guideline, VHA/DOD guideline	41.3	AMDA Guideline (2003), VHA/DOD guideline (2010)	ND	25.9			
					2815 Control				96		ND	ND			
20	Giron MS et al., [27]	2001	Sweden	>81	188 Mental health disease	P	Medical chart	Swedish National Formulary	82.9	Swedish Physicians' Desk Reference (1998)	ND	26.6			4.6
					6532				**65.2**		**86.4**	**22.5**	**50**	**NA**	

[a]At the end of the table, the prevalence of PIM and DDI is reported as the weighted mean (in bold).

Footnote: Prospective (P), Retrospective (R), Mean (M), Median (m), Threshold (t), Severe (S), Moderate (M), not apply (NA), not Determined (ND).

Source: Bories, M., Bouzillé, G., Cuggia, M., & Le Corre, P. Drug–Drug Interactions in Elderly Patients with Potentially Inappropriate Medications in Primary Care, Nursing Home and Hospital Settings: A Systematic Review and a Preliminary Study. Pharmaceutics. 2021; 13(2):266. https://doi.org/10.3390/pharmaceutics13020266.

When two drugs combine antagonistically, the overall effect is smaller than it would be if they were additive; when they interact synergistically, the overall effect is larger. The isobole is a term used to describe the continuum of drug concentrations across different drug pair combinations (X in combination with Y). An isoeffect line for a chosen probability of effect is called an isobole. The 50% isobole line is a typical example of an isobole. It shows every possible pairing of two-drug effect-site concentrations that could produce an effect with a 50% chance of occurring (Table 2.3).

More clinical interest is derived from other isoboles. For instance, the concentration pairs required to guarantee a 95% probability of unresponsiveness are represented by the 95 percent isobole for loss of responsiveness. Comparably, the concentration pairs with a low probability of that effect (i.e., the majority of patients would respond) are represented by the 5 percent isobole. It is ideal to dose an anesthetic to achieve a probability of effect that is slightly above but not significantly beyond the 95 percent isobole when creating an anesthetic dosing regimen. Three-dimensional anesthetic drug interactions are characterized by mathematical models that have been developed by several researchers. Known as response surface models, these models contain a probability estimate of the overall effect along with effect-site concentrations for every drug. The propofol-remifentanil interaction for loss of responsiveness, as reported by Bouillon and associates, is an example. The response surface displays the entire isobole range for remifentanil-propofol for loss of responsiveness, ranging from 0% to 100%. The response surface model is commonly represented by two plot types: the topographic plot and the three-dimensional plot. The vertical and horizontal axes of the topographic plot show the drug concentrations and provide a top-down view of the response surface. Selected isobole lines (i.e., 5 percent, 50 percent, and 95 percent) are used to illustrate the drug effect. (Youngs and Shafer, 1999)

Many anesthetic effects, such as responses to verbal and tactile stimuli, painful stimuli, hemodynamic or respiratory effects, and alterations in electrical brain activity, have led to the development of response surface models. For instance, response surface models have been created for tracheal intubation, laryngoscopy, esophageal instrumentation, and loss of response to the insertion of a laryngeal mask airway18 for specific combinations of anesthetic medications. Despite the abundance of response surface models, there are some gaps in the models that cover all typical anesthetic drug combinations and different types of stimuli seen in the perioperative setting (Table 2.4 and 2.5).

Table 2.4. *A Review of the Prevalence (%) of PIM and DDI (Total, Severe and Moderate) and Polymedication (Mean or Median) in Elderly Patients Primary Care Settings*[a]

	Author	Year	Country	Age (Mean, Median or Treshold)	Sample Size	Study Style P–R	Source of Data (Medical Chart–Database)	PIM Criteria	Prevalence of PIM (% Patients with at least 1 PIM)	DDI Checkers (Access Date or Version)	Prevalence of DDI (% of Patients)				Polymedication (Mean or Median Number of Medications)
											All Risk Rating	Severe and Moderate Risk Rating	Severe	Moderate	
1	Bobrova et al. [34]	2019	Finland	84.6	208	R	Database (PharmaService's documentation system ANJA)	EU [7], PIM list	73	INXBASE (2017)	ND	ND	2.4	50	5.9
2	Vatcharavongvan et al. [35]	2019	Thailand	70.5 (m)	400	R	Medical chart	Beers Criteria (2015), STOPP/START, Winit–Watjana Beers Criteria (2015) STOPP/START	75.3 59 40.3	2015 Beers criteria	NA	16	NA	NA	11(m)
3	Toivo et al. [36]	2019	Finland	81.6 84.0	65 64	P	Medical chart	Winit–Watjana Beers criteria (2015)	66.8 93.9 90.6	SFINX (2018)	ND ND	ND ND	10.8 1.6	ND ND	10.4 9.8
4	Stuhec et al. [37]	2019	Slovenia	77.5	91	R	Medical chart	PRISCUS	ND	Lexicomp (version 4.0.1 and 4.0.2)	ND	ND	54.9	ND	13.8
5	Patel R et al. [38]	2018	USA	>65 (t)	703	P	Medical chart	Beers criteria (2015)	29	Beers criteria (2015)	NA	7.7	NA	NA	5.7
6	Novaes PH et al. [39]	2017	Brazil	73.8 (>60)	368	R	Medical chart	Beers criteria (2012) STOPP (2015)	42.1 46.2	Medscape Drug Interaction Checker (2016)	72.3	ND	17.9	ND	4.46
7	Hanlon JT et al. [40]	2017	USA	73.6	3055	R	Database (Health ABC study)	Beers criteria (2015)	34.0	Panel of 70 DDI used for the study (2017)	ND	25.1	ND	ND	NA
8	Marín-Gorricho R et al. [41]	2017	Spain	85.2	103	R	Medical chart	STOPP/START (2014)	81.6	CheckTheMeds (2017)	57.3	ND	ND	ND	7.4
9	Bazargan M et al. [42]	2016	USA	73.5	400	R	Interview	Beers criteria (2012)	69.5	Healthline drug interaction checker (2015)	ND	ND	52.75	ND	NA
10	Popovic B et al. [43]	2014	Croatia	77	29418	R	Database (Croatian Health Insurance Fund database)	Mimica Matanović and Vlahović-Palčevski (2012)	62.4	Panel of 49 potentially serious DDI used for the study (2014)	ND	ND	ND	ND	NA
11	Tora H et al. [44]	2014	Sweden	75.8	180059	R	Database (Swedish national prescription repository)	Swedish National Board of Health and Welfare	30.8	First Databank's DDI module (2013)	ND	38.6	ND	ND	10.4
12	Steinman MA et al. [45]	2014	USA	75	462405	R	Database (Merged VA database-Medicare Program)	Beers criteria (2012)	26.0	Lexicomp (2013)	ND	30.2	4.4	30	NA
13	Lund BC et al. [46]	2013	USA	75.8	1549824	R	Database (VA database)	Zhan criteria (adapted from 1997 Beers criteria)	17.9	Hansten PD, Horn JR. Applied Therapeutics Inc. (1998)	NA	3.75	NA	NA	5.5
14	Koper D et al. [47]	2013	Austria	76.4	169	P	medical chart	Fick criteria 2003 (updated Beers Criteria) PRISCUS	16.5 37.3	Lexicomp (2012)	ND	59.2	2.4	58	9.1
15	Haasum Y et al. [23]	2012	Sweden	75.6	1260843	R	Database (Swedish Prescribed Drug Register SPDR)	Swedish National Board of Health and Welfare	11.6	Swedish Physicians' Desk Reference (2010)	ND	ND	3.2	ND	4.3
16	Halvorsen KH et al. [24]	2011	Norway	83.0	8268	R	Database (Norwegian prescription database)	NORGEP	24.6	DRUID (2011)	57	ND	2	10	5.7
17	Ghadimi H et al. [48]	2011	Iran	73.0	2041	R	Medical chart	Fick criteria 2003 (updated Beers Criteria)	30.3	Swedish Physicians' Desk Reference (2009)	ND	14.3	2.4	13.1	4.4
18	Pozzi C et al. [49]	2010	Italy	73.0	1022	R	Database (ICARe Dicomano Study database)	Beers Criteria (1991)	9.0	Micromedex (2009)	ND	ND	7.2	ND	2.2
19	Johnell K et al. [50]	2009	Sweden	81.0	645429	R	Database (Swedish Prescribed Drug Register SPDR)	Swedish NationalBoard of Health and Welfare	22.5	Swedish Physicians' Desk Reference (2009)	ND	ND	6.9	ND	6.8

	Author	Year	Country	Age (Mean, Median or Treshold)	Sample Size	Study Style P–R	Source of Data (Medical Chart–Database)	PIM Criteria	Prevalence of PIM (% Patients with at least 1 PIM)	DDI Checkers (Access Date or Version)	Prevalence of DDI (% of Patients)				Polymedication (Mean or Median Number of Medications)
											All Risk Rating	Severe and Moderate Risk Rating	Severe	Moderate	
20	Chrischilles EA et al. [51]	2009	USA	>68 (t)	626	P	Database (Iowa medicare beneficiaries)	Beers Criteria (1997)	51.4	Hansten PD, Horn JR. Applied Therapeutics Inc. (1998)	NA	5.8	NA	NA	8.5
21	Haider SI et al. [52]	2009	Sweden	80.9	626258	R	Database (Swedish Prescribed Drug Register SPDR)	Swedish National Board of Health and Welfare	34.6	Swedish Physicians Desk Reference (2007)	ND	25	ND	ND	5.8
22	Lapi F et al. [53]	2009	Italy	72.7 77.7	568	R	Database (ICARe Dicomano study database)	Beers Criteria (1991)	9.1 5.1	Micromedex (2008)	ND ND	20.1 30.5	4.7 5.6	ND ND	NA NA
23	Johnell K et al. [54]	2008	Sweden	>75 (t)	122413 606692	R	Database (Swedish Prescribed Drug Register SPDR)	Swedish National Board of Health and Welfare	40.3 13.6	Swedish Physicians' Desk Reference (2007)	ND ND	ND ND	8.8 3.7	ND ND	9.4 4.6
24	Johnell K et al. [55]	2007	Sweden	82	732228	R	Database (Swedish Prescribed Drug Register SPDR)	Swedish National Board of Health and Welfare	16.5	Swedish Physicians' Desk Reference (2007)	ND	ND	4.1	ND	5.4
25	Bregnhøj L et al. [56]	2007	Denmark	76.6	212	R	Database (Drug subsidy system of Danish pharmacies)	MAI	84	Hansten and Horn (2004)	NA	0.6	NA	NA	7.6
26	Cannon KT et al. [57]	2006	USA	78	786	R	Medical chart	Beers criteria (1997)	31	Multidisciplinary Medication Management (M3) Project criteria (2005)	NA	NA	10	NA	8.0
27	Zhan C et al. [58]	2005	USA	> 65 (t)	70203	R	Database (National Ambulatory Medical Care Survey NAMCS)	1997 Beers criteria, Mac Leod 1997, Panel expert 50 drug-disease *combinations*	2.58	1997 Beers criteria, Mac Leod 1997, Panel expert 6 drug-drug combinations	NA	0.76	NA	NA	NA
28	Azoulay L et al. [59]	2003	Iran	72.6	3000	R	Medical chart	Beers criteria (1997)	27.6	Micromedex (Drug–Reax vol. 114)	9.5	ND	ND	ND	3.7
29	Tamblyn R et al. [60]	2003	Canada	75.4 75.3	6284 6276	P	Medical chart	McLeod 1997	31.8 33.3	McLeod (1997)	NA NA	2.6 2.4	NA NA	NA NA	NA NA
30	Schmader K et al. [61]	1994	USA	69.8	208	R	Medical chart	MAI	14	MAI (1994)	NA	0	NA	NA	NA
					7,872,649				**19.1**		**45.3**	**14.65**	**4.4**	**29.6**	
31	Courlet P [62]	2019	Switzerland	71	122 HIV	P	Database (Swiss HIV cohort study)	Beers criteria (2015)	31	University of Liverpool drug interaction checker, Up-to-Date database (2017)	11	ND	ND	ND	4
32	Lund BC et al. [63]	2017	USA	>66	19318 Cancer	R	Database (SEER Medicare)	Beers criteria (2012)	37.3	Micromedex (2017)			5	3.2	
33	Oesterhus R et al. [64]	2017	Norway	77	251 Mental health disease	R	Database (DemWest study)	NORGEP	14	Norwegian drug interaction database (2014, Norwegian medicines agency)	41		1.6	36	4
34	Wucherer D et al. [65]	2017	Germany	79.8	446 Mental health disease	R	Database (Dementia DelpHi–MV study)	PRISCUS	22.9	ABDA (2017)	ND	ND	3.8	34.8	6.4
35	Yazdanshenas H et al. [66]	2016	USA	>65	187 Pain	R	Medical chart	Beers criteria (2012)	83	Healthline (2015)	60	ND	ND	ND	
36	Suehs B.T. et al. [67]	2016	USA	>65	66275 Overactive bladder	R	Medical chart	Beers criteria (2012)	31.1	Beers criteria (2012)		14.3 (anticholinergic DDI)			
37	Dionne PA et al. [68]	2013	Canada	73.8	744 Overactive bladder	R	Database (ESA survey)	Fick criteria 2003 (updated Beers Criteria)	22	Micromedex (2012)	15	ND	ND	ND	
38	Gallagher [69]	2001	USA	88	146 Heart Failure	R	Medical chart	Beers criteria (1997)	8.2	Panel of DDI used for the study (1999)	ND	44.5	ND	ND	8
					87,489				**32.4**		**26.1**	**14.4**	**4.9**	**4.3**	

[a]At the end of the table, the prevalence of PIM and of DDI is reported as the weighted mean (in bold).

Footnote: Prospective (P), Retrospective (R), Mean (M), Median (m), Threshold (t), Severe (S), Moderate (M), not Apply (NA), not Determined (ND)

Source: Bories, M., Bouzillé, G., Cuggia, M., & Le Corre, P. Drug–Drug Interactions in Elderly Patients with Potentially Inappropriate Medications in Primary Care, Nursing Home and Hospital Settings: A Systematic Review and a Preliminary Study. Pharmaceutics. 2021; 13(2):266. https://doi.org/10.3390/pharmaceutics13020266.

Table 2.5. *A Review of the Prevalence (%) of PIM and DDI (Total, Severe and Moderate) and Polymedication (Mean or Median) in Elderly Patients In Hospital Settings*[a]

	Author	Year	Country	Age (Mean, Median or Treshold)	Sample Size	Study Style P–R	Source of Data (Medical Chart—Database)	PIM Criteria	Prevalence of PIM (% Patients with at least 1 PIM)	DDI Checkers (Access Date or Version)	Prevalence of DDI (% of Patients)				Polymedication (Mean or Median Number of Medications)
											All Risk Rating	Severe and Moderate Risk Rating	Severe	Moderate	
1	Al-Azayzih A et al. [70]	2019	Jordan	73.2	4622	R	Medical chart	Beers criteria (2015)	62.5	Beers criteria (2015)	NA	1.6	NA	NA	NA
2	Ertuna E et al. [71]	2019	Turkey	80.3	91	R	Medical chart	Beers criteria (2015), STOPP/START	24.17	RxMediaPharma Interactive Drug Database (2018)	40.12		ND	ND	8.17
3	De Oliveira S.B.V. et al. [72]	2018	Brazil	76 (m) > 60 yrs	170	P	Medical chart	Beers criteria (2015)	44.7	Micromedex (2017)	55.3		ND	ND	11 (m)
4	Colombo F. et al. [73]	2018	Italy	77 (m)	122	P	Medical chart	EU [7]–PIM list	69.6	Micromedex (2017)	78.7		26,1	50,1	7 (m)
5	Ruiz-Millo O. et al. [74]	2018	Spain	81.1	162	P	Medical chart	Beers Criteria (2015) STOPP/START	72,6 90.7	Micromedex (2017)		80,2	51,9	48,1	12.2
6	Saqib A et al. [75]	2018	Pakistan	> 60 (t)	432	R	Medical chart	Beers criteria (2015)	48.3	Drugs.com interaction checker (2017), Stockley's drug interaction checker (2017)	61.8		6.9	74,3	4.74
7	Gutiérrez-Valencia M et al. [76]	2017	Spain	88.3	200	R	Medical chart	Beers criteria (2012) 2015 STOPP	68.5 71	BOT Plus tool (2016)	82.5		24	66.5	9.1
8	Franchi C et al. [77]	2016	Italy	83.7 83.8	347 350	P	Medical chart	Beers criteria (2012), START/STOPP, MAI, IPET	39.1 44.7	INTERcheck (2013)	91.4 85.6		58.3 53.9		5.7 6.3
9	De Melo DL et al. [78]	2016	Brazil	73.7 (>60)	316	P	Medical chart	Beers criteria (2015)	85.8	Micromedex (2014)	44.5		19.9		5.73
10	Grion AM et al. [79]	2016	Italy	86.5	100 449	P	Medical chart	STOPP/START	53 54	Micromedex (version 2.0)			38 37		6 6
11	Salwe K et al. [80]	2016	India	71.6	100	R	Medical chart	Beers criteria (2012)	6.3	Drugs.com interaction checker (2013)	52.7		3.7	40,4	7.6
12	Matanovic SM et al. [81]	2014	Croatia	>65 (t)	454	R	Medical chart	Beers criteria (2012) Suzana Matanović & Vlahović-Palčevski self screening tool	57.9 44.1	Matanović & Vlahović-Palčevski self screening tool (2014)	32.8		ND	ND	5.3
13	Franchi C et al. [82]	2014	Italy	82.8 81.6	39 39	P	Medical chart	Beers criteria (2012)	25.6 17.95	Italian Formulary Guida all uso dei farmaci (2013)	56.4		12.8	51.3	6 (m)
14	Ghibelli S et al. [83]	2013	Italy	81.3 81.1	74 60	P	Medical chart	Beers criteria (2012)	39.1 41.7	INTERcheck (2013)	76.9 90.5	86.5	15.4 37,8	66.7 48,6	7 (m) NA
15	Bakken MS et al. [21]	2012	Norway	84.7	133	P	Medical chart	NORGEP	22.6	DRUID (2011)	85 54.9	73.3	45 0	28,3 8.3	NA 6.0
16	Siqueira JS et al. [84]	2012	Brazil	77.5 (m)	62	R	Medical chart	Fick criteria 2003 (updated Beers Criteria)	34	Micromedex (2011)	77		23,9	49,3	11
17	Trivalle C et al. [85]	2010	France	83.6	526	P	Medical chart	Beers criteria (1997)	13	Vidal (2005)	6		ND	ND	9.4
18	Schuler J et al. [86]	2008	Austria	>75 (t)	543	R	Medical chart	Beers criteria (1997)	30.1	Medis Software (2008)		65.8			7.5
19	Nixdorff N et al. [87]	2008	USA	75	124	P	Medical chart	Fick criteria 2003 (updated Beers Criteria)	34.6	Lexicomp (2007)	26.6		ND	ND	8.6

	Author	Year	Country	Age (Mean, Median or Treshold)	Sample Size	Study Style P–R	Source of Data (Medical Chart—Database)	PIM Criteria	Prevalence of PIM (% Patients with at least 1 PIM)	DDI Checkers (Access Date or Version)	Prevalence of DDI (% of Patients)				Polymedication (Mean or Median Number of Medications)
											All Risk Rating	Severe and Moderate Risk Rating	Severe	Moderate	
20	Radosevic N et al. [88]	2008	Croatia	65.9	225	R	Medical chart	Fick criteria 2003 (updated Beers Criteria)	25	Fick criteria 2003 (updated Beers Criteria)	NA	22.2	NA	NA	5.78
21	Saltvedt I et al. [89]	2005	Norway	81.8	127	R	Medical chart	Beers criteria (1997)	10	DRUID (1999), Hansten PD, Horn JR. Applied Therapeutics Inc. (2000)	44		0	ND	4 (m)
				82.4	127				9		52		0	ND	4 (m)
22	Fillenbaum GG et al. [90]	2004	USA	>65 (t)	3237	R	Database (Established Populations for Epidemiologic Studies of the Elederly (EPESE))	Beers criteria (1997)	21.3	Beers criteria (1997)	NA	13.3	NA	NA	NA
23	Frank C et al. [91]	2001	Canada	77.8	120	R	Medical chart	Beers criteria (1997)	7.4	Clinidata Drug Interactions program (1996)	NA	10.6	NA	NA	NA
					14,127				**44.6**		**53.8**	**12.9**	**26.9**	**54.4**	
24	Jorgensen TL [92]	2020	Denmark	>70 (t)	1294 Cancer	R	Database (Danish Gynaecological Cancer Database (DGCD))	EU [7]–PIM list (PIM A)	48.6	Micromedex (2019), Lexicomp (2019)	ND	38.6	ND	ND	
								EU [7]–PIM list (PIM B)	33.8						
25	Hong S et al. [93]	2020	South Korea	75	301 Cancer	P	Database (Korean Cancer Study Group PC13-09)	2015 Beers criteria	45.5	Lexicomp (2019)		30.6	1,5	28,5	4.7
26	Lavan A [94]	2019	Ireland	72.5	186 Cancer	P	Medical chart	STOPP/START	73.1	Stockley's interaction checker (2019)			50.5	ND	7
27	Graf J et al. [95]	2018	Germany	71	1508 COPD	R	Database (COPD cohort COSYCONET)	PRISCUS	10.2	AiD-Klinik system Heidelberg University Medical Center (2017)			4.3	6.4	5
28	Leger DY et al. [96]	2018	France	81.5	122 Cancer	P	Medical chart	Laroche	34.4	Theriaque (2016), e-Vidal (2016)	71.3		3.3	13.9	6.6
29	Alkan A et al. [97]	2017	Turkey	70	159 Cancer inpatients	R	Medical chart	2012 Beers Criteria	48.4	Lexicomp (2016)		47.2			
					286 Cancer outpatients				14.2			28.3			
30	Rougé Bugat ME et al. [98]	2017	France	83.3	106 Cancer	R	Medical chart	Laroche, START tool	61.3	Panel of DDI used for the study (2016)	16		ND	ND	6.67
31	Vrijkorte E et al. [99]	2017	Netherlands	> 65 (t)	60 Cancer	P	Medical chart	Oncostrip	78	Oncostrip (2016)	12		ND	ND	ND
32	Parian A et al. [100]	2015	USA	70	190 Inflammatory Bowel Disease patients	R	Medical chart	2012 Beers Criteria	35	Micromedex (2014)	73.7		ND	ND	6
33	Jarchow AA & Mangoni AA [101]	2013	UK	84	148 Gastric diseases	R	Medical chart	NICE, British National Formulary, SIGN	99.3	British National Formulary (2009)	56.5		ND	ND	7
					5654				**35.0**		**53.5**	**37.4**	**7.9**	**10.3**	

[a]*At the end of the table, the prevalence of PIM and of DDI is reported as the weighted mean (in bold).*

Footnote: Prospective (P), Retrospective (R), Mean (M), Median (m), Threshold (t), Severe (S), Moderate (M), not Apply (NA), not Determined (ND).

Source: Bories, M., Bouzillé, G., Cuggia, M., & Le Corre, P. Drug–Drug Interactions in Elderly Patients with Potentially Inappropriate Medications in Primary Care, Nursing Home and Hospital Settings: A Systematic Review and a Preliminary Study. Pharmaceutics. 2021; 13(2):266. https://doi.org/10.3390/pharmaceutics13020266.

2.3. Special Populations

The right dose of anesthetic is determined by taking into account various factors such as the patient's medical history and demographics. These variables include age, gender, body habit, long-term alcohol, benzodiazepine, or opioid exposure, the existence of kidney, liver, heart, or lung disease, and the degree of blood loss or dehydration.

The kinetics and dynamics of anesthetic drugs can be significantly impacted by each of them. While the effects of certain patient characteristics, such as obesity, on the behavior of anesthetic drugs have been studied, the effects of other patient characteristics, such as chronic opioid exposure, are still difficult to evaluate. To describe the pharmacokinetics and pharmacodynamics in a few distinct special populations, the results are succinctly summarized.

2.3.1. Influence of Obesity on Anesthetic Drugs

There is a global obesity epidemic, and patients who are overweight often require surgery and anesthesia. As a result, anesthesia professionals need to be aware of how anesthesia interacts with obesity pharmacologically. Manufacturer dosage guidelines are typically expressed in kilograms of actual total body weight (TBW). However, because they are afraid of giving obese patients an excessive dose (a 136-kg patient does not require twice as much drug as a patient of the same height who weighs 68 kg), anesthesia providers rarely use mg/kg dosing in obese patients.

In order to prevent overdosing or underdosing in this patient population, researchers have created a number of weight scalars. Lean body mass (LBM), ideal body weight (IBW), and fat-free mass (FFM) are a few of these scalars. The formulas used to estimate these weight scalars are shown in Table 2.6. Samples of the resulting scaled weight for an obese person and a lean person are shown in Table 2.7. Weight scalars generally aim to match the dosage regimens needed for patients with obesity to those needed for patients with normal body sizes. Since these scaled weights are typically lower than TBW in patients with obesity, they aid in avoiding the overuse of medications. For both bolus (mg/kg) and infusion (mg/kg/h) dosing, as well as target-controlled infusions (TCIs), scaled weights have been used in lieu of TBW.

Table 2.6. *Common Weight Scalars*

Scalars[a]	Equations
Ideal body weight	Male: 50 kg + 2.3 kg for each 2.54 cm (1 inch) over 152 cm (5 feet) Female: 45.5 kg + 2.3 kg for each 2.54 cm (1 inch) over 152 cm (5 feet)
Lean body mass	Male: $1.1 \times TBW - 128 \times (TBW/Ht)^2$ Female: $1.07 \times TBW - 148 \times (TBW/Ht)^2$
Fat-free mass[19]	Male: $(9.27 \times 10^3 \times TBW)/(6.68 \times 10^3 + 216 \times BMI)$ Female: $(9.27 \times 10^3 \times TBW)/(8.78 \times 10^3 + 244 \times BMI)$
Pharmacokinetic mass[20,21]	$52/(1+[1.196.4 \times e^{-0.025\ TBW} - 53.66]/100$ (fentanyl only)
Modified fat-free mass[22 23]	$FFM+0.4^b(TBW - FFM)$

[a]Superscript numbers in this column indicate references at the end of the chapter.

[b]The dose/kg using IBW, TBW, or FFM in an obese person are all less than the dose/kg using TBW in a nonobese patient.

BMI, Body mass index; FFM, fat-free mass; Ht, height in centimeters; IBW, ideal body weight; LBM, lean body mass; MFFM, modified fat-free mass; TBW, total body weight in kg.

Table 2.7. *Dosing Weights Based on Various Dosing Scalars*

Dosing Scalar	Dosing Weight,176-cm(6-foot)-Tall Male	
	68kg BMI=22	185kg BMI=60
Total body weight (TBW)	68	185
Ideal body weight (IBW)	72	72
Lean body mass (LBM)	56	62
Fat-free mass (FFM)	55	88
Modified fat-free mass (MFFM)	60	127

BMI, Body mass index (kg/m^2).

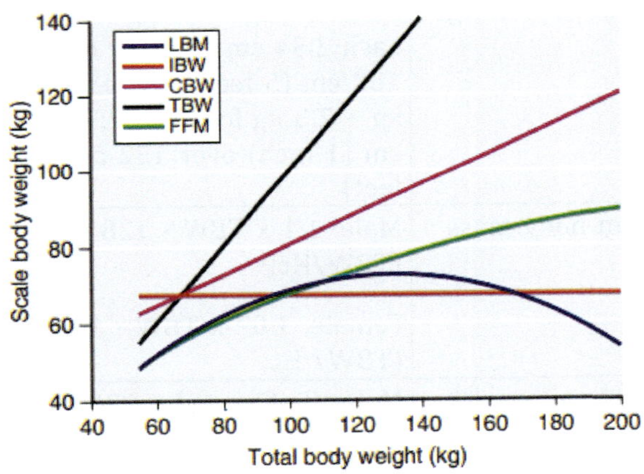

Figure 2.14. *Scaled weights as a function of total body weight (TBW). Key points in this plot: IBW remains the same regardless of the TBW, and LBM starts to decline for weight increases above 127 kg. CBW, Corrected body weight; FFM, fat-free mass; IBW, ideal body weight; LBM, lean body mass (for a 40-year-old man, 176 cm tall).*

Source: From Miller RD, Cohen NH, Eriksson LI, et al., eds. Miller's Anesthesia. 8th ed. Philadelphia: Saunders Elsevier; 2015:Fig. 24.31.

The effects of obesity on the pharmacologic properties of some IV anesthetics, such as propofol, remifentanil, and fentanyl, as well as the drawbacks of using weight scalers for both bolus and continuous infusion dosage (Figure 2.14).

2.3.1.1. Propofol

The impact of obesity on the pharmacokinetics of propofol is not fully understood. Obese patients typically have higher plasma drug concentrations with mg/kg dosing than normal patients with less adipose mass because their blood typically distributes more to non adipose tissues than to adipose tissues. Additionally, the increased liver volume and liver blood flow linked to obesity (as well as increased cardiac output) result in an increase in propofol clearance. Whereas variations in clearance probably have an impact on concentrations during and after infusions, changes in distribution volumes probably have an impact on concentration peaks with bolus dosage. Studies have been conducted on different weight scalars for propofol bolus and continuous infusion dosage.

Dosing Scalars for Propofol

Figure 2.15 shows simulations of an infusion using different weight scalars. The models forecast the effect-site concentrations of propofol after a 60-minute infusion (167 μg/kg/min) in a male patient who is 176 cm (6 feet) tall and weighs both 185 kg and 68 kg. Peak plasma concentrations in lean and obese individuals differ if dosing is based on TBW. With the infusion, the other weight scalars result in substantially lower concentrations.

Of the various dosing scalars that are available, the authors suggest TBW or corrected body weight (CBW) for infusions and LBM24 for bolus dosing (i.e., during induction). Other weight scalars—most concerning for LBM—are likely to produce insufficient dosage for continuous infusions. When TBW is used to dose continuous infusions, there is one issue to consider. Drug accumulation is expressed as μg/kg/min. However, previous research refutes this theory. Servin and associates used TBW and CBW to conduct pharmacokinetic analyses of the administration of propofol to patients who were normal weight and obese. The definition of the CBW was the IBW plus 0.4 × (TBW – IBW).

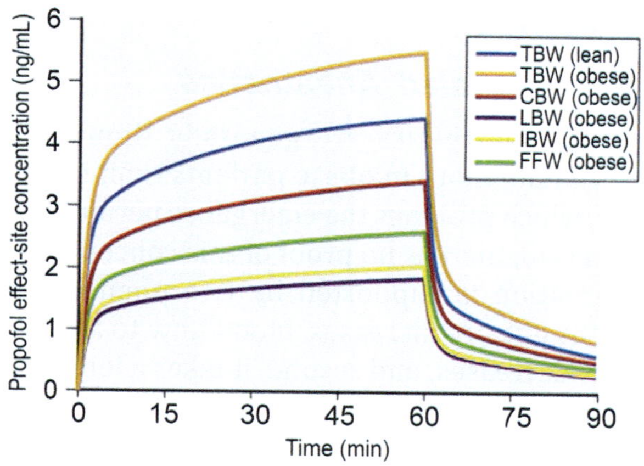

Figure 2.15. *Simulations of propofol plasma concentrations that result from a 60-minute infusion (10 mg/kg/h [167 µg/kg/min]) to a 40-year-old man who is 176 cm tall. Simulations include the following dosing weights: total body weights (TBW) of 68 kg and 185 kg (body mass indices of 22 and 60, respectively) and scaled weights for the 185-kg weight to include Servin's corrected body weight (CBW), lean body mass (LBM), ideal body weight (IBW), and fat-free mass (FFM). Key points: At the 185-kg weight, when dosed to TBW, the infusion leads to high propofol concentrations, whereas when dosed to IBW or LBM, the infusion leads to low propofol concentrations. When the 185-kg individual is dosed using CBW, it best approximates the propofol concentrations that result from TBW in a lean individual.*

Source: From Miller RD, Cohen NH, Eriksson LI, et al., eds. Miller's Anesthesia. 8th ed. Philadelphia: Saunders Elsevier; 2014:Fig. 24.32.

In the two groups, they discovered comparable concentrations at eye-opening, and in the obese patients, there was no propofol buildup. Reports, however, indicate that patients who are morbidly obese may not receive enough infusions based on CBW guidelines for dosage.

Other Sedatives

The effects of other sedatives, such as midazolam, ketamine, etomidate, and barbiturates, on obese patients are poorly understood. Bolus doses should presumably be based on TBW, even though they haven't been clinically validated in obese patients. Using different dosing scales will result in insufficient effect. On the other hand, IBW should receive doses from continuous infusion rates.

2.3.1.2. Opioids

Remifentanil

Remifentanil's distribution volume and clearance in lean and obese patients are similar, primarily because of its fast metabolism by nonspecific esterases in obese patients. Similar to propofol, some scaled weights have been investigated by researchers in an attempt to maximize bolus dose, continuous infusions, and TCIs.

2.3.1.3. Dosing Scalars

As described with propofol, simulation is used to predict remifentanil effect-site concentrations and analgesic effect for a variety of scaled weights in a 174-cm-tall obese (185 kg, BMI of 60) individual and lean (68 kg, BMI of 22) individual. Several key points are illustrated in these simulations:

- For an obese patient, dosing scaled to FFM or IBW resulted in almost identical remifentanil effect-site concentrations as in the lean patient dosed according to TBW. Unlike propofol, dosing remifentanil to CBW (red line) leads to higher plasma concentrations compared to levels achieved when dosing to TBW in a lean individual.

- Dosing scaled to LBM in the obese individual resulted in lower effect-site concentrations than those in a lean individual dosed according to TBW.
- Dosing the obese individual to TBW was excessive. All dosing scalars, except LBM, provided effect-site concentrations associated with a high probability of analgesia.

In patients who are morbidly obese, LBM has significant drawbacks, as shown in Figure 2.15. First, compared to the other dosing scalars, administering remifentanil to LBM results in plasma concentrations with a low probability of effect. Second, when a person is overweight (BMI greater than 40), their LBM actually gets smaller as their TBW increases, making it useless. FFM, a modified LBM, solves the issue of extremely low dosing weight. Suitable effect-site concentrations are also provided by IBW in this simulation; however, this may not always be the case if a weight scalar based solely on patient height is used.

2.3.1.4. Fentany

Though fentanyl is widely used in clinical settings, not much research has been done on how obesity impacts the pharmacokinetics of the drug. When TBW rises, published fentanyl pharmacokinetic models typically overestimate fentanyl concentrations. Researchers have looked into ways to alter demographic information (such as height or weight) to enhance predictions made with published models. One of the numerous fentanyl kinetic models that are currently available can be made more predictive by using a modified weight known as the pharmacokinetic mass.

2.3.1.5. Other Opioids

For opioids other than fentanyl and remifentanil, even less data is available regarding the influence of obesity on drug behavior. Sufentanil's volume of distribution increases linearly with TBW, according to research on obese patients, and its clearance was similar in lean and obese subjects. For continuous infusions, they advise "prudently reduced" dosing and bolus dosing with TBW.

2.3.1.6. Inhaled Anesthetics

Volatile anesthetics are generally thought to accumulate more in obese patients than in lean ones, which prolongs the emergence period. That being said, there is no proof of this concept. This observation is supported by two phenomena: first, as obesity increases, blood flow to adipose tissue decreases; and second, it takes a long time to fill adipose tissue with volatile anesthetics.

2.3.2. Influence of Increasing Age on Anesthetic Drug Pharmacology

One of the most important covariates to take into account when creating an anesthetic plan is age. Remifentanil and propofol can both be used as prototypes to study how age affects anesthetic drug behavior, similar to how obesity works. There is a quantitative description of how age affects remifentanil and propofol. Elderly patients need less remifentanil to achieve an opioid effect. In older patients, pharmacodynamic changes predominate, though pharmacokinetic changes may also be involved in the efficacy of lower dosages. One can conduct simulations to investigate the potential impact of age on dosage, using models of pharmacokinetics and pharmacodynamics that have been previously constructed from measurements taken across a broad age range. To attain equipotent doses in individuals aged 20 and 80, for instance, the dose for the latter should be lowered by fifty-five percent. When it comes to propofol, an analogous analysis suggests lowering the dosage for an 80-year-old by 65% in comparison to a 20-year-old. In particular, the mechanisms underlying the pharmacodynamic changes remain unclear.

Reduced cardiac output could be one reason for pharmacokinetic behavior to change. The reduced cardiac output in the elderly causes slower circulation and more drug mixing. High peak concentrations, decreased drug delivery to metabolic organs, and decreased clearance could result from this. Propofol, thiopental, and etomidate are just a few examples of intravenous anesthetics with slower clearance and smaller volumes of distribution. In addition to alterations in cardiac output brought on by aging, other comorbid conditions can also impair cardiovascular function. Because of this, anesthesia professionals frequently take into account a patient's "physiologic" age rather than depending only on their chronological age. A significant dosage reduction might not be necessary for some elderly patients, such as those with normal body habitus, good exercise tolerance, and no significant coexisting diseases. (Youngs and Shafer, 1999)

A Closer Look

Inhaled Anesthetics in Clinical Use

Inhaled anesthetics have revolutionized modern medicine by providing a safe and effective means of inducing unconsciousness during surgical procedures. These agents are administered through inhalation, allowing for rapid onset and precise control of anesthesia depth. The primary classes of inhaled anesthetics include volatile liquids and gases such as halothane, isoflurane, sevoflurane, and desflurane. Each agent possesses unique pharmacokinetic and pharmacodynamic properties, influencing their clinical use.

Halothane, once widely used, has been largely replaced by newer agents due to its hepatotoxicity and potential for arrhythmias. Isoflurane, characterized by its rapid induction and emergence, remains a cornerstone in anesthesia practice, particularly in long-duration surgeries. Sevoflurane, known for its pleasant odor and minimal airway irritation, is commonly utilized in pediatric and outpatient settings. Desflurane, with its low solubility and rapid recovery profile, is favored for ambulatory surgery and cases requiring swift emergence.

The choice of inhaled anesthetic depends on various factors, including the patient's age, medical history, surgical procedure, and preferences of the anesthesia provider. Inhalational agents offer advantages such as titratability, rapid adjustment of anesthesia depth, and easy administration via standard anesthesia circuits. Additionally, their reversible nature allows for prompt recovery postoperatively, minimizing the risk of residual effects.

However, inhaled anesthetics are not without risks. They can depress cardiovascular and respiratory function, necessitating vigilant monitoring during administration. Adverse effects such as hypotension, respiratory depression, and malignant hyperthermia may occur, albeit rarely. Careful patient selection and meticulous dose titration are essential to mitigate these risks and ensure patient safety.

In recent years, there has been a growing interest in balanced anesthesia techniques, which combine inhaled agents with intravenous medications to optimize anesthesia outcomes. This approach allows for reduced doses of inhaled anesthetics, potentially minimizing their side effects while enhancing overall anesthetic efficacy. Furthermore, adjunctive medications such as opioids, benzodiazepines, and neuromuscular blockers may be utilized to complement the effects of inhaled agents, providing tailored anesthesia tailored to individual patient needs.

Advancements in anesthesia delivery systems, including closed-circuit anesthesia machines and vaporizers with precise concentration control, have further enhanced the safety and efficiency of inhaled anesthetic administration. These technologies enable the delivery of precise concentrations of inhaled agents while minimizing environmental pollution and waste.

Inhaled anesthetics play a crucial role in modern anesthesia practice, offering rapid induction, reversible unconsciousness, and precise control of anesthesia depth. Despite their risks, when administered judiciously and in conjunction with careful monitoring and adjunctive medications, inhaled anesthetics provide safe and effective anesthesia for a wide range of surgical procedures. Continued research and technological innovation will further refine their clinical utility, ensuring optimal outcomes for patients undergoing anesthesia.

Summary

- Pharmacokinetics describes the relationship between drug dose and drug concentration in plasma or at the site of drug effect over time. The processes of absorption, distribution, and elimination (metabolism and excretion) govern this relationship.
- Compartmental models have no physiologic correlate. They are built by using mathematical expressions fit to concentration over time data and then reparameterized in terms of volumes and clearances.
- The terminal phase is often called the "elimination phase" because the primary mechanism for decreasing drug concentration during the terminal phase is elimination of drug from the body.
- Biophase refers to the time delay between changes in plasma concentration and drug effect. Biophase accounts for the time required for drug to diffuse from the plasma to the site of action plus the time required, once drug is at the site of action, to elicit a drug effect.
- To create a pharmacodynamic model, the hysteresis loop is collapsed using modeling techniques that account for the lag time between plasma concentrations and the observed effect. These modeling techniques provide an estimate of the lag time, known as the $t_{½}k_{e0}$, and an estimate of the effect-site concentration (Ce) associated with a 50% probability of drug effect (C_{50}).
- An average clinical anesthetic rarely consists of one drug but rather a combination of drugs to achieve desired levels of hypnosis, analgesia, and muscle relaxation. Hypnotics, analgesics, and muscle relaxants all interact with one another such that each drug, when administered in the presence of other drugs, rarely behaves as if it were administered alone.
- Response surface models have been developed for a variety of anesthetic effects including responses to verbal and tactile stimuli, painful stimuli, hemodynamic or respiratory effects, and changes in electrical brain activity.
- The influence of obesity on propofol pharmacokinetics is not entirely clear. Generally, in obese patients, the blood distributes more to nonadipose than to adipose tissues, resulting in higher plasma drug concentrations in obese patients with mg/kg dosing than in normal patients with less adipose mass.

References

1. Albertin, A., Poli, D., La Colla, L., et al. (2007). Predictive performance of "Servin's formula" during BIS-guided propofol-remifentanil target-controlled infusion in morbidly obese patients. *British Journal of Anaesthesia, 98*(1), 66–75.
2. Anderson, B. J., & Holford, N. H. (2009). Mechanistic basis of using body size and maturation to predict clearance in humans. *Drug Metabolism & Pharmacokinetics, 24*(1), 25–36.
3. Arden, J. R., Holley, F. O., & Stanski, D. R. (1986). Increased sensitivity to etomidate in the elderly: Initial distribution versus altered brain response. *Anesthesiology, 65*(1), 19–27.

4. Avram, M. J., Krejcie, T. C., & Henthorn, T. K. (1990). The relationship of age to the pharmacokinetics of early drug distribution: The concurrent disposition of thiopental and indocyanine green. *Anesthesiology, 72*(3), 403–411.

5. Bouillon, T. W., Bruhn, J., Radulescu, L., et al. (2004). Pharmacodynamic interaction between propofol and remifentanil regarding hypnosis, tolerance of laryngoscopy, bispectral index, and electroencephalographic approximate entropy. *Anesthesiology, 100*(6), 1353–1372.

6. Cortinez, L. I., Anderson, B. J., Penna, A., et al. (2010). Influence of obesity on propofol pharmacokinetics: Derivation of a pharmacokinetic model. *British Journal of Anaesthesia, 105*(4), 448–456.

7. Cortinez, L. I., Gambús, P., Trocóniz, I. F., et al. (2011). Obesity does not influence the onset and offset of sevoflurane effect as measured by the hysteresis between sevoflurane concentration and bispectral index. *Anesthesia & Analgesia, 113*(1), 70–76.

8. Doufas, A. G., Bakhshandeh, M., Bjorksten, A. R., et al. (2004). Induction speed is not a determinant of propofol pharmacodynamics. *Anesthesiology, 101*, 1112–1121.

9. Duffull, S. B., Dooley, M. J., Green, B., et al. (2004). A standard weight descriptor for dose adjustment in the obese patient. *Clinical Pharmacokinetics, 43*(16), 1167–1178.

10. Egan, T. D., Muir, K. T., Hermann, D. J., et al. (2001). The electroencephalogram (EEG) and clinical measures of opioid potency: Defining the EEG-clinical potency relationship ("fingerprint") with application to remifentanil. *International Journal of Pharmaceutics & Medicine, 15*(1), 11–19.

11. Greenblatt, D. J., Abernethy, D. R., Locniskar, A., et al. (1984). Effect of age, gender, and obesity on midazolam kinetics. *Anesthesiology, 61*(1), 27–35.

12. Heyse, B., Proost, J. H., Schumacher, P. M., et al. (2012). Sevoflurane-remifentanil interaction: Comparison of different response surface models. *Anesthesiology, 116*(2), 311–323.

13. Homer, T. D., & Stanski, D. R. (1985). The effect of increasing age on thiopental disposition and anesthetic requirement. *Anesthesiology, 62*, 714–724.

14. Hudson, R. J., Bergstrom, R. G., Thomson, I. R., et al. (1989). Pharmacokinetics of sufentanil in patients undergoing abdominal aortic surgery. *Anesthesiology, 70*, 426–431.

15. Hughes, M. A., Glass, P. S., & Jacobs, J. R. (1992). Context-sensitive half-time in multicompartment pharmacokinetic models for intravenous anesthetic drugs. *Anesthesiology, 76*(3), 334–341.

16. Igarashi, T., Nagata, O., Iwakiri, H., et al. (2002). Two cases of intraoperative awareness during intravenous anesthesia with propofol in morbidly obese patients. *Masui, 51*(11), 1243–1247.

17. Janmahasatian, S., Duffull, S. B., Ash, S., et al. (2005). Quantification of lean body weight. *Clinical Pharmacokinetics, 44*(10), 1051–1065.

18. Johnson, K. B., Syroid, N. D., Gupta, D. K., et al. (2008). An evaluation of remifentanil-propofol response surfaces for loss of responsiveness, loss of response to surrogates of painful stimuli, and laryngoscopy in patients undergoing elective surgery. *Anesthesia & Analgesia, 106*(2), 471–479.

19. Kern, S. E., Xie, G., White, J. L., & Egan, T. D. (2004). A response surface analysis of propofol-remifentanil pharmacodynamic interaction in volunteers. *Anesthesiology, 100*(6), 1373–1381.

20. Krejcie, T. C., & Avram, M. J. (1999). What determines anesthetic induction dose? It's the front-end kinetics, doctor! *Anesthesia & Analgesia, 89*(3), 541–544.

21. Krejcie, T. C., Avram, M. J., Gentry, W. B., et al. (1997). A recirculatory model of the pulmonary uptake and pharmacokinetics of lidocaine based on analysis of arterial and mixed venous data from dogs. *Journal of Pharmacokinetics and Biopharmaceutics, 25*, 169–190.

22. La Colla, L., Albertin, A., La Colla, G., et al. (2009). No adjustment vs. adjustment formula as input weight for propofol target-controlled infusion in morbidly obese patients. *European Journal of Anaesthesiology, 26*(5), 362–369.

23. La Colla, L., Albertin, A., La Colla, G., et al. (2010). Predictive performance of the "Minto" remifentanil pharmacokinetic parameter set in morbidly obese patients ensuing from a new method for calculating lean body mass. *Clinical Pharmacokinetics, 49*(2), 131–139.

24. LaPierre, C. D., Johnson, K. B., Randall, B. R., et al. (2011). An exploration of remifentanil-propofol combinations that lead to a loss of response to esophageal instrumentation, a loss of responsiveness, and/or onset of intolerable ventilatory depression. *Anesthesia & Analgesia, 113*(3), 490–499.

25. Lee, S., Kim, B. H., Lim, K., et al. (2012). Pharmacokinetics and pharmacodynamics of intravenous dexmedetomidine in healthy Korean subjects. *Journal of Clinical Pharmacy and Therapeutics, 37*, 698–703.

26. Lesser, G. T., & Deutsch, S. (1967). Measurement of adipose tissue blood flow and perfusion in man by uptake of 85Kr. *Journal of Applied Physiology, 23*(5), 621–630.

27. Manyam, S. C., Gupta, D. K., Johnson, K. B., et al. (2006). Opioid-volatile anesthetic synergy: A response surface model with remifentanil and sevoflurane as prototypes. *Anesthesiology, 105*(2), 267–278.

28. Mertens, M. J., Engbers, F. H., Burm, A. G., & Vuyk, J. (2003). Predictive performance of computer-controlled infusion of remifentanil during propofol/remifentanil anesthesia. *British Journal of Anaesthesia, 90*(2), 132–141.

29. Minto, C. F., Schnider, T. W., & Shafer, S. L. (1997). Pharmacokinetics and pharmacodynamics of remifentanil. II. Model application. *Anesthesiology, 86*(1), 24–33.

30. Minto, C. F., Schnider, T. W., Egan, T. D., et al. (1997). Influence of age and gender on the pharmacokinetics and pharmacodynamics of remifentanil. I. Model development. *Anesthesiology, 86*(1), 10–23.

31. Rodeheffer, R. J., Gerstenblith, G., Becker, L. C., et al. (1984). Exercise cardiac output is maintained with advancing age in healthy human subjects: Cardiac dilatation and increased stroke volume compensate for a diminished heart rate. *Circulation, 69*(2), 203–213.

32. Schnider, T. W., Minto, C. F., & Shafer, S. L. (1999). The influence of age on propofol pharmacodynamics. *Anesthesiology, 90*(6), 1502–1516.

33. Schnider, T. W., Minto, C. F., Gambus, P. L., et al. (1998). The influence of method of administration and covariates on the pharmacokinetics of propofol in adult volunteers. *Anesthesiology, 88*(5), 1170–1182.

34. Schwartz, A. E., Matteo, R. S., Ornstein, E., et al. (1991). Pharmacokinetics of sufentanil in obese patients. *Anesthesia & Analgesia, 73*(6), 790–793.

35. Scott, J. C., & Stanski, D. R. (1987). Decreased fentanyl and alfentanil dose requirements with age: A simultaneous pharmacokinetic and pharmacodynamic evaluation. *Journal of Pharmacology and Experimental Therapeutics, 240*(1), 159–166.

36. Servin, F., Farinotti, R., Haberer, J. P., & Desmonts, J. M. (1993). Propofol infusion for maintenance of anesthesia in morbidly obese patients receiving nitrous oxide: A clinical and pharmacokinetic study. *Anesthesiology, 78*(4), 657–665.

37. Shibutani, K., Inchiosa Jr., M. A., Sawada, K., & Bairamian, M. (2004). Accuracy of pharmacokinetic models for predicting plasma fentanyl concentrations in lean and obese surgical patients: Derivation of dosing weight ("pharmacokinetic mass"). *Anesthesiology, 101*(3), 603–613.

38. Shibutani, K., Inchiosa Jr., M. A., Sawada, K., & Bairamian, M. (2005). Pharmacokinetic mass of fentanyl for postoperative analgesia in lean and obese patients. *British Journal of Anaesthesia, 95*(3), 377–383.

39. Stanski, D. R., & Maitre, P. O. (1990). Population pharmacokinetics and pharmacodynamics of thiopental: The effect of age revisited. *Anesthesiology, 72*(3), 412–422.

40. Upton, R. N., Ludbrook, G. L., Grant, C., & Martinez, A. M. (1999). Cardiac output is a determinant of the initial concentrations of propofol after short-infusion administration. *Anesthesia & Analgesia, 89*(3), 545–552.

41. Wilkinson, G. R., & Shand, D. G. (1975). Commentary: A physiological approach to hepatic drug clearance. *Clinical Pharmacology & Therapeutics, 18*, 377–390.

42. Williams, T. F. (1987). Aging or disease? *Clinical Pharmacology & Therapeutics, 42*(6), 663–665.

Chapter 3

INHALED ANESTHETICS

Contents

Introduction

Inhaled anesthetics represent a cornerstone in modern medicine, revolutionizing the landscape of surgical procedures and patient care. These compounds, administered via inhalation, induce a reversible loss of sensation and consciousness, facilitating painless surgical interventions. The advent of inhaled anesthetics marked a significant advancement in anesthesia practice, offering safer, more controllable means of achieving unconsciousness during surgery compared to earlier methods.

One of the most notable attributes of inhaled anesthetics is their rapid onset and offset of action, allowing for precise control over the depth and duration of anesthesia. This characteristic is particularly advantageous in tailoring anesthesia to individual patient needs, minimizing the risk of prolonged unconsciousness or delayed recovery. The pharmacological properties of inhaled anesthetics vary widely, encompassing a spectrum of potency, solubility, and physicochemical characteristics. This diversity enables anesthesiologists to select agents tailored to specific patient requirements, taking into account factors such as age, medical history, and the nature of the surgical procedure. Despite their widespread use and efficacy, inhaled anesthetics are not devoid of risks and side effects. Potential adverse effects include respiratory depression, cardiovascular instability, and postoperative cognitive dysfunction, necessitating vigilant monitoring and appropriate management strategies.

Continuous research and development efforts aim to enhance the safety and efficiency of inhaled anesthetics, with ongoing exploration of novel compounds and delivery techniques. Additionally, advancements in pharmacogenomics offer insights into individual variability in drug response, paving the way for personalized anesthesia regimens.

Inhaled anesthetics represent a cornerstone of modern anesthesia practice, providing indispensable support for a wide range of surgical interventions. With ongoing advancements in pharmacology and technology, the field continues to evolve, promising further improvements in patient safety and outcomes. (Eger, 1963; Eger, 1974; Eger, 1985; Eger, 1993; Eger, 2000).

Orientation and Directional Terms

Term	Definition	Illustration
Nitrous Oxide	Nitrous oxide is an odorless, colorless, non-flammable gas. While nitrous oxide is not flammable, it will support combustion to the same extent as oxygen. It leads to a state of euphoria, explaining its nickname, 'laughing gas.' Nitrous oxide is the least potent inhalational anesthetic.	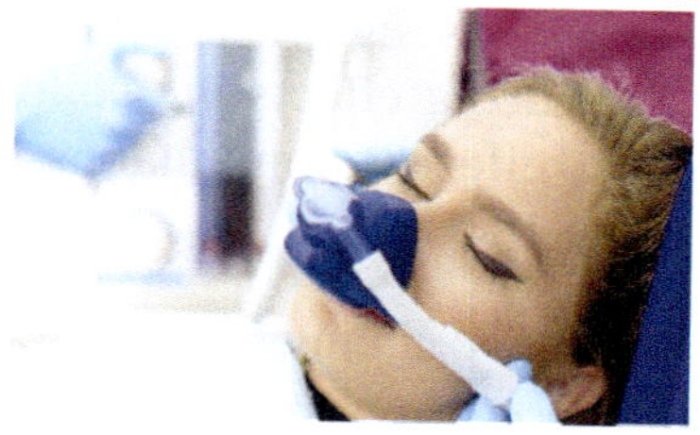
Methoxyflurane	Methoxyflurane is an ether in which the two groups attached to the central oxygen atom are methyl and 2,2-dichloro-1,1-difluoroethyl. It has a role as an inhalation anaesthetic, a non-narcotic analgesic, a hepatotoxic agent and a nephrotoxic agent.	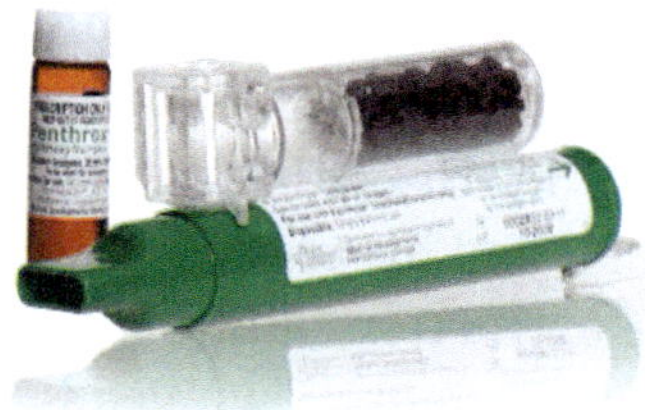
Pharmacokinetics	Pharmacokinetics (PK) is the study of how the body interacts with administered substances for the entire duration of exposure. This is closely related to but distinctly different from pharmacodynamics, which examines the drug's effect on the body more closely.	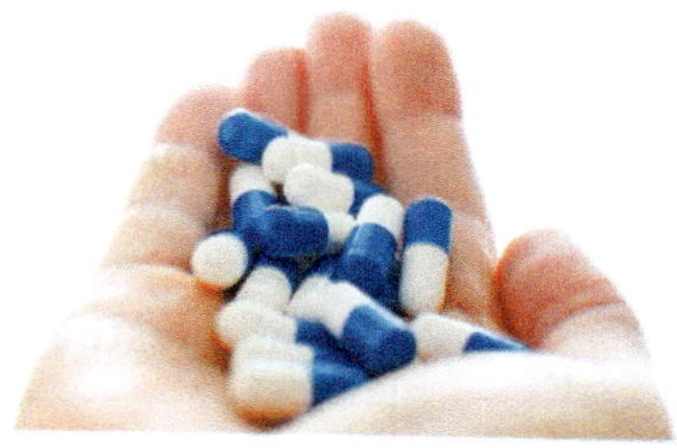
Alveolar Partial Pressure	This alveolar partial pressure of oxygen is the driving force for the diffusion of oxygen across the alveolar membranes, through pulmonary capillary walls, and into the arteriolar blood flow and erythrocytes for transport throughout the body into peripheral tissues.	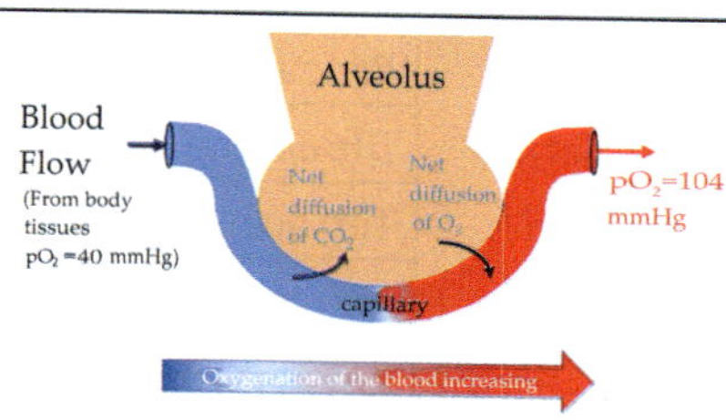
Anesthetic Breathing System	Anesthesia breathing systems serve as a conduit to deliver anesthetic and other gases to a patient. Various designs of breathing systems have been created to serve this function. One method of classifying anesthesia breathing systems is based on how gas flows: open, semi-open, semi-closed, and closed systems.	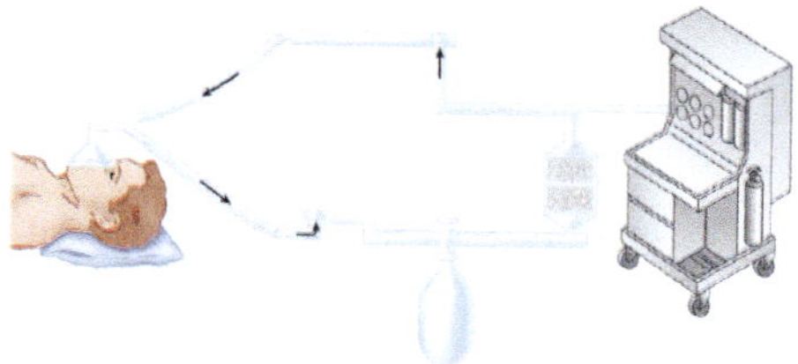

3.1. The First Inhaled Anesthetics

3.1.1. Nitrous Oxide

Nitrous oxide has significant medical uses, especially in surgery and dentistry, for its anaesthetic and pain-reducing effects. Its colloquial name, "laughing gas," coined by Humphry Davy, is due to the euphoric effects upon inhaling it, a property that has led to its recreational use as a dissociative anaesthetic.

The English chemist, writer, and Unitarian minister Joseph Priestley created nitrous oxide gas for the first time in 1772. Twenty-seven years later, Sir Humphry Davy used nitrous oxide to relieve pain in the teeth. Though he had a suspicion that nitrous oxide might be used to reduce pain during surgery, it wasn't until 42 years later that a 29-year-old dentist named Horace Wells used it on himself and discovered that it did so. It was during a public exhibition in Hartford, Connecticut, in 1842 that he first observed the hypnotic and analgesic effects of nitrous oxide. Wells himself had his teeth extracted by another dentist the following day. Wells had very little pain during the extraction, and he went on to learn how to make nitrous oxide so that he could give it to his own patients. Two years later, he set up a demonstration of nitrous oxide administration for painless dental surgery at Massachusetts General Hospital. This demonstration proved to be partially unsuccessful and led to Wells' discredit (Table 3.1). (Figures 3.1 and 3.2).

Table 3.1. *An Example Timeline*

Local anesthetics	Year of synthesis	Introduction in clinic
Cocaine	1860	1884
Procaine	1904	1905
Dibucaine	1925	1930
Tetracaine	1928	1932
Lidocaine	1943	1947
Chloroprocaine	1950	1952
Mepivacaine	1956	1957
Prilocaine	1959	1960
Bupivacaine	1957	1963
Etidocaine	1971	1972
Ropivacaine	1957	1997
Levobupivacaine	1972	1999

Source: From M. Whizar-Lugo, V., L. Íñiguez-López, K., C. Cárdenas-Maytorena, A., & D. Ramírez-Puerta, C. (2020). Local Anesthetics. IntechOpen. doi: 10.5772/intechopen.93643.

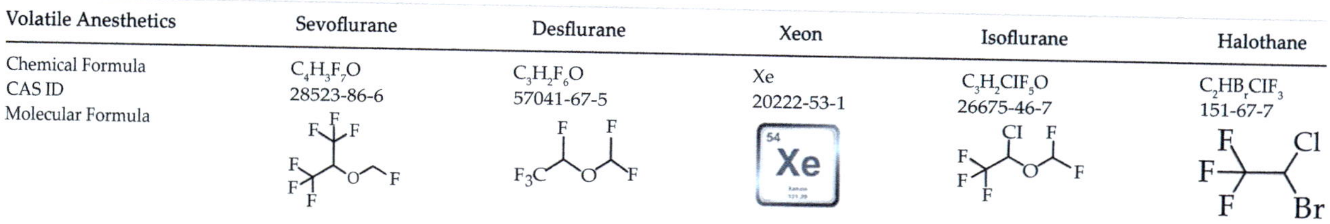

Figure 3.1. *Molecular structures of potent volatile anesthetics. Halogenated volatile anesthetics are liquids at room temperature. Among the volatile anesthetics, halothane is an alkane derivative, whereas all the others are derivatives of methyl ethyl ether. Isoflurane is the chemical isomer of enflurane.*

Source: Wang J, Cheng C-s, Lu Y, Sun S and Huang S (2021) Volatile Anesthetics Regulate Anti-Cancer Relevant Signaling. Front. Oncol. 11:610514. doi: 10.3389/fonc.2021.610514.

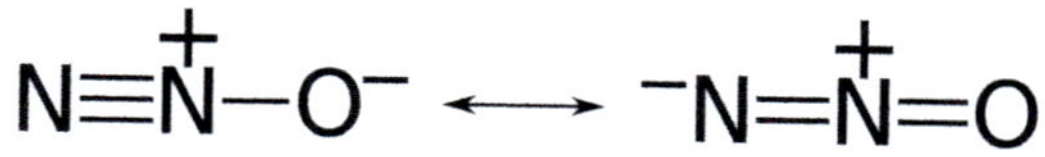

Figure 3.2. *Molecular structure of nitrous oxide. Nitrous oxide is a linear molecule existing in two resonance structures. Dots denote nonbonding electrons.*

Source: By WhiteTimberwolf, Ben Mills (PNG version) - Own work, Public Domain, https://commons.wikimedia.org/w/index.php?curid=9507167.

3.1.2. Diethyl Ether

Diethyl ether, or simply ether, is an organic compound with the chemical formula $(CH_3CH_2)_2O$, also written as $C_4H_{10}O$ or $(C_2H_5)_2O$, sometimes abbreviated as Et_2O. It is a colourless, highly volatile, sweet-smelling ("ethereal odour"), extremely flammable liquid. It belongs to the ether class of organic compounds. It is commonly used as a solvent in laboratories and as a starting fluid for some engines. It was formerly used as a general anesthetic, until non-flammable drugs were developed, such as halothane. It has been used as a recreational drug to cause intoxication.

Boston dentist William Morton discovered that diethyl ether had effects akin to nitrous oxide when used in "ether frolics," where ether was breathed for its inebriating properties. Similar to Wells, Morton used ether in his dental practice. On October 16, 1846, also known as "ether day," he demonstrated the anesthetic qualities of ether at the Massachusetts General Hospital. Unlike the disaster that was Wells, Morton's demonstration was warmly welcomed. The Boston Medical and Surgical Journal quickly published the outcomes of effective ether anesthetics. Despite the fact that Crawford Long used diethyl ether on a patient in 1842—four years before Morton—he kept his findings to himself, and as a result, diethyl ether's ability to induce anesthesia has historically been attributed to Morton.

Table 3.2. *This Table Provides all LIDO-Containing Medications Approved by the FDA, along with their Concentrations, their Compositions, and Concentrations.*

Drug Name	Drugs in Its Composition	Application Method	Concentration (%)
Lidocaine	Lidocaine	Topical	5
Lidocaine and Prilocaine	Lidocaine; Prilocaine	Topical	2.5; 2.5
Lidoderm	Lidocaine	Topical	5
Oraqix	Lidocaine; Prilocaine	Periodontal	2.5; 2.5
Pliaglis	Lidocaine; Tetracaine	Topical	7; 7
Versatis	Lidocaine	Topical	700 mg
Xylocaine	Lidocaine	Topical	5
Xylocaine	Lidocaine hydrochloride	Injectable	0.5 to 2
Xylocaine	Lidocaine hydrochloride	Topical	2
Zingo	Lidocaine; Hydrochloride	Intradermal	0.5 mg
ZTLIDO	Lidocaine	Topical	1.8

Source: Silva A, Mourão J, Vale N. A Review of the Lidocaine in the Perioperative Period. Journal of Personalized Medicine. 2023; 13(12):1699. https://doi.org/10.3390/jpm13121699.

3.1.3. Chloroform

Chloroform is an organochloride with the formula $CHCl_3$ and a common solvent. It is a very volatile, colorless, strong-smelling, dense liquid produced on a large scale as a precursor to refrigerants and PTFE. Chloroform is a trihalomethane that serves as a powerful general anesthetic, euphoriant, anxiolytic, and sedative when inhaled or ingested, for this reason, Chloroform was used as an inhalational anesthetic between the 19th century and the first half of the 20th century. It is miscible with many solvents but it is only very slightly soluble in water (only 8 g/L at 20°C).

Chloroform was created by Scottish obstetrician James Simpson; it did not have the long induction, flammability, or postoperative nausea associated with diethyl ether. While diethyl ether dominated medical practice in North America, chloroform quickly gained popularity as an inhaled anesthetic in England. Regretfully, chloroform has been linked to multiple cases of hepatotoxicity and a number of inexplicable intraoperative deaths of otherwise healthy patients.

3.1.4. Inhaled Anesthetics between 1920 and 1940

Between 1920 and 1940, significant advancements were made in the field of inhaled anesthetics, leading to the development of safer and more effective agents. During this period, two notable inhaled anesthetics emerged: ethylene and cyclopropane. Ethylene, introduced in the 1920s, was non-flammable and provided rapid induction of anesthesia, but it had a narrow therapeutic range and caused significant postoperative nausea and vomiting. Cyclopropane, introduced in the 1930s, became popular due to its rapid onset and potency. Despite being highly flammable, cyclopropane offered excellent muscle relaxation and analgesia, which made it a valuable tool in surgeries. Another significant development during this period was the refinement of nitrous oxide use, which was often combined with other agents to enhance its anesthetic effects and reduce risks. The advancements in these anesthetics were driven by a growing understanding of their pharmacodynamics and pharmacokinetics, as well as improvements in delivery systems, such as the introduction of more precise vaporizers and better methods for administering mixed gases. These innovations between 1920 and 1940 laid the foundation for modern anesthesia, significantly improving the safety and effectiveness of surgical procedures.

3.2. Fluorine Chemistry and Modern Inhaled Anesthetics

Fluorine chemistry has played a pivotal role in the development of modern inhaled anesthetics, revolutionizing the field by enhancing the safety, efficacy, and control of these agents. The introduction of fluorinated hydrocarbons in the mid-20th century marked a significant breakthrough. These compounds, including halothane, enflurane, isoflurane, desflurane, and sevoflurane, demonstrated superior properties compared to their predecessors.

Halothane, introduced in the 1950s, was one of the first fluorinated anesthetics and quickly gained popularity due to its potency and rapid onset. However, its potential for hepatotoxicity and cardiac arrhythmias necessitated the search for safer alternatives. This led to the development of enflurane and isoflurane in the 1970s, both of which offered better cardiovascular stability and less hepatotoxicity. Isoflurane, in particular, became widely used due to its favorable safety profile and ease of use.

The advancements continued with the introduction of desflurane and sevoflurane in the 1990s. Desflurane is known for its rapid induction and emergence, making it ideal for outpatient procedures. Sevoflurane, with its low blood-gas partition coefficient, allows for smooth and rapid induction and recovery, making it particularly suitable for pediatric anesthesia. Both agents exhibit excellent controllability and minimal side effects, largely due to the presence of fluorine atoms in their chemical structures.

Fluorine's unique properties, such as high electronegativity and the ability to form strong carbon-fluorine bonds, contribute to the stability, non-flammability, and low solubility of these anesthetics in blood, enhancing their safety and effectiveness. The evolution of fluorinated anesthetics underscores the profound impact of fluorine chemistry on modern medicine, offering anesthesiologists a range of agents that provide precise control over anesthesia with improved patient outcomes.

3.2.1. Halothane

In 1956, halothane was first used in clinical settings and quickly gained popularity. It was nonflammable, had a pleasant smell, was less harmful to organs, and its pharmacokinetic qualities allowed for a much quicker induction of anesthesia and emergence than ether, among its many advantages over the older anesthetics. Unfortunately, reports of fulminant hepatic necrosis following halothane anesthesia started to surface after the drug had been used commercially for four years. These patients did not appear to have other obvious causes of liver damage. The need to find alternative volatile anesthetics arose from the problem of unpredictable liver damage. Additionally, halothane makes the myocardium more susceptible to the dysrhythmogenic effects of catecholamines.

3.2.2. Methoxyflurane

In 1960, methylflurane was initially used in clinical settings. Studies verifying a dose-related nephrotoxicity due to the inorganic fluoride produced by this anesthetic's metabolism followed reports of renal failure with methoxyflurane anesthesia within the first ten years of its introduction.

3.2.3. Enflurane

In clinical settings, enflurane was first used in 1972. Not only did it not cause hepatotoxicity like halothane, but it also did not cause the heart to become sensitive to catecholamines. The electroencephalogram (EEG) may show seizure activity in response to enflurane, though, as it was converted to inorganic fluoride during metabolism. This is particularly true when high dosages and hypocapnia are present.

3.2.4. Isoflurane

In clinical settings, isoflurane was first used extensively in 1980. Dysrhythmias of the heart were not linked to it. It has been found that isoflurane is less toxic than halothane and enflurane because it is not metabolized as quickly. When it comes to surgical anesthesia and awakening, isoflurane facilitated a quicker onset than its predecessors.

3.2.5. Sevoflurane and Desflurane

Sevoflurane and desflurane were first synthesized in the late 1960s and 1970s, respectively, and are the only halogenated compounds with fluorine. Due to their high cost and challenging synthesis, neither was promptly taken into consideration for commercial application. Their creation was reexamined in the 1980s due to the realization that an increasing amount of anesthetic procedures were being performed in an outpatient setting and that medications that were only halogenated with fluorine were less soluble in blood and tissues, enabling quicker awakening and recuperation. (Eger, 1963; Eger, 1974; Eger, 1985; Eger, 1993; Eger, 2000).

3.3. Mechanism of Action

At many levels of biologic organization, such as their site of action within the central nervous system, the molecules they interact with, and the nature of this biologic interaction, the question of how inhaled anesthetics produce the anesthetic state can be addressed. Measuring the effects of anesthetics is necessary to provide answers to these questions. Although inhaled anesthetics have been used for nearly 160 years to provide surgical anesthesia, the term "anesthetic state" is not universally recognized. An operational definition of amnesia for intraoperative events and immobility in response to surgical stimulation has proven useful for experimental purposes.

3.3.1. Measurable Characteristics

Amnestic effects and immobility are two measurable and common features of all inhaled anesthetics. The minimum alveolar concentration (MAC) of anesthetic needed to impede movement to a surgical incision in 50% of patients is used to quantify immobility. It is challenging to confirm whether amnesia or awareness is present. Even though analgesia is a component of the anesthetic state, it is also impossible to quantify in a patient who is unconscious and unable to move. Measures of pain substitutes (i.e., elevated heart rate or systemic arterial blood pressure) imply that anesthetics inhaled through the nose do not block the feeling of pain. In small doses, some inhaled anesthetics have hyperalgesic (pain-enhancing) effects. Nitrous oxide, which raises skeletal muscle tone, demonstrates that skeletal muscle relaxation is a main effect of inhaled anesthetics that is frequently, but not always, present.

3.3.1.1. Immobility

The determination of MAC in decerebrate animals shows that strong inhaled anesthetics primarily cause immobility by acting on the spinal cord. Nitrous oxide may inhibit nociceptive input in the dorsal horn of the spinal cord by activating descending noradrenergic pathways that originate in the periaqueductal gray matter brainstem, according to studies conducted on rodents.

3.3.1.2. Amnestic Effects

Supraspinal structures such as the amygdala, hippocampus, and cortex are considered highly probable targets for the amnestic effects of anesthetics.

3.3.1.3. Central Nervous System Depression and Ion Channels

By acting on ion channels, which control the nervous system's electrical activity, inhaled anesthetics cause depression of the central nervous system. Inhaled anesthetics most likely work by increasing the activity of inhibitory ion channels and inhibiting the activity of excitatory ion channels in order to produce anesthesia. The neuron becomes hyperpolarized when inhibitory ion channels are activated. When chloride anions enter neurons via glycine or γ-aminobutyric acid A (GABAA) receptors, or when potassium cations are effluxed out of neurons via potassium ion channels, hyperpolarization ensues. By stopping the entry of positive charges into the neuron, blocking the activity of excitatory ion channels stops the neuron from depolarizing (i.e., the flow of sodium ions via sodium channels or N-methyl d-aspartate [NMDA] receptors. The release of neurotransmitters may also be impacted by anesthetics, and this effect may be partially mediated by ion channels that control neurotransmitter release.

3.4. Physical Properties

Inhalation anesthetics can be classed as either vapors or gases. According to this classification a gas exists in the gaseous state at room temperature and sea-level pressure, while a vapor exists as a liquid under similar standard conditions.

3.4.1. Molecular Structure

All of the current inhaled anesthetics are halogenated hydrocarbons, except for nitrous oxide. Because halothane doesn't have the same ether moiety as isoflurane, sevoflurane, and desflurane, it can cause ventricular cardiac dysrhythmias. The only difference between isoflurane and desflurane is one chlorine atom in place of one fluorine atom. Increased resistance to metabolism and stability are conferred by fluorine substitution.

3.4.2. Vapor Pressure and Delivery

Nitrous oxide exists as a gas at ambient temperature, although it becomes a liquid at higher pressures. The remaining inhaled anesthetics are liquids at ambient temperatures.

3.4.2.1. Variable-Bypass Vaporizers

Provided by variable-bypass vaporizers (Tec 4, 5, and 7; North American Draeger 19n and 20n), halothane, sevoflurane, and isoflurane are administered. Two streams of fresh gas are introduced into the variable-bypass vaporizer, one of which contacts a liquid anesthetic reservoir (sump) and the other of which avoids it. The saturated vapor pressure of the anesthetic controls how much of it gets saturated in the gas stream that passes through the sump. The gas leaving the sump needs to be diluted by gas that hasn't come into contact with the volatile anesthetics because they produce clinically useful anesthesia at partial pressures much lower than that of their saturated vapor pressure in the first place. The relative flow, or how much anesthetic is in the gas leaving the vaporizer, determines the concentration of anesthetic. , splitting ratio) of new gas passing via the bypass channel as opposed to the sump channel. When the clinician modifies the vaporizer's dial or electronic control, the anesthetic output concentration that emerges from the device is controlled. Temperature-compensated variable-bypass vaporizers maintain a consistent output across a broad temperature range and are calibrated for each specific anesthetic based on its unique vapor pressure. A vaporizer that is tilted or overfilled may accidentally release an excessive amount of anesthetic vapor into the bypass channel, which could result in an overdose.

The Datex-Ohmeda Aladin Cassette Vaporizer is a single electronically controlled vaporizer that is used in the Datex-Ohmeda Anesthesia Delivery Unit (ADU) machines. The sump is housed within interchangeable, magnetically coded cassettes that are used to deliver halothane, enflurane, isoflurane, sevoflurane, and desflurane. The bypass is housed within the ADU. The Aladin uses a central processing unit's (CPU) activity to control output concentration through variable bypass.

The concentration setting, flowmeters, internal pressure and temperature sensors, and other sources provide input to the CPU, which then controls a flow control valve at the vaporizing chamber's outlet. One-way check valves are intended to close in the event that the pressure in the cassette (sump) surpasses the bypass chamber pressure, which would happen if the room temperature rose above 22.8% C while desflurane was being administered. This prevents the retrograde flow of anesthetic saturated gas back into the ADU and consequent anesthetic overdose.

3.4.2.2. Heated Vaporizer

Desflurane has a vapor pressure of 700 mm Hg at 20° C at sea level, which is almost boiling at room temperature. When it is delivered using a variable-bypass vaporizer, the concentrations can vary greatly. Because of this, the anesthesia provider uses a specially designed vaporizer (Tec 6, Datex-Ohmeda) to accurately measure and deliver desflurane vapor following adjustments of the concentration dial. The vaporizer heats desflurane gas to 2 atm of pressure. The desflurane output concentration from the Tec 6 is constant across a range of barometric pressures, in contrast to the variable-bypass vaporizers. Consequently, unless an adjustment is made to account for the higher altitude, the partial pressure of desflurane at high altitudes will be lower than at sea level at a given Tec 6 vaporizer setting and output (volume percent) concentration. This could result in an underdosing of the anesthetic: required vaporizer setting = (desired vaporizer setting at sea level × 760 mm Hg)/ local barometric pressure (in mm Hg). A higher output, on the other hand, is possible with variable-bypass vaporizers. However, partial pressure—rather than volume percent—is the quantitative measure of anesthetic activity that is pharmacologically significant. As a result, for the same vaporizer setting, a higher altitude will produce a greater anesthetic output; however, the anesthetic impact and delivered partial pressure will be the same in both locations.

3.4.3. Economic and Environmental Considerations

The amount of volatile liquid used and, in turn, the cost of the anesthetic delivery are directly influenced by the fresh gas flow rate. Elevated fresh gas flows (at or beyond minute ventilation) reduce the likelihood of rebreathing and facilitate quicker equilibration between inspired and CNS partial pressures. However, using nonrebreathing flows results in anesthetic loss to the surrounding air and should only be done for a short while—typically during anesthetic induction—or in situations where light sedation and impending surgical stimulation are anticipated.

Concerns and knowledge about the role that inhaled anesthetic release plays in total greenhouse gas emissions and climate change are growing. The distinct infrared absorption spectrum and atmospheric lifetime gas of each anesthetic seem to have an influence on the environment. The estimated atmospheric lifetimes of inhaled anesthetics, such as nitrous oxide, desflurane, sevoflurane, and isoflurane, vary significantly, with 114, 10, 3.6, and 1.2 years, respectively. Different infrared absorbance spectra correspond to different compounds; desflurane, for example, has a higher carbon dioxide equivalent impact than sevoflurane. While the relationship between inhaled anesthetics and global climate change is still up for debate, there are a few points that need to be taken into account. First, cost and release to the environment will be balanced by using low fresh gas flows (0.5-2 L/min). Secondly, the creation of systems for recovering and reusing anesthetics has the potential to reduce environmental impact and save costs.

3.4.4. Stability

The breakdown of anesthetics through metabolism or interaction with carbon dioxide absorbents (particularly when desiccated) can result in the production of multiple compounds that may be hazardous.

3.4.4.1. Metabolism and Degradation

The inorganic fluoride that is produced by methyloxyflurane was previously the cause of the occasional occurrence of nephrotoxicity, or high-output renal failure, following extended anesthesia. After extended exposure, Compound A (fluoromethyl-2,2-difluoro-1-[trifluoromethyl] vinyl ether), which is created when sevoflurane breaks down, and a related compound made from halothane are nephrotoxic to animals. Extended use of sevoflurane during anesthesia at low fresh gas flows (1 L/min) in humans causes compound A exposure sufficient to cause temporary proteinuria, enzymuria, and glycosuria; however, elevated serum creatinine concentrations and long-term detrimental effects on renal function are not observed. However, the sevoflurane package insert advises limiting low fresh gas flow (<2L/min) to fewer than two MAC hours (i.e., sevoflurane anesthesia (MAC concentration × administration time).

3.4.4.2. Carbon Dioxide Absorbents and Exothermic Reactions

The state (temperature and hydration) and chemical composition of the absorbent, fresh gas flow rates, minute ventilation, and—above all—the anesthetic itself are factors that affect how much volatile anesthetic degrades when exposed to carbon dioxide absorbents. All volatile anesthetics, regardless of temperature, degrade and produce carbon monoxide when conventional carbon dioxide absorbents containing sodium and potassium hydroxide are fully desiccated.

This is true even though desflurane and isoflurane remain highly stable in hydrated carbon dioxide absorbents up to temperatures of over 60° C. Elevated fresh gas flow rates, particularly those surpassing standard minute ventilation, hasten the desiccation process of the absorbent material, which in turn causes expedited degradation. The absorbent temperature may rise significantly due to the exothermic nature of degradation.

Absorbent canister temperatures can rise to extremely high levels due to the exothermic reaction between the volatile anesthetics (particularly sevoflurane) and desiccated carbon dioxide absorbent. An explosion and fire in the anesthetic circuit or canister could result from the temperature rise. By implementing strategies that guarantee the preservation of sufficient hydration in the carbon dioxide absorbent, the remote risk of fire and explosion from exothermic reactions can be completely eliminated. Regular absorbent changes, limiting fresh gas flow rates during anesthesia, adjusting fresh gas flow on unattended anesthesia machines, and replacing the absorbent when unsure of its hydration). Carbon dioxide absorbents that are sold commercially have reduced or no monovalent bases (i.e., potassium hydroxide and sodium hydroxide) do not significantly degrade when exposed to volatile anesthetics, even in cases where absorbent hydration is present. (Eger, 1963; Eger, 1974; Eger, 1985; Eger, 1993; Eger, 2000).

3.5. Relative Potency of Inhaled Anesthetics

The most common way to compare the relative potency of different inhaled anesthetics is to look at the amount needed to stop 50% of patients from moving after a surgical incision. The MAC is the dose (a single point on a dose-response curve). Ninety-five percent of patients should not move in response to incision at 1.2. MAC of the inhaled anesthetic, and 99 percent of patients should not move in response to incision at 1.3. MAC of the inhaled anesthetic due to the standard deviation in the MAC being roughly 10 percent. While MAC is impacted by some factors, gender, the length of the procedure, and anesthesia have no bearing on it.

MAC makes it possible to compare anesthetic potencies (see Table 3.2); in patients with comparable body temperatures and ages, 1.15 percent isoflurane and 6 percent desflurane are equally effective at preventing movement in response to a surgical incision. Surprisingly, the MAC values of various inhaled anesthetics add up. When it comes to stopping movement in response to an incision, for instance, 0.5. MAC of nitrous oxide given in conjunction with 0.5. MAC of isoflurane has the same effect as 1 MAC of any inhaled anesthetic (reflecting anesthetic-induced inhibition of reflex responses at the level of the spinal cord). It is likely that a greater anesthetic concentration at the brain is required to stop movement in response to a surgical incision than the MAC.

There is likely more variation in the anesthetic dose needed to cause amnesia than there is in the MAC. In 50% of the volunteers, the alveolar concentration of isoflurane that inhibited recall of a verbal stimulus was 0.20 MAC, while in 95% of the volunteers, it was 0.40 MAC. The minimum concentration that prevents recall has a standard deviation that is roughly half of the mean value, assuming a standard normal distribution of dose-response (0.1. MAC). By using standard normal curves, we can determine that, in order to prevent recall of verbal stimulus, 1 in 100,000 subjects with the highest anesthetic requirement would require a concentration of 4.27 standard deviations (SD) above the mean, or greater than 0.627 MAC. It is important to exercise caution when extrapolating this value to the surgical setting, as the dose needed to prevent recall of painful rather than verbal stimulation may be significantly higher. The ratio of concentration required to suppress consciousness and prevent recall versus that required to prevent motor response to surgical incision (as indicated by MAC) varies slightly between potent inhaled anesthetics individually and significantly between potent inhaled anesthetics combined versus nitrous oxide. When given 0.45 MAC of isoflurane, volunteers did not show recall; however, recall did occur when given as much as 0.6. MAC of nitrous oxide. (Eger, 1963; Eger, 1974; Eger, 1985; Eger, 1993; Eger, 2000).

3.6. Pharmacokinetics of Inhaled Anesthetics

The pharmacokinetics of inhaled anesthetics involve the processes of absorption, distribution, metabolism, and excretion, which collectively determine their onset, duration, and recovery from anesthesia. Upon inhalation, these agents are absorbed through the alveoli into the bloodstream, driven by the partial pressure gradient between the alveoli and blood. The speed of induction and recovery is influenced by the blood-gas partition coefficient; agents with lower coefficients, such as desflurane and sevoflurane, are less soluble in blood and equilibrate more rapidly, leading to quicker onset and emergence. Distribution throughout the body is rapid due to the high lipid solubility of these anesthetics, allowing them to cross cell membranes and reach the brain efficiently. Metabolism of inhaled anesthetics varies; for instance, sevoflurane undergoes more significant hepatic metabolism compared to desflurane and isoflurane, which are largely excreted unchanged. The excretion of these agents primarily occurs through the lungs, with the anesthetic being eliminated by exhalation. Factors such as cardiac output, alveolar ventilation, and the solubility of the anesthetic in tissues and blood play critical roles in their pharmacokinetics, influencing the overall effectiveness and safety profile during anesthesia administration.

An inhaled anesthetic can be delivered from the anesthetic machine to its site of action, the brain, by controlling the inspired partial pressure (Pi), which is the same as the concentration [%] when referring to the gas phase. A stable and ideal brain partial pressure (Pbr) of the anesthetic is the main goal of inhaled anesthesia. Every tissue, including the brain, adjusts to the partial pressure of the inhaled anesthetic that is carried to them by the arterial blood (Pa).

Likewise, the blood equilibrates with the alveolar partial pressure (Pa) of the anesthetic:

$$P_A \rightleftarrows Pa \rightleftarrows Pbr$$

Sustaining a steady and ideal Pa turns into a helpful, albeit indirect, way to manage the Pbr. Because the Pa of an inhaled anesthetic reflects its Pbr, it can be used as a measure of equal potency, an index of anesthetic depth, and a reflection of the rate of induction and recovery from anesthesia. The anesthesia provider can expertly control and modify the amount of inhaled anesthetic administered to the brain by knowing the factors that determine the Pa and the Pbr.

3.6.1. Factors That Determine the Alveolar Partial Pressure

Input (delivery) into the alveoli less absorption (loss) of the drug from the alveoli into the pulmonary arterial blood yields the Pa and, eventually, the Pbr of an inhaled anesthetic. The inhaled anesthetic's input is determined by the anesthetic breathing system's properties, alveolar ventilation ($\dot{V}_A$), and P_i. The solubility, cardiac output (CO), and alveolar-to-venous partial pressure difference ($P_A - P_v$) all affect how well the inhaled anesthetic is absorbed. The P_A is determined by the simultaneous action of these six factors. P_A is not substantially affected by percutaneous anesthetic loss or metabolism during the induction or maintenance of anesthesia.

3.6.1.1. Inspired Anesthetic Partial Pressure

When an inhaled anesthetic is first administered, a high Pi is required. As evidenced by the rate at which the Pa increases, this initial high Pi (i.e., input) accelerates the induction of anesthesia and counteracts the effect of uptake into the blood. The concentration effect is the name given to this Pi effect. Clinically, nitrous oxide is most likely the only gas that can produce the range of concentrations required to produce a concentration effect. Pi should be lowered over time to correspond with the declining anesthetic uptake as blood uptake declines. In order to maintain a consistent and ideal Pbr, the anesthesia provider must decrease the Pi in proportion to the time that the uptake decreases. For instance, the Pa and depth of anesthesia as indicated by the Pbr would gradually rise as the anesthetic's blood absorption decreased over time if the Pi were kept constant (input constant).

3.6.1.2. Second Gas Effect

A separate phenomenon that happens apart from the concentration effect is the second gas effect. The second gas effect is the capacity of large-volume uptake of one gas (first gas) to quicken the rate of increase of the Pa of a companion gas (second gas) administered concurrently. For instance, nitrous oxide's initial large volume uptake speeds up the uptake of companion gases like oxygen and volatile anesthetics. The early phase of nitrous oxide administration is accompanied by a brief (10%) increase in Pao_2, which is indicative of the second gas effect of nitrous oxide on oxygen. We refer to this rise in PaO2 as alveolar hyperoxygenation. The second gas effect can be explained by the increased tracheal inflow of all inhaled gases (i.e., first and second gases) and concentration of the second gases in a smaller lung volume (i.e., concentrating effect) due to the high-volume uptake of the first gas. Despite being founded on established pharmacokinetic principles, the clinical significance of the second gas effect is questionable (Figure 3.3).

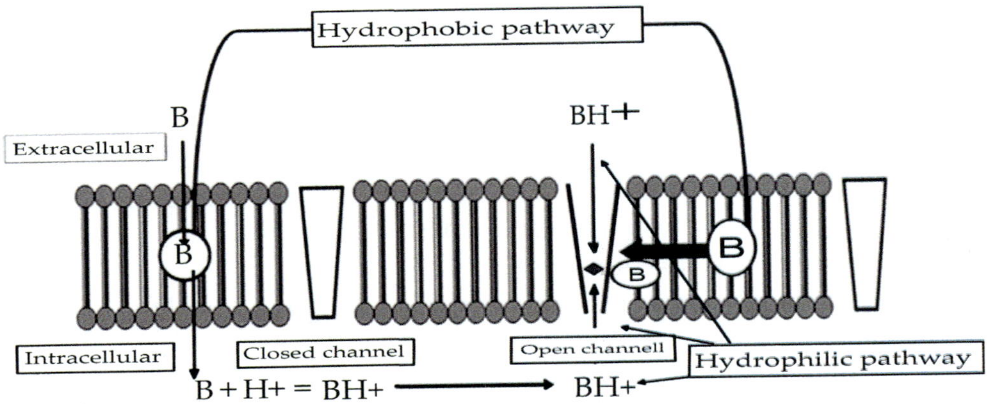

Figure 3.3. *Arrival pathways of LAs to the sodium channel. The hydrophobic pathway refers to the passage of LAs in their neutral (lipophilic) form that easily penetrate the cell membrane. Once in the cell membrane, the LA (B) expands it and by mechanical effect closes the sodium channel. This same neutral form of LA penetrates the cell, where it is protonized by incorporating an H+, (BH+ cationic form) that easily reaches the internal gate of the sodium channel and attaches to segment 6 of domains 3 and 4, activating the closure of the sodium channel. The hydrophilic pathway exemplified in the right portion of the scheme illustrates how a cationic LA (BH+) penetrates through and is fixed in the sodium channel.*

Source: M. Whizar-Lugo, V., L. Íñiguez-López, K., C. Cárdenas-Maytorena, A., & D. Ramírez-Puerta, C. (2020). Local Anesthetics. IntechOpen. doi: 10.5772/intechopen.93643.

3.6.1.3. Alveolar Ventilation

Similar to P_i, elevated $\dot{V}_A$ encourages the intake of inhaled anesthetics to counteract blood uptake. The overall result is a faster rate of anesthesia induction and Pa increase. Hypoventilation, as one might expect, has the opposite effect and slows the induction of anesthesia. The rate at which the P_A increases is accelerated by controlled lung ventilation that causes hyperventilation and reduced venous return because of increased input (i.e., elevated V_A) and reduced absorption (i.e., reduced CO). Because of this, there may be a greater chance of anesthetic overdose during controlled lung ventilation. Therefore, when switching from spontaneous to controlled lung ventilation, it may be appropriate to reduce the P_i of volatile anesthetics to maintain a P_A that is comparable to that of spontaneous ventilation. Reduced cerebral blood flow is another result of hyperventilation due to the corresponding decline in $Paco_2$. It is plausible that a reduction in the amount of anesthetic delivered to the brain would counteract the effect of an increased anesthetic input on the rate of increase of the P_A. Theoretically, coronary blood flow might stay constant, resulting in myocardial depression from increased anesthetic input and cerebral blood flow preventing the concurrent onset of central nervous system depression.

3.6.1.4. Anesthetic Breathing System

The anesthetic breathing system's volume, the solubility of the inhaled anesthetics in the rubber or plastic parts of the system, and the gas inflow from the anesthetic machine are characteristics that affect the rate at which the P_A increases. The anesthetic breathing system's volume functions as a buffer to delay the P_A attainment.

This buffer effect is eliminated by the anesthetic machine's high gas intake. The rate at which the P_A increases is initially slowed by the solubility of inhaled anesthetics in the parts of the anesthetic breathing system. Elution of the anesthetics occurs at the end of an anesthetic, which slows the rate at which the P_A decreases due to the reversal of the partial pressure gradient in the anesthetic breathing system.

3.6.1.5. Solubility

Partition coefficients indicate the solubility of inhaled anesthetics in blood and tissues. The distribution ratio that describes how the inhaled anesthetic splits into two phases at equilibrium—that is, when the partial pressures are equal—is called a partition coefficient. For instance, when the partial pressures of the inhaled anesthetic in these two phases are the same, a blood-gas partition coefficient of 10 indicates that the concentration of the anesthetic is 10 in the blood and 1 in the alveolar gas. Temperature affects partition coefficients. For instance, when a liquid's temperature drops, a gas's solubility in the liquid increases. Partition coefficients are given for 37° C unless otherwise indicated.

Blood-Gas Partition Coefficient

Due to its high blood solubility, an inhaled anesthetic must dissolve (i.e., be absorbed) in a significant amount of blood before reaching equilibrium with the gas phase. The solubility of the anesthetic in the blood determines the size of what can be thought of as a pharmacologically inactive reservoir—the blood.

Before the P_A equilibrates with the P_A, a significant amount of anesthetic must dissolve in the blood when the blood-gas partition coefficient is high. Clinically, raising the P_i can partially counteract the effect of high blood solubility on the rate at which the P_A increases. Low blood solubility means that the anesthetic must dissolve in the blood in very small amounts before equilibrium is reached, resulting in a fast rate of increase in the P_A as well as the P_A and Pbr.

Tissue-Blood Partition Coefficients

Tissue-blood partition coefficients determine the time necessary for equilibration of the tissue with the P_A (Figure 3.4).

By computing a time constant for each tissue—that is, the ratio of the amount of inhaled anesthetic that can dissolve in the tissue to the tissue blood flow—it is possible to predict this time. For a volatile anesthetic like isoflurane, the brain-blood partition coefficients translate into time constants of roughly three to four minutes. Any tissue, including the brain, needs at least three-time constants to fully equilibrate with the PA. This is the reasoning behind keeping this volatile anesthetic's P_A constant for ten to fifteen minutes and then presuming that the Pbr is comparable. Less soluble anesthetics like desflurane, sevoflurane, and nitrous oxide have time constants of roughly two minutes, and full equilibration takes about six minutes (i.e., three-time constants).

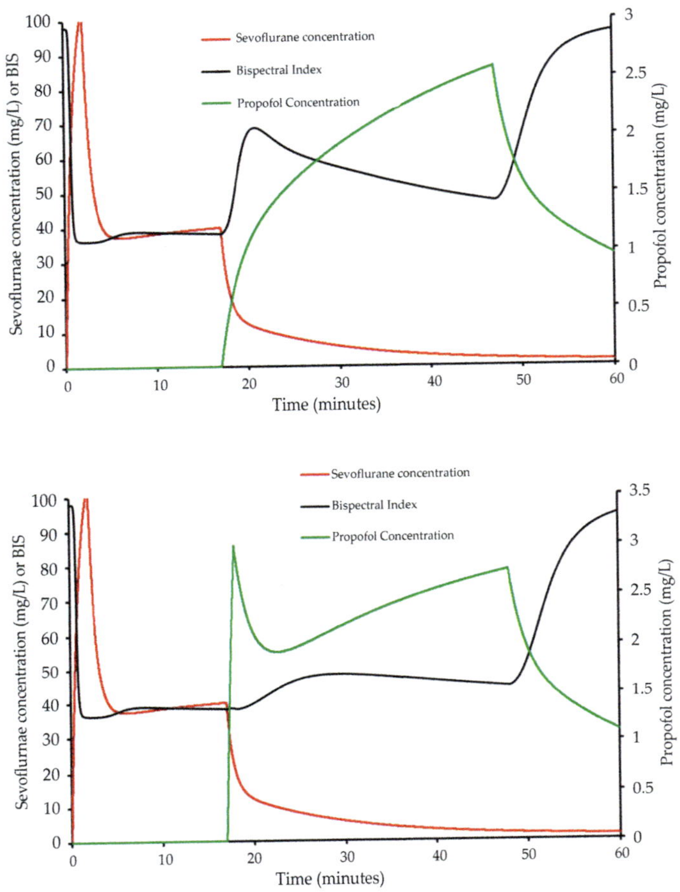

Figure 3.4. *Inhalational induction with 8% sevoflurane was followed after 2 min with 2% inhaled sevoflurane to maintain a bispectral index of 40. Cessation of sevoflurane caused a rapid increase in the bispectral index if only a propofol infusion of 10 mg/h/kg was administered (upper panel). That BIS was maintained at an acceptable score (40–60) if a modest dose of propofol 1 mg/kg was given before propofol infusion.*

Source: *Morse JD, Cortinez LI, Anderson BJ. Pharmacokinetic Pharmacodynamic Modelling Contributions to Improve Paediatric Anaesthesia Practice. Journal of Clinical Medicine. 2022; 11(11):3009. https://doi.org/10.3390/jcm11113009.*

Anesthetic Transfer by Intertissue Diffusion

There is mounting evidence that suggests some anesthetic uptake might happen directly from tissues with lower to higher anesthetic affinity, rather than through blood flow to different tissues (i.e., from adipose to lean tissues), such as the junction of omental fat and viscera (refer to "Context-Sensitive Half-Time"). Sevoflurane and isoflurane are absorbed more readily by larger individuals and animals with presumably larger lean-fat surface area interfaces. Since the bulk fat compartment receives relatively little blood flow and is relatively large, it is unlikely that transfer to bulk fat by blood flow during an anesthetic of a duration of less than 12 to 24 hours will explain these differences.

Nitrous Oxide and Methionine Synthase Inactivation

Among anesthetics, nitrous oxide is distinct because it inhibits the enzyme methionine synthase, which controls the metabolism of folate and vitamin B12. While many patients may not experience any noticeable effects from the enzyme inactivation, those who already have a vitamin B12 deficiency or an underlying critical illness may experience neurologic or hematologic consequences. When homocysteine levels in the blood are elevated, it is linked to a higher risk of adverse coronary events because it needs functional methionine synthase to convert to methionine. When compared to patients who did not receive nitrous oxide during a carotid endarterectomy, those who did have significantly higher homocysteine levels and a higher frequency of myocardial ischemia episodes.

Nitrous Oxide Transfer to Closed Gas Spaces

Nitrous oxide has a blood-gas partition coefficient (0.46) that is 34 times higher than that of nitrogen (0.014). Since nitrogen cannot exit an air-filled cavity and enter the blood 34 times faster than nitrous oxide can, this indicates a differential solubility.

The volume or pressure of the air-filled cavity rises as a result of this preferential transfer of nitrous oxide. The gas space expands when nitrous oxide enters an air-filled cavity with a compliant wall (such as intestinal gas, pneumothorax, pulmonary blebs, or air embolism). On the other hand, pressure rises when nitrous oxide enters an air-filled space with a noncompliant wall (such as the middle ear, cerebral ventricles, or supratentorial subdural space). The P_A of nitrous oxide, blood flow to the air-filled cavity, and length of nitrous oxide administration all affect how much the volume or pressure increases in the air-filled cavity. A seventy-five percent nitrous oxide inhalation doubles the volume of a pneumothorax in ten minutes in an animal model. Nitrous oxide administration is contraindicated in the event of a closed pneumothorax.

If a patient has a history of chest trauma, such as rib fractures, decreasing pulmonary compliance during nitrous oxide administration may indicate nitrous oxide-induced expansion of an undetected pneumothorax. Similar to this, nitrous oxide causes the air bubbles linked to venous air embolism to rapidly expand. A venous air embolism or pneumothorax expands quickly, whereas nitrous oxide causes a slow increase in the volume of intestinal gas. If the procedure is brief, it doesn't really matter if patients receiving intra-abdominal surgery are given nitrous oxide. Nonetheless, it might be wise to advise against nitrous oxide inhalation at concentrations higher than 50% before surgery if bowel gas volume is elevated (for example, due to bowel obstruction). Even during lengthy procedures, the bowel gas volume would, at most, double if this recommendation were followed.

3.6.1.6. Cardiac Output

The CO removes some anesthetic from the alveoli, influencing uptake into the pulmonary arterial blood and, consequently, P_A. High CO levels, such as those brought on by anxiety, cause more rapid uptake, which slows down the rate at which the P_A increases and the induction of anesthesia. A low CO (such as shock) accelerates the rate at which the P_A rises because the blood absorbs less oxygen to counteract the input. It's a common clinical perception that patients in shock can be quickly put into anesthesia.

Shunt

An intracardiac or intrapulmonary shunt placed from right to left slows the induction of anesthesia. This slowing is a result of the dilutional effect of blood that has been shunted and does not contain anesthetic on the anesthetic partial pressure of blood that is being drawn from ventilated alveoli. The decrease in Pao_2 in the presence of a right-to-left shunt is caused by a similar mechanism. A left-to-right shunt causes the delivery of venous blood to the lungs with a higher partial pressure of anesthetic than that of venous blood that has passed through the tissues (e.g., arteriovenous fistula, volatile anesthetic-induced increases in cutaneous blood flow). Consequently, the dilutional effect of a right-to-left shunt on the P_A is counteracted by a left-to-right tissue shunt. Only when a right-to-left shunt is concurrently present can the impact of a left-to-right shunt on the rate of increase in the P_A be observed. Similarly, in the absence of a left-to-right shunt, the dilutional effect of a right-to-left shunt is greatest. Taking everything into account, it doesn't seem likely that a right-to-left shunt would have a clinically noticeable effect (Table 3.3).

Table 3.3. *Physical and Chemical Characteristics and Relative Potency of some Local Anesthetics**

	Physico-Chemical Characteristics				Relative Potency in Different Blocks		
Anesthetic	pKa	Ionized % at pH 7.4	Partition Coefficient	% Protein Binding	Epidural	Spinal	Peripheral Nerve
· Bupivacaine	8.1	83	3420	95	4	9.6	3.6
· Levobupivacaine	8.1	83	3420	97	4	9.6	3.6
· Etidocaine	7.7	66	7317	94	2	6.7	0.7
· Lidocaine	7.9	76	366	64	1	1	1
· Mepivacaine	7.6	61	130	77	1	1	2.6
· Prilocaine	7.9	76	129	55	1	¿	0.8
· Ropivacaine	8.1	83	775	94	4	4.8	3.6
· Chloroprocaine	8.7	95	810	—	0.5	—	—
· Procaine	8.9	97	100	6	—	—	—
· Tetracaine	8.5	93	5822	94	—	—	—

Source: M. Whizar-Lugo, V., L. Íñiguez-López, K., C. Cárdenas-Maytorena, A., & D. Ramírez-Puerta, C. (2020). Local Anesthetics. IntechOpen. doi: 10.5772/intechopen.93643.

Wasted Ventilation

Since there is no dilutional effect on the P_A, ventilation of nonperfused alveoli has no effect on the rate of induction of anesthesia. The creation of a difference between the P_A and P_A of the inhaled anesthetic is the main result of wasted ventilation. A comparable process accounts for the frequently noted distinction between end-tidal Pco_2 and $Paco_2$.

Alveolar-to-Venous Partial Pressure Differences

The tissue uptake of inhaled anesthetics is reflected by the P_A-P_v. Less than 10% of body mass is made up of highly perfused tissues, such as the brain, heart, kidneys, and liver, yet these tissues receive approximately 75% of CO. These heavily perfused tissues thus quickly acclimate to the P_A. A narrow $P_A - P_v$, or roughly 75% of the returning venous blood, is at the same partial pressure as the P_A after three-time constants (6 to 12 minutes for inhaled anesthetics). Thus, after 6 to 12 minutes, there is a significant decrease in the uptake of volatile anesthetics from the alveoli, as indicated by a narrowing of the $P_i - P_A$ difference. In order to maintain a constant P_A in the face of decreased uptake, the inhaled concentrations of volatile anesthetics should be reduced after this point. Skeletal muscle and fat represent about 70% of the body mass but receive less than 25% of the CO (Figure 3.5).

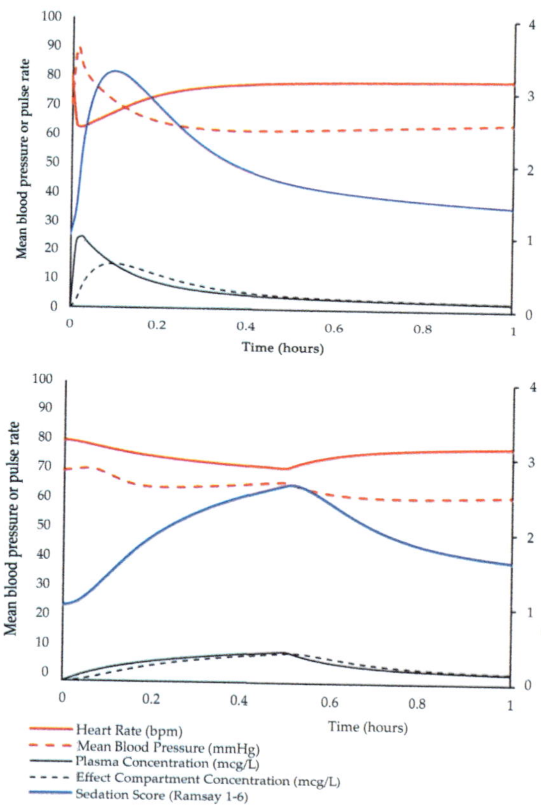

Figure 3.5. *A simulation of dexmedetomidine demonstrating plasma concentration and haemodynamic effects when given intravenously to a 5-year-old child. The upper panel shows effects when the drug was given as a rapid intravenous bolus of 0.49 µg/kg. The lower panel shows concentration and haemodynamic changes after a larger dose of 0.57 µg/kg was administered as an infusion over 15 min. A similar level of sedation is achieved at 15 min, but slow infusion does not have the same magnitude of blood pressure and heart rate changes observed with rapid infusion.*

Source: Morse JD, Cortinez LI, Anderson BJ. Pharmacokinetic Pharmacodynamic Modelling Contributions to Improve Paediatric Anaesthesia Practice. Journal of Clinical Medicine. 2022; 11(11):3009. https://doi.org/10.3390/jcm11113009.

These tissues continue to act as inactive reservoirs for anesthetic uptake for several hours. Equilibration of fat with inhaled anesthetics in the arterial blood is probably never achieved.

3.6.2. Recovery from Anesthesia

The rate at which the P_A falls over time is known as the recovery rate from anesthesia. Recovery is similar to induction of anesthesia in many ways. For instance, the rate at which the P_A falls is determined by V''_A, solubility, and CO.

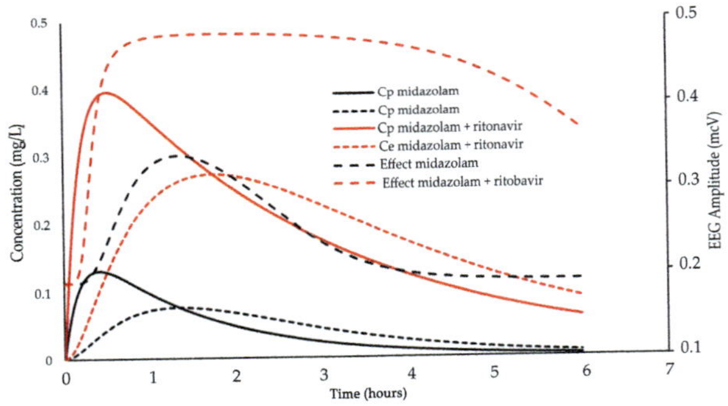

Figure 3.6. *A child was given midazolam 0.5 mg/kg orally. The effect compartment concentration (Ce) is linked to plasma concentration by a rate constant (keo). The simulation shows the impact of increased bioavailability (2.7-fold) and slower clearance (assumed 50% reduction). Electroencephalographic amplitudes in the 11.5 to 30 Hz (beta) frequency band were used as an effective measure. Not only is the electroencephalographic effect prolonged due to slower clearance, but a ceiling effect is also achieved because of higher concentrations.*

Source: Morse JD, Cortinez LI, Anderson BJ. Pharmacokinetic Pharmacodynamic Modelling Contributions to Improve Paediatric Anaesthesia Practice. Journal of Clinical Medicine. 2022; 11(11):3009. https://doi.org/10.3390/jcm11113009.

The lungs are ventilated in order to eliminate the anesthetic after it has been stopped being administered. Anesthetic is subsequently moved from the tissues—including the brain—into the alveoli as the alveolar partial pressure drops. The anesthetic will be transferred back into the tissues, including the brain, if hypoventilation or the use of fresh gas flows low enough to allow rebreathing to occur. This will delay the patient's recovery (Figure 3.6).

3.6.2.1. How does Recovery Differ from Induction of Anesthesia?

Anesthesia recovery is not the same as induction of anesthesia in that there is no concentration effect on recovery (the P_i cannot be less than zero), anesthetic tissue concentrations vary at the beginning of recovery, and metabolism may play a role in the rate at which the P_A decreases.

Tissue Concentrations

When the partial pressure gradient is reversed at the end of anesthesia by bringing the P_i down to zero or close to it, the tissue concentrations of the inhaled anesthetics act as a reservoir to keep the P_A constant. The length of anesthesia and the anesthetics' solubility in different tissue compartments determine how tissue storage affects a patient. For example, with soluble anesthetics (like isoflurane), the amount of time it takes to recover is directly proportional to the length of anesthesia; however, with poorly soluble anesthetics (like sevoflurane and desflurane), the effect of the length of administration on recovery time is negligible. When anesthesia is induced, all tissues have the same zero concentration of anesthetic at the beginning; this is in contrast to the varying concentrations of anesthetics in different tissues at the end of anesthesia.

Metabolism

The possible influence of metabolism on the rate of decrease in P_A at the end of anesthesia is a significant distinction between induction of anesthesia and recovery from anesthesia. In this sense, the rate at which the highly lipid-soluble methoxyflurane's P_A decreases is primarily determined by metabolism. While V_A is primarily responsible for the rate of decrease in the P_A of less lipid-soluble isoflurane, desflurane, and sevoflurane, metabolism also plays a significant role in the rate of decrease in the P_A of halothane.

Context-Sensitive Half-Time

The duration of administration (the "context") and the inhaled anesthetic's solubility in blood and tissues determine the pharmacokinetics of the drug's elimination from the body. Similar to intravenous anesthetics, context-sensitive decrement times (i.e., the amount of time needed for anesthetic concentrations in the central nervous system to drop to a fraction of what they were before) can be found for volatile anesthetics using computer simulations. Every tissue compartment in the body is required for the kinetic modeling to function (i.e., blood, muscle, fat, vessel-rich group), the proportionate blood flow that each compartment receives, the relative sizes of each compartment, and the solubility of each individual anesthetic in the tissue that makes up each compartment. Equilibration refers to the anesthetic's continuous absorption during administration until the tissue concentration approaches the alveolar concentration. The balance of anesthetic concentration between the alveoli and a small compartment with high blood flow (less than 10% of body mass) (i.e., kidneys, brain, and heart) transpire in a comparatively brief amount of time (10 to 15 minutes). On the other hand, anesthesia equilibration in bigger chambers with lower relative blood flow (i.e., bulk fat, and skeletal muscle) happens over a longer time frame (hours), as the anesthetic absorbs. Less than five minutes are required for a fifty percent drop in the anesthetic concentrations of isoflurane, desflurane, and sevoflurane, and this time does not increase noticeably as anesthesia is prolonged. This is presumably a reflection of the first stage of elimination, which is mostly determined by $\dot{V}A$. Larger differences between different inhaled anesthetics are revealed by determining other decrement times (≥80%), particularly as the duration of the anesthetic increases. Because simulation does not take into account the anesthetic that is transferred from lean to fatty tissues by intertissue diffusion, it may underestimate the uptake of anesthesia, particularly with more soluble anesthetics. Before a patient regains coordinated protective functions, such as the ability to breathe and swallow, all anesthetics must be completely removed, with the exception of very small dosages (less than what is required for patients to obey orders). Patients undergoing surgery who were given a longer duration of anesthesia and a more soluble anesthetic (sevoflurane as opposed to desflurane) needed more time to recover their ability to swallow. When given small doses of sevoflurane and isoflurane while awake, awake subjects show decreased chemical ventilatory drive and pharyngeal dyscoordination (Figure 3.7).

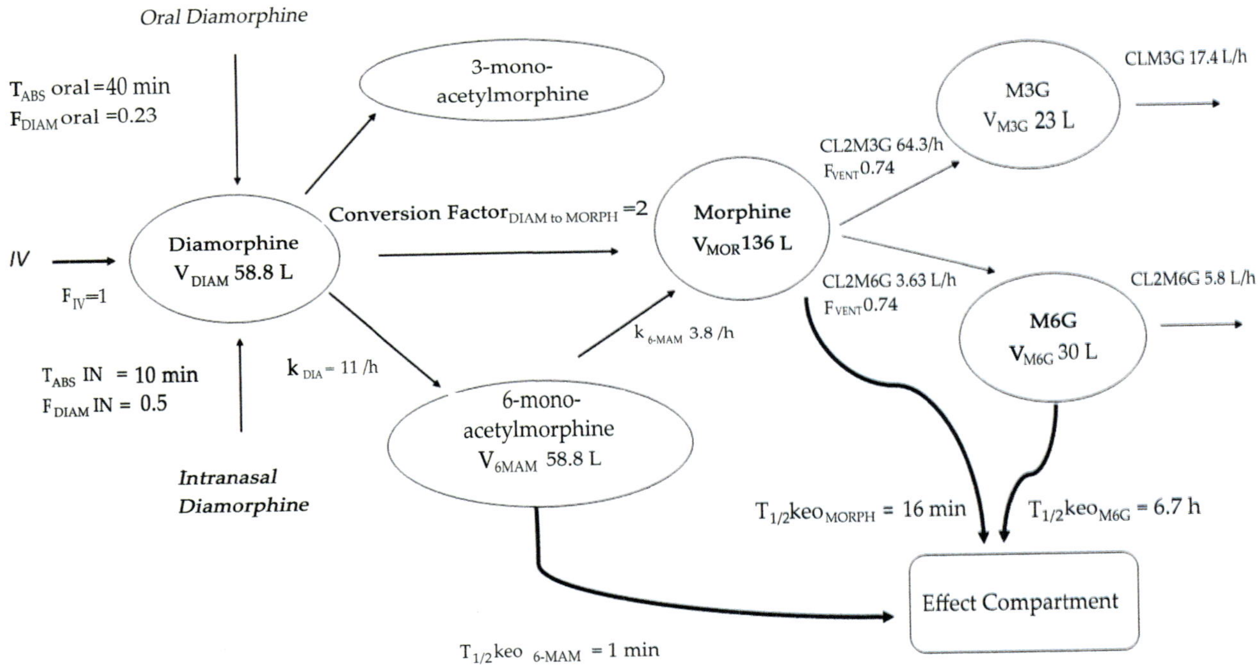

Figure 3.7. *The diagram shows the metabolite flow of diacetylmorphine, 6-mono-acetylmorphine, morphine and morphine glucuronide metabolites. Diamorphine absorption is described in terms of absorption half-times (TABS) and relative bioavailability (FDIAM) by oral or intranasal (IN) routes. Rate constants (kDIA, k6-MAM)) describe the flow between metabolites. Clearance of morphine 3-glucuronide (M3G) and morphine 6-glucuronide (M6G) are driven by renal function. The delay between active metabolites (6-MAM, morphine, M6G) and the effect compartment is described using equilibration half-times (T1/2keo).*

Source: Morse JD, Cortinez LI, Anderson BJ. Pharmacokinetic Pharmacodynamic Modelling Contributions to Improve Paediatric Anaesthesia Practice. Journal of Clinical Medicine. 2022; 11(11):3009. https://doi.org/10.3390/jcm11113009.

3.6.2.2. Diffusion Hypoxia

After nitrous oxide is administered, patients may experience diffusion hypoxia if they are permitted to breathe room air. When the gas is no longer inhaled, a high-volume initial leakage of nitrous oxide from the blood into the alveoli can cause the Pao_2 to fall. When the patient's lungs are fully supplied with oxygen after receiving nitrous oxide, diffusion hypoxia is avoided.

3.6.3. Feasibility of Inhaled Anesthetic Use for Sedation in ICU

The AnaConDa (Anaesthetic Conserving Device, Sedana Medical AB, Uppsala, Sweden) is a device that helps the intensive care unit (ICU) administer inhaled anesthesia (isoflurane, sevoflurane). Syringe pumps are used to inject liquid anesthetic into a chamber that is attached to the breathing circuit between the Y-piece and the endotracheal tube. A porous plastic rod inside the chamber receives a very slow delivery of liquid anesthetic from the syringe. There, the liquid evaporates and combines with newly drawn gas from the circuit's inspiratory limb. A charcoal filter that absorbs and retains about 90% of the exhaled anesthetic is used to filter out exhaled gas. The absorbed anesthetic mixes with the fresh gas in the charcoal filter as the inspiratory flow is subsequently directed through it. Strong inhaled anesthetics are being used outside of the operating room for postsurgical patients in the intensive care unit (ICU), and there is mounting evidence to support this use being both possible and potentially beneficial. The anesthetic delivery device's placement between the tracheal tube and circuit causes increased dead space and work of breathing, which poses challenges to the use of inhaled anesthesia in the ICU. Another issue is the loss of anesthetic to the environment during frequent tracheal tube suctioning, and there is uncertainty about the availability of the right equipment and caregivers with the necessary technical expertise.

3.7. Effects on Organ Systems

3.7.1. Circulatory Effects

Similar circulatory effects are produced by inhaled anesthetics at equipotent concentrations, particularly in human volunteers when the anesthesia is being maintained. On the other hand, surgical patients might react differently than volunteers in good health. For instance, variables like age extremes, coexisting diseases, non-optimal intravascular volume status, surgical stimulation, and concurrent medication use may change, reduce, or magnify the responses predicted by data collected from healthy volunteers.

3.7.1.1. Responses during Maintenance of Anesthesia

Mean Arterial Pressure

In a dose-dependent manner, mean arterial pressure (MAP) falls with increasing concentrations of enflurane, desflurane, sevoflurane, isoflurane, and halothane. The decrease in MAP, except for halothane, is mainly due to a decrease in systemic vascular resistance (SVR) as opposed to a decrease in CO. Halothane, on the other hand, reduces MAP partially or completely by lowering CO, while SVR remains mostly unaltered. Measurements of SVR in patients undergoing cardiopulmonary bypass perfusion and receiving desflurane, sevoflurane, and isoflurane corroborate these findings. Part of the volatile drug is replaced with nitrous oxide to reduce the dose-related decrease in SVR. Unlike the other inhaled anesthetics, nitrous oxide either causes a mild increase in MAP or leaves it unchanged.

Heart Rate

Patients' and volunteers' heart rates rise in response to stepwise increases in the administered concentrations of isoflurane, desflurane, and sevoflurane, albeit at varying rates (Table 3.4).

Isoflurane raises heart rate in a linear, dose-dependent manner at as low as 0.25 MAC. When desflurane concentrations are less than 1 MAC, there is a slight increase in heart rate. The heart rate increases in a dose-dependent, linear fashion above 1 MAC for desflurane concentrations. Heart rate does not rise in the presence of sevoflurane until the concentration surpasses 1.5 milliampere-ciclopane (MAC), in contrast to desflurane and isoflurane. However, tachycardia is brought on by 8 percent sevoflurane induction, also known as single-breath induction, in patients undergoing controlled hyperventilation, including adults. This tachycardia could be brought on by stimulation of the sympathetic nervous system linked to epileptiform brain activity.

Table 3.4. *The Impact of Anesthetic Drugs on Inflammatory Expression and Cellular Pathways Activity*

Author	Anesthetic Drug	Study Type	Comments
Gyires et al.	Morphine	in vivo	↓ edema; ↓ bradykinin activity; no influence on edema induced by histamine;
Sacerdote et al.	Morphine	in vivo	↓ inflammatory response; ↑ activation of mu-opioid receptors;
Planas et al.	Liposomal morphine	in vivo	↓ inflammatory edema; ↑duration of effects by encapsulation;
Joris et al.	Morphine	in vivo	↓ vascular inflammation; ↓ vascular permeability;
Honore et al.	Morphine	in vivo	↓ edema; ↓ Fos-like immunoreactive activity;
Jin et al.	Endomorphin-1 (Endogenous ligand for mu opioid receptor)	in vivo	↓ peripheral edema; ↓ activity of Fos-like immunoreactive expression;
Fletcher et al.	Morphine	in vivo	↓ inflammation; ↓ edema;
Walker et al.	Kappa-opioid drugs	in vivo	↓ adhesion molecules; ↓ TNF expression; ↓ expression of inflammation cascade;
Hu et al.	Sufentanil	in vivo	↑ super oxide dismutase (SOD) activity; ↑ catalase (CAT) activity; ↑ glutathione peroxidase (GSH-Px) activity; ↓ malondialdehyde (MDA) expression; ↓ Nuclear factor erythroid 2—related factor 2 (Nrf2) expression; ↓ inflammation and oxidative stress;
Rahimi et al.	Morphine	in vivo	↓ neuroinflammation via opioid receptors; ↑ neurobehavioral function after traumatic brain injury; ↓ blood brain barrier (BBB) leakage;

Author	Anesthetic Drug	Study Type	Comments
Zhou et al.	Sufentanil	in vivo	↓ Activating transcription factor 4 (AFT4) expression; ↓ liver inflammation; ↓ apoptosis injury induced by ischemia–reperfusion injury;
Hofbauer et al.	Remifentanil	in vitro	↓ endothelial cell adhesion molecule; ↓ polymorphonuclear neutrophils migration;
Lei et al.	Remifentanil	in vitro	↑ cardiomyocytes protection against oxidative stress; ↓ PKCβ expression; ↓ autophagy activity;
Zhao et al.	Remifentanil	in vivo	↓ NF-kB expression; ↓ TNF-α expression; ↓ IAM-1 expression; ↑ protective effect against ischemia–reperfusion injury syndrome;
Hyejin et al.	Remifentanil	in vitro	↓ human neutrophils activations induced by lipopolysaccharide (LPS); ↑ anti-inflammatory effects;
Maeda et al.	Remifentanil	in vivo	↓ IL-6 expression in mouse brain; ↓ inflammation in cerebral tissue;
Hasegawa et al.	Remifentanil	in vivo	↓ inflammation expression caused by surgical stress;
Lu et al.	Ketamine	in vitro	↓ NMDA receptors activity; ↓ calmodulin-dependent protein kinase 2 (CAMK2) activity; ↓ NF-kB phosphorylation and nuclear translocation; ↑ protective against inflammation induced by LPS;
Wu et al.	Propofol	in vitro	↑ NMDA expression; ↑ Ca^{2+} accumulation; ↓ NF-kB phosphorylation; ↓ LPS- induced pro-inflammatory cytokine;

Author	Anesthetic Drug	Study Type	Comments
Inada et al.	Propofol	in vitro	↓ production of TNF-α and IL-6; ↓ production of neutrophil chemokines; ↑ anti-inflammatory effects;
Zhao et al.	Propofol	in vitro	↓ activity of NLR family pyrin domain containing 3 (NLRP3); ↓ inflammation and apoptosis mechanisms;
Plachinta et al.	Isoflurane	in vivo	↓ TNF-α activity; ↓ acidosis; ↓ damage to the vascular endothelium associated with LPS-induced inflammation; ↑ vascular protection during inflammation;
Wang et al.	Isoflurane	in vitro	↑ microRNA-9-3p expression; ↓ activity of fibronectin type III domain containing 3B (FNDC3B); ↑ protection against hepatic ischemia–reperfusion injury;
Lu et al.	Isoflurane	in vivo	↓ caspase-11, IL-1β and IL-18 expression; ↓ intracellular Ca^{2+} accumulation; ↑ protection against inflammation-induced by liver ischemia/ reperfusion injury;
Zhang et al.	Isoflurane	in vitro	↓ heme-oxygenase-1 (HO1) activity; ↓ redox, inflammation and apoptosis expression in sepsis- induced brain damage;
Lv et al.	Sevoflurane	in vivo	↑ neuro-inflammation and apoptosis by activation of cholinergic anti-inflammatory pathway;

Author	Anesthetic Drug	Study Type	Comments
Ngamsri et al.	Sevoflurane	in vivo	↓ neutrophil expression in peritoneal lavage; ↑ protection against peritonitis- induced sepsis in rats; ↑ expression of hypoxia- inducible factor 1α and adenosine A2B receptor in liver, intestine and lung;
Wang et al.	Sevoflurane	in vivo	↓ allergic airway inflammation; ↓ Th2 expression and NLRP3 activity;
Shen et al.	Sevoflurane	in vivo	↓ acute lung inflammation in ovalbumin-induced allergic mices; ↑ protection against airway remodeling in mouse; ↓ VEGF and TGF-β1 activity in lung tissues;
Wang et al.	Sevoflurane	in vivo	↑ inflammation of microglia in hippocampus of neonatal rats; ↓ activity of WNT/β-catenin/CaMKIV pathway;

Source: Ritiu SA, Rogobete AF, Sandesc D, Bedreag OH, Papurica M, Popovici SE, Toma D, Ivascu RI, Velovan R, Garofil DN, et al., The Impact of General Anesthesia on Redox Stability and Epigenetic Inflammation Pathways: Crosstalk on Perioperative Antioxidant Therapy. Cells. 2022; 11(12):1880. https://doi.org/10.3390/cells11121880.

The propensity of desflurane to increase blood flow (i.e., MAP and heart rate) is reduced by giving an opioid (fentanyl), β-adrenergic blocker (esmolol), and extending the duration of anesthesia (10 to 15 minutes). The addition of nitrous oxide to partially replace the desflurane does not lessen the dose-related increase in heart rate observed at desflurane concentrations greater than 1 MAC. Similar to halothane, isoflurane, sevoflurane, and desflurane reduce baroreceptor responses in a concentration-dependent way. Rather than a reflex baroreceptor activity response to decreased MAP, desflurane causes a brief increase in heart rate above 1 MAC. This increase is caused by sympathetic nervous system stimulation (Figure 3.8).

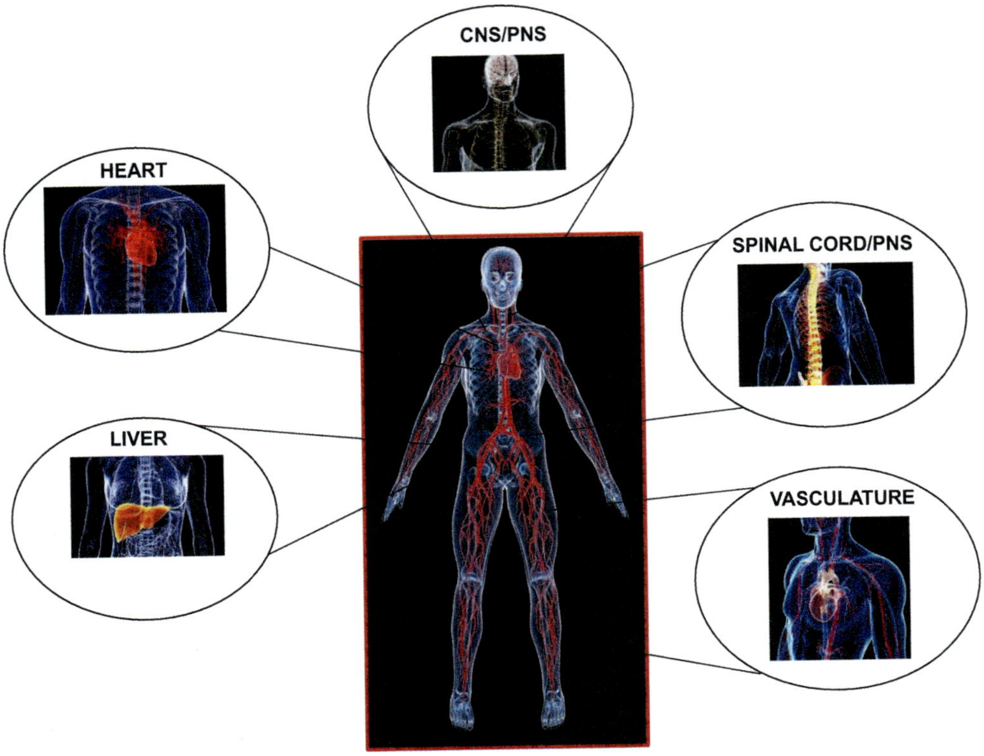

Figure 3.8. *The effects of anesthetics.*

Source: Constantinides C and Murphy K (2016) Molecular and Integrative Physiological Effects of Isoflurane Anesthesia: The Paradigm of Cardiovascular Studies in Rodents using Magnetic Resonance Imaging. Front. Cardiovasc. Med. 3:23. doi: 10.3389/fcvm.2016.00023.

Cardiac Index

In healthy young adults, desflurane, sevoflurane, or isoflurane administered at a variety of concentrations has little effect on the cardiac index. Desflurane causes slight increases in the left ventricular circumferential shortening velocity and ejection fraction when compared to awake measurements, according to transesophageal echocardiography data.

Circulatory Effects with Rapid Concentration Increase

Desflurane does not raise heart rate or mean arterial pressure at concentrations below 1 MAC. When opioids, adrenergic blockers, or other analgesic adjuncts are not present, sudden increases in inspired desflurane concentrations above 1 MAC result in brief circulatory stimulation. Similar effects on an elevated heart rate and blood pressure can also be somewhat elicited by isoflurane. Increases in plasma norepinephrine and adrenaline concentrations as well as sympathetic nervous system activity accompany the hemodynamic stimulation observed with abruptly increased desflurane and isoflurane concentrations. A rapid drop in heart rate is linked to an inspired sevoflurane concentration increase from 1 MAC to 1.5. MAC (Table 3.5).

Table 3.5. *Published Trials of General Anesthetic Agents for Cranial Procedures.*

Authors and Year	Surgical Procedure	Comparison	Findings
Aken et al., 1990 [35]	Unspecified cranial procedure	Balanced anesthesia (loading thiopental and fentanyl + maintenance fentanyl, droperidol, thiopental, and isoflurane in nitrous oxide, $n = 20$) vs. TIVA (loading propofol + alfentanil infusion, n = 20)	During induction, TIVA had a significantly greater hemodynamic stability. Balance anesthesia was associated with a significantly longer emergence time than TIVA.
Hemelrijck et al., 1991 [30]	Craniotomy for resection of brain tumor	Propofol ($n = 20$) vs. thiopental ($n = 20$)	Postoperative return to orientation time was shorter in the propofol group (7 +/− 5 min vs. 27 +/− 23 min).
Ornstein et al., 1993 [36]	Craniotomy for resection of supratentorial lesion	Anesthetic maintenance via desflurane ($n = 12$) vs. isoflurane (n = 12)	CBF values were non-significantly different as measured at 1 MAC and 1.5. MAC concentrations for both desflurane and isoflurane ($p > 0.05$), as well as at 1.25 MAC as measured in $n = 15$ patients (p > 0.05).
Talke et al., 1996 [37]	Hypophysectomy	Propofol ($n = 10$) vs. loading propofol + maintenance desflurane ($n = 10$) vs. loading propofol + maintenance isoflurane (n = 10)	Minimum CPP was significantly lower in desflurane ($p < 0.05$) and isoflurane ($p < 0.05$) groups compared to propofol-only control. Minimum SBP was significantly lower in desflurane ($p < 0.05$) and isoflurane (p < 0.05) compared to propofol-only control.
Artru et al., 1997 [38]	Unspecified cranial procedure	Anesthetic maintenance via sevoflurane ($n = 8$) and isoflurane (n = 6) following induction via mannitol	Neither sevoflurane or isoflurane significantly altered ICP, and both decreased middle cerebral artery flow velocity (Vmca). Notably, decreased Vmca with sevoflurane was related to decreased CPP at 0.5. MAC ($p < 0.05$), and increased CVRe at 1.0 and 1.5. MAC ($p < 0.05$). The CPP decreased from baseline at 0.5, 1.0, and 1.5. MACs of isoflurane (p < 0.05).

Authors and Year	Surgical Procedure	Comparison	Findings
Hoffman et al., 1998 [39]	Craniotomy for unspecified pathology	Thiopental induction (*n* = 10) vs. desflurane (n = 10)	Neither thiopental nor desflurane changed tissue gases or pH, but desflurane increased PO_2 70% ($p < 0.05$), whereas thiopental decreased PO_2 30% during temporary brain artery occlusion.
Talke et al., 1999 [40]	Transsphenoidal Hypophysectomy	Anesthetic maintenance via propofol (*n* = 10) vs. sevoflurane (*n* = 20)	Sevoflurane increased lumbar CSF pressure and decreased CPP and systolic blood pressure following infusion while propofol did not affect lumbar CSF pressure, CPP, nor systolic blood pressure.
Talke et al., 2002 [33]	Craniotomy for resection of supratentorial lesion	Propofol (*n* = 20) vs. isoflurane (n = 20)	Emergence time to eyes opening was not different between anesthetic agents ($p > 0.05$). There was no difference in occurrence of hypertension ($p > 0.05$).
Iwata et al., 2003 [41]	Unspecified intracranial surgery	Propofol (*n* = 13) vs. sevoflurane (*n* = 13)	There was no difference in the rate of temperature decrease and recovery in induced hypothermia ($p < 0.05$).
Fraga et al., 2003 [42]	Craniotomy for resection of supratentorial lesion	Inhalation of isoflurane (*n* = 30) vs. desflurane (n = 30) following induction via fentanyl, thiopental, and vecuronium maintained with 60% nitrous oxide in oxygen	There were no significant differences between MAP, ICP, and CPP between use of desflurane and isoflurane, but notable decreases ($p < 0.05$) in both groups from baseline values with regard to MAP and CPP. The ratio between the cerebral metabolic oxygen requirement and cerebral blood flow decreased significantly for both groups as well.
Petersen et al., 2003 [31]	Craniotomy for resection of supratentorial tumor	Propofol (*n* = 41) vs. isoflurane (*n* = 38) vs. sevoflurane (n = 38)	No differences in ICP or CPP between anesthetic agents ($p > 0.05$).
Günes et al., 2005 [43]	Unspecified intracranial procedure	Anesthetic maintenance via propofol (*n* = 39) vs. dexmedetomidine (*n* = 39)	Systolic blood pressure and MAP were not different between the two agents. Extubation time was shorter for propofol ($p < 0.05$). Analgesic requirements were higher for propofol ($p = 0.013$).

Authors and Year	Surgical Procedure	Comparison	Findings
Magni et al., 2005 [32]	Supratentorial craniotomy for unspecified pathology	Propofol (n = 64) vs. sevoflurane (n = 64)	Emergence time was not different between anesthetic agents. Occurrence of hypertension was higher in propofol than sevoflurane use (p = 0.0046), and hypotension was higher in propofol than sevoflurane (p = 0.02).
Sekimoto et al., 2006 [44]	Craniotomy for resection of brain tumor	Anesthetic maintenance via halothane vs. isoflurane vs. sevoflurane after induction via propofol/fentanyl/nitrous oxide	Halothane, isoflurane, and sevoflurane were all found to reduce systolic blood pressure, but only sevoflurane and isoflurane decreased train-of-four ratios significantly at 1.0. MAC (p < 0.001). Amplitudes of transcranial motor-evoked potentials were reduced by isoflurane and sevoflurane at 0.5. MACs, but not halothane, reflecting the reduced extent of the neuromuscular blockade initiated by halothane.
Djian et al., 2006 [45]	Unspecified intracranial procedure	Remifentanil vs. sufentanil in combination with propofol for maintenance of anesthesia	Remifentanil was associated with the need for less adjustments with regard to hemodynamic stability (p = 0.037), greater use of morphine (p = 0.01), and higher intraoperative opioid costs. However, there was no significant differences in extubation times between groups.
Bhagat et al., 2008 [46]	Craniotomy for unspecified pathology	Anesthetic maintenance via propofol (n = 50) vs. isoflurane (n = 50)	Hypertension occurrence and MAP change were not different between the two agents. Emergence time was higher for propofol (p = 0.008).

Authors and Year	Surgical Procedure	Comparison	Findings
Bonhomme et al., 2009 [47]	Unspecified intracranial procedure	Propofol ($n = 30$) vs. sevoflurane ($n = 31$)	Propofol was associated with higher occurrence of intraoperative hypertension ($p < 0.001$) and sevoflurane was associated with higher occurrence of intraoperative hypotension ($p = 0.015$).
Ali et al., 2009 [48]	Resection of pituitary tumor	Propofol ($n = 30$), isoflurane ($n = 30$), sevoflurane (n = 30)	Emergence time was significantly longer with use of isoflurane ($p < 0.001$). Hypertension occurrence was higher in isoflurane than in propofol or sevoflurane, and higher in sevoflurane than propofol ($p < 0.001$). Hypotension was not difference between anesthetics (p = 0.36).
Bilotta et al., 2009 [49]	Craniotomy for resection of supratentorial lesion	Sevoflurane ($n = 28$) vs. desflurane (n = 28)	Significant delays in cognitive "awakening" for obese and overweight patients receiving sevoflurane-based anesthesia as compared to those receiving desflurane-based anesthesia as measured by post-operative short orientation memory concentration test scores at 15 and 30 min ($p < 0.005$, $p < 0.005$) as well as with the Rancho Los Amigos scale (p < 0.005)
Güneş et al., 2009 [71]	Craniotomy for resection of supratentorial lesion	Anesthetic maintenance with dexmedetomidine in addition to sevoflurane ($n = 30$), desflurane ($n = 30$), and isoflurane (n = 30)	MAP was elevated following intubation for all groups. Rates of eyes opening and responsiveness following verbal commands were lower in desflurane–dexmedetomidine than in other groups (p = 0.001).

Authors and Year	Surgical Procedure	Comparison	Findings
Magni et al., 2009 [72]	Craniotomy for resection of supratentorial lesion	Anesthetic maintenance via sevoflurane ($n = 60$) vs. desflurane (n = 60)	Mean emergence was similar between the two groups, but extubation and recovery time were lower ($p < 0.001$) in the desflurane group. Hemodynamic stability differences were non-significant between the two groups.
Lauta et al., 2010 [50]	Craniotomy for resection of supratentorial lesion	Anesthetic maintenance via propofol ($n = 153$) vs. sevoflurane ($n = 149$)	Propofol was associated with a significantly longer emergence time to eyes opening ($p < 0.014$. Sevoflurane was associated with higher occurrence of hypotension (p < 0.0167).
Yildiz et al., 2011 [51]	Craniotomy for resection of supratentorial lesion	Anesthetic maintenance via desflurane ($n = 35$) vs. isoflurane (n = 35)	Heart rate was not different between the two agents. MAP was higher for desflurane ($p < 0.05$). Extubation time and eyes opening time was shorter for desflurane (p < 0.05).
Ghoneim et al., 2015 [52]	Craniotomy for resection of supratentorial tumors	Anesthetic maintenance via isoflurane ($n = 20$) vs. sevoflurane ($n = 20$) vs. desflurane (n = 20)	Emergence times were significantly shorter for desflurane or sevoflurane than with isoflurane in pediatric patients following a craniotomy for supratentorial tumors.
Hernandez et al., 2015 [53]	Craniotomy for hematoma	Anesthetic maintenance via propofol ($n = 20$) or sevoflurane ($n = 20$)	SSEPs amplitudes and latencies were not different between the two agents. TceMEPs amplitudes were higher for propofol ($p < 0.05$). Latencies were shorter in the propofol group ($p < 0.05$).
Goettel et al., 2016 [54]	Awake craniotomy for unspecified pathology	Dexmedetomidine ($n = 25$) vs. propofol ($n = 25$)	There were no differences in level of sedation (OAA) ($p = 0.13$). There were no differences in intraoperative hypertension ($p = 0.60$), hypotension ($p = 0.50$), or complications ($p = 0.99$). There was no difference in postoperative complications ($p > 0.05$).

Authors and Year	Surgical Procedure	Comparison	Findings
Gokcek et al., 2016 [55]	Unspecified intracranial procedure	Anesthetic maintenance via sevoflurane ($n = 25$) vs. desflurane (n = 25)	Emergence time and time to eyes opening were higher with sevoflurane ($p < 0.001$).
Lin et al., 2016 [56]	Resection of supratentorial lesion	Anesthetic maintenance via propofol ($n = 31$) vs. dexmedetomidine ($n = 31$)	NIHSS-positive change was higher in propofol than dexmedetomidine ($p < 0.001$). Focal neurologic deficits were higher in propofol than dexmedetomidine ($p < 0.05$).
Rajan et al., 2016 [57]	Craniotomy or transsphenoidal approach for resection of brain tumor	Dexmedetomidine ($n = 68$) vs. remifentanil ($n = 71$)	Dexmedetomidine was associated with significantly lower postoperative MAP ($p < 0.001$). Dexmedetomidine was associated with significantly longer emergence time to open eyes ($p < 0.001$).
Thongrong et al., 2017 [58]	Craniotomy for unspecified pathology	Anesthetic maintenance via fentanyl ($n = 30$) vs. dexmedetomidine ($n = 30$) after propofol induction	Dexmedetomidine infusions reduced adverse effects, with signs of effectively controlled systolic blood pressure one minute prior to skull pin insertion ($p < 0.05$), as well as during skull pin insertion ($p < 0.01$) in comparison to fentanyl. Similarly, dexmedetomidine infusions were related to reduced adverse hypertensive and hypotensive responses in patients.
Bhardwaj et al., 2018 [59]	Surgical clipping for aneurysmal subarachnoid hemorrhage	Propofol ($n = 35$) vs. desflurane (n = 35)	There was no difference in blood loss ($p < 0.05$), hypotension ($p < 0.05$), hypertension ($p < 0.05$), or emergence time for eyes opening ($p < 0.05$).
Gracia et al., 2018 [60]	Unspecified intracranial procedure	Anesthetic induction via propofol ($n = 20$) vs. thiopental ($n = 20$)	There was no difference in heart rate ($p > 0.05$). MAP was significantly higher in thiopental groups ($p < 0.05$). Systolic and diastolic blood pressure was significantly lower in thiopental groups ($p < 0.05$).

Authors and Year	Surgical Procedure	Comparison	Findings
Molina et al., 2018 [61]	Craniotomy for resection of tumor	Propofol–remifentanil (*n* = 105) for asleep sedation vs. conscious sedation with dexmedetomidine (*n* = 75)	Patients sedated with dexmedetomidine used less opiates, antihypertensive drugs, and had a lower postoperative duration and length of stay (all $p < 0.001$).
Xinyan et al., 2018 [62]	Awake craniotomy for unspecified pathology	Dexmedetomidine (*n* = 20), propofol (*n* = 20), etomidate (*n* = 20)	There was no significant difference in perioperative wake up duration ($p > 0.05$) and postoperative emergence time ($p > 0.05$). The rate of adverse events was lower in dexmedetomidine than propofol and etomidate ($p < 0.05$). The rate of adverse events was lower in propofol than etomidate ($p < 0.05$).
Khallaf et al., 2019 [63]	Craniotomy for hematoma	Anesthetic maintenance via propofol (*n* = 20) vs. dexmedetomidine (*n* = 20)	Tachycardia, bradycardia, and hypertension occurrences were not different between the two agents. IPP and CPP changes were not different between the two agents. Hypotension occurrences were higher in the propofol group ($p = 0.024$).
Preethi et al., 2021 [64]	Craniotomy for hematoma	Anesthetic maintenance via propofol (*n* = 45) vs. isoflurane	Change in heart rate, systolic blood pressure, diastolic blood pressure, and MAP were not different between the two agents. Brain relaxation was higher for propofol ($p < 0.05$). ICP was higher for isoflurane (p = 0.01).
Balasubramanian et al., 2021 [65]	Surgical clipping/ endovascular coiling for aneurysmal subarachnoid hemorrhage	Propofol (*n* = 8) vs. isoflurane (*n* = 8) vs. sevoflurane (*n* = 8), vs. desflurane (n = 8)	There was no significant difference found between anesthetic on levels of CSF caspase-3 levels.

Source: *Nguyen A, Mandavalli A, Diaz MJ, Root KT, Patel A, Casauay J, Perisetla P, Lucke-Wold B. Neurosurgical Anesthesia: Optimizing Outcomes with Agent Selection. Biomedicines. 2023; 11(2):372. https://doi.org/10.3390/biomedicines11020372.*

The heart rate and blood pressure may double over the baseline in a minute if end-tidal desflurane concentration is increased stepwise from 4% to 8%. Little doses of esmolol, clonidine, or opioids significantly reduce the blood pressure and heart rate responses to a stepwise increase in desflurane concentration. The heart rate and mean arterial pressure drop minimally when the fast increase in end-tidal desflurane concentration from 4% to 8% is repeated after 30 minutes, indicating that the receptors regulating these changes in circulation become accustomed to repeated stimulation. Abrupt increases in sevoflurane, halothane, or enflurane concentrations up to 2 MAC do not cause vascular stimulation. Because they are not pungent, sevoflurane and halothane are commonly administered by inhalation to produce anesthesia. Myocardial contractility is decreased when children are given halothane, but not sevoflurane, during the induction of anesthesia. Myocardial contractility is reduced in adults when anesthesia is maintained with 1 MAC of sevoflurane or halothane with 67 percent nitrous oxide. When used in conjunction with controlled ventilation, sevoflurane may momentarily elevate heart rate in adults.

Administration with Nitrous Oxide and Oxygen Versus 100% Oxygen

When given in combination with oxygen and nitrous oxide, desflurane, isoflurane, and sevoflurane reduce the heart rate, pulmonary artery pressure, and central venous pressure in a dose-dependent manner. These results are in line with those obtained when each volatile anesthetic is given in oxygen alone. Direct comparison shows that when desflurane is given in oxygen instead of nitrous oxide at roughly equivalent MAC multiples, there is a more marked diminution of MAP, SVR, cardiac index, and LVSWI as well as a faster heart rate and greater CO.

3.7.1.2. Myocardial Conduction and Dysrhythmogenicity

The heart is not predisposed to premature ventricular extrasystoles by isoflurane, sevoflurane, or desflurane. On the other hand, especially when catecholamines are present, halothane does make the myocardium more susceptible to premature ventricular extrasystoles; this relationship is exacerbated in cases of hypercarbia. It is likely that inhaled anesthetics suppress ventricular dysrhythmias by extending the effective refractory period during myocardial ischemia.

The choice of inhaled anesthetic influences the occurrence of reflex bradydysrhythmias that may result from vagal stimulation. Children anesthetized with sevoflurane, compared with halothane, exhibit fewer episodes of decreased heart rate or sinus node arrest in response to surgical traction on the ocular muscles.

QT Interval

The electrocardiogram's QT interval is extended by inhaled anesthetics. Sevoflurane should not be administered to patients who have been diagnosed with congenital long QT syndrome (LQTS), despite the lack of systematic comparisons of the relative propensity of each anesthetic to prolong the QT interval. Sevoflurane and propofol, two anesthetics that prolong the QT interval in children, do not, however, increase transmural dispersion of repolarization, a measurement of the variable rates at which myocardial cells repolarize during phases 2 and 3 of the action potential. In susceptible patients, the clinical significance of QT prolongation with sevoflurane and other inhaled anesthetics is unknown. The primary treatment for patients with LQTS is β-adrenergic blockade. All contemporary inhaled anesthetics have been safely used to sedate patients with known long QTS while they are also taking β-adrenergic blocking medications. Patients undergoing halothane anesthesia have experienced multiple malignant intraoperative arrhythmias, which were later linked to undiagnosed LQTS. Notably, none of these patients had been administered β-blocking medication.

3.7.1.3. Patients with Coronary Artery Disease

Many trials on patients undergoing coronary artery bypass surgery or at risk for coronary artery disease have not been able to show a difference in the outcome between groups receiving anesthetic techniques that are administered intravenously (fentanyl or sufentanil) versus those that are inhaled (desflurane). Neither have the results show a difference between groups receiving one type of inhaled anesthetic versus another (desflurane vs. Isoflurane in contrast to sevoflurane. isoflurane. Efforts to rule out the possibility of coronary steal, a condition in which a patient with vulnerable anatomy experiences localized myocardial ischemia due to coronary vasodilatation, were unfounded due to isoflurane's ability to dilate small-diameter coronary arteries. Rather than causing damage to the heart, volatile anesthetics shield it from harm and maintain its functionality following an ischemic insult.

Anesthetic Preconditioning

The benefits of volatile anesthetics in preventing myocardial ischemia are attributed to a process known as anesthetic preconditioning, rather than a favorable change in the myocardial oxygen supply-demand ratio. Research indicates that in situations where regional perfusion is impaired, volatile anesthetics protect the myocardium. When compared to patients receiving propofol, patients undergoing coronary artery bypass graft (CABG) surgery experienced a lower incidence of abnormally elevated troponin levels when maintained with 0.2 to 1 MAC of desflurane or sevoflurane. A lower frequency of postoperative myocardial infarction was observed when sevoflurane was administered throughout the entire CABG surgery as opposed to just during the prebypass or postbypass period. Similarly, a lower risk of myocardial infarction was observed when prebypass or postbypass administration was combined with propofol anesthesia.

Mechanisms of Ischemic Preconditioning

The basic defense mechanism known as ischaemic preconditioning is found in every tissue in every species. In ischemic preconditioning, the myocardium is protected against irreversible or reversible damage with a subsequent prolonged ischemic insult by exposure to one or more brief episodes of ischemia. After a brief ischemic episode, the myocardium is protected for two different periods of time. The first phase lasts for one to two hours following the conditioning session before ending. The benefit resurfaces 24 hours later and may extend for up to three days during the second period. The critical process that bestows the protective activity is the opening of mitochondrial ATP-sensitive potassium channels (KATP), which is brought about by the binding of different ligands to G protein-coupled receptors. KATP channels are essential to the protective effects of volatile anesthetics, which either improve ischemic preconditioning or directly protect the heart.

3.7.2. Ventilation Effects

As the concentration of the anesthetic increases, breathing frequency increases and tidal volume decreases when using inhaled anesthetics. The reduced tidal volume results in a comparatively higher percentage of dead space ventilation in comparison to alveolar ventilation, even though minute ventilation is largely preserved. At higher anesthetic concentrations, gas exchange becomes less effective, and $Paco_2$ rises in direct proportion to anesthetic concentration. Strong anesthetics have comparable effects at specific

MAC multiples. The rise in $Paco_2$ at deeper levels of anesthesia may be lessened by substituting 60% of the nitrous oxide with an equivalent amount of volatile anesthetic. Subjects receiving 1.7. MAC of desflurane in oxygen experience apnea due to a dose-related blunting of carbon dioxide responsiveness in both volunteers and patients breathing desflurane (and other volatile anesthetics). Patients undergoing surgery may experience a less marked blunting of ventilation with inhaled anesthetics when compared to volunteers, which may be due to the stimulatory effect of surgery on breathing. All volatile anesthetics reduce the stimulation of the ventilator brought on by arterial hypoxemia. (Eger, 1963; Eger, 1974; Eger, 1985; Eger, 1993; Eger, 2000)

3.7.2.1. Chest Wall Changes

The chest wall's conformational changes brought on by inhaled anesthetics may have an impact on ventilatory mechanics. The diaphragm's cephalad displacement and the rib cage's inward displacement are caused by increased expiratory muscle activity, which ultimately lowers functional residual capacity. When spontaneous ventilation is allowed, atelectasis happens more frequently and preferentially in the dependent regions of the lung.

3.7.2.2. Hypoxic Pulmonary Vasoconstriction

Although there is some inhibition of hypoxic pulmonary vasoconstriction, inhaled anesthetics change the flow of blood through the lungs. For instance, patients receiving one-lung ventilation under isoflurane versus desflurane and sevoflurane versus propofol anesthesia exhibit comparable arterial oxygenation levels.

3.7.2.3. Airway Resistance

Inhaled anesthetics have minimal bronchodilating effects in the absence of bronchoconstriction. After tracheal intubation, volunteers respond better to isoflurane, halothane, and sevoflurane than to nitrous oxide and thiopental. Smokers experience a slight, temporary increase in airway resistance following tracheal intubation and desflurane anesthesia, while nonsmokers experience no change in airway resistance following these procedures, compared with a slight decrease with sevoflurane. Variations in gas density may mediate some or all of the changes in airway resistance.

3.7.2.4. Airway Irritant Effects

The ability of inhaled anesthetics to irritate airways varies (i.e., tendency). Over a wide range of concentrations, nitrous oxide, halothane, and sevoflurane are nonpungent and cause little to no irritation. Because desflurane and isoflurane are pungent, they may irritate the respiratory tract at concentrations higher than one milliampere-hour (MAC). This is especially true when no intravenous medication (such as opioids or sedative-hypnotics) is present to lessen the sensation of pungency. The most common choice when an inhaled induction of anesthesia is required is sevoflurane or halothane. Nevertheless, compared to sevoflurane or propofol, desflurane and isoflurane can be given to surgical patients via a laryngeal mask airway without increasing the likelihood of airway irritation (such as coughing, breath holding, laryngospasm, and arterial oxygen desaturation). This is because maintenance usually does not call for a concentration above 1 MAC (i.e., nonirritating concentrations).

3.7.3. Central Nervous System Effects

3.7.3.1. Cerebral Blood Flow

When nitrous oxide is given without the use of volatile anesthetics, cerebral vasodilatation and blood flow are both increased. There is a slight increase in the cerebral metabolic rate for oxygen ($CMRO_2$). These effects are countered by the coadministration of opioids, barbiturates, or propofol (but not ketamine). Changes in $Paco_2$ do not cause cerebral vascular responsiveness to be eliminated by inhaled anesthetics. Desflurane, sevoflurane, halothane, and isoflurane all lower $CMRO_2$. These volatile anesthetics cause cerebral vasodilatation in normocapnic humans at concentrations greater than 0.6. MAC. On cerebral blood flow, there is a biphasic dose-dependent effect. At 0.5. MAC, cerebral blood flow remains relatively constant due to the counteracting effect of the decrease in $CMRO_2$. Vasodilating effects dominate at concentrations above 1 MAC, and cerebral blood flow rises, particularly if systemic blood pressure is kept at awake levels. When compared to isoflurane, sevoflurane, or desflurane, halothane causes a comparatively larger increase in cerebral blood flow.

3.7.3.2. Intracranial Pressure

All volatile anesthetics cause an increase in intracranial pressure at doses greater than one MAC, and at concentrations lower than one MAC, autoregulation—the adaptive mechanism that maintains cerebral blood flow in awake patients over a wide range of systemic arterial pressures—is compromised. Patients receiving 1 MAC of isoflurane or desflurane during a craniotomy for supratentorial tumors exhibit a decrease in cerebral perfusion pressure and an arteriovenous oxygen difference for oxygen, but not an intracranial pressure change. On the other hand, patients receiving 1 MAC of desflurane, isoflurane, or sevoflurane during pituitary tumor resection exhibit slight increases in intracranial pressure and a decrease in cerebral blood flow. Compared to patients receiving 1 MAC of desflurane or isoflurane without nitrous oxide, neurosurgical patients receiving 50% nitrous oxide plus 0.5. MAC of these drugs appear to exhibit greater levels of brain relaxation. Changes in $Paco_2$ do not cause cerebral vascular responsiveness to be eliminated by inhaled anesthetics.

3.7.3.3. Evoked Potentials

In a dose-dependent manner, nitrous oxide and all volatile anesthetics decrease the amplitude and lengthen the latency of somatosensory evoked potentials. At 1 MAC of volatile anesthetic alone or above 0 MAC when given with 50% nitrous oxide, evoked potentials can be eliminated. The reliability of motor-evoked potential monitoring may be compromised by low concentrations of volatile anesthetics (0.2 to 0.3. MAC), though multipulse stimuli can mitigate some of the effects.

3.7.3.4. Electroencephalographic Effects

The EEG exhibits distinctive, dose-dependent changes when exposed to volatile anesthetics. Increased amplitude and synchrony are indicative of a deeper level of anesthesia from waking. As depth increases, electrical silence periods start to take up a larger percentage of the time (burst suppression). On the EEG, this isoelectric pattern is predominant between 1.5 and 2.0. MAC. Particularly when administered at higher dosages or in conjunction with controlled hyperventilation, sevoflurane and enflurane have the potential to cause epileptiform activity on the EEG. Children have been observed to exhibit seizure-like behavior during sevoflurane induction, however it is unclear what this means clinically.

3.7.4. Neuromuscular Effects

Volatile anesthetics increase the effectiveness of neuromuscular blocking medications and cause dose-related relaxation of the skeletal muscles. When using desflurane anesthesia as opposed to sevoflurane or isoflurane, the relaxant effect of rocuronium is enhanced more; however, when using any volatile anesthetic, skeletal muscle relaxation is enhanced more than when using intravenous anesthetics (e.g., propofol plus fentanyl). The removal of volatile anesthetic improves neuromuscular blockade recovery. More so than an equipotent decrease in isoflurane concentration, a desflurane concentration reduction to 0.25 MAC promotes the reversal of neuromuscular block following vecuronium administration.

3.7.5. Malignant Hyperthermia

Malignant hyperthermia (MH) is still a potentially fatal anesthesia-related complication. It is an inherited condition characterized by elevated metabolism of skeletal muscle that is brought on by the use of volatile anesthetics, particularly succinylcholine and/or halothane. All strong inhaled volatile anesthetics have the potential to cause mixed hallucinations (MH), but research on desflurane, sevoflurane, and potentially isoflurane indicates a lower risk than halothane. It seems that men are more likely than women to experience a clinical MH episode. Of all MH reactions, 52.1 percent occur in the pediatric population. Muscle rigidity, elevated temperature, tachycardia, and elevated end-tidal carbon dioxide levels are indicators of metabolic hypermetabolism (MH). Due to increased diagnostic awareness, early detection with end-expired carbon dioxide, decreased use of strong anesthetic triggers, and the administration of medications that attenuate fulminant episodes of MH, more recent cases of MH have been less severe. The mainstays of care are treating potentially fatal electrolyte imbalances like hyperkalemia, stopping the use of volatile anesthetics and succinylcholine right away, and starting intravenous dantrolene treatment right away.

3.7.6. Hepatic Effects

Hepatic injury after anesthesia may be categorized as severe (immune-mediated) or mild.

3.7.6.1. Immune-Mediated Liver Injury

After anesthesia with halothane, isoflurane, sevoflurane, or desflurane, there may be severe liver damage. Massive hepatic necrosis in this severe form can be fatal or require liver transplantation. This serious injury has an immunologic mechanism that necessitates prior exposure to a volatile anesthetic. Trifluoroacetate is created by the oxidative metabolism of halothane, isoflurane, and desflurane by cytochrome P-450 enzymes. Hepatocyte proteins can bind covalently to trifluoroacetate. Hepatocyte moieties containing trifluoroacetyl can function as haptens, substances that the body identifies as foreign and against which the immune system produces antibodies. Any anesthetic that can produce trifluoroacetate, later on, could cause an immunological reaction that would result in severe hepatic necrosis. After being metabolized, sevoflurane yields hexafluoroisopropanol, a substance lacking trifluoroacetate's antigenic properties.

3.7.6.2. Mild Liver Injury

Halothane administration may result in a clinically mild form of liver injury. This more prevalent entity's primary feature is a slight increase in serum transaminase levels. This mild type of liver damage may be more likely to happen following concurrent reductions in hepatic blood flow and related decreases in oxygen delivery to the liver. It is thought to be mediated by the reductive metabolism of halothane.

3.7.6.3. History of Prior Anesthesia-Related Hepatic Dysfunction

Volatile anesthetics are probably not harmful to patients with preexisting hepatic disease unrelated to anesthesia, although they are often not given to patients who have previously experienced unexplained symptoms of hepatic dysfunction after inhaling anesthesia.

3.7.7. Renal Effects

The first volatile anesthetic that was nonflammable to be used in clinical settings was methyloxyflurane. Renal damage was linked to its use. Further analysis indicates that the damage is most likely caused by its extensive metabolism, specifically to dichloroacetic acid and inorganic fluoride from O-demethylation. However, there is no correlation between renal injury and the generation of fluoride resulting from the metabolism of other strong inhaled anesthetics, such as sevoflurane. (Eger, 1963; Eger, 1974; Eger, 1985; Eger, 1993; Eger, 2000).

A Closer Look

Malignant Hyperthermia

Malignant hyperthermia (MH) is a rare but potentially life-threatening condition triggered by certain drugs used during anesthesia, particularly in susceptible individuals. It is characterized by a rapid and uncontrolled increase in body temperature, muscle rigidity, and metabolic abnormalities. MH is most commonly associated with the use of volatile anesthetic agents like halothane and the muscle relaxant succinylcholine.

The exact mechanism of MH involves an abnormal response of skeletal muscle cells, particularly the sarcoplasmic reticulum, to triggering agents. In susceptible individuals, exposure to triggering agents leads to uncontrolled release of calcium ions within muscle cells, resulting in sustained muscle contraction, increased metabolism, and excessive heat production.

The classic signs of MH typically manifest shortly after exposure to triggering agents and include muscle rigidity, rapid increase in body temperature (hyperthermia), tachycardia (rapid heartbeat), tachypnea (rapid breathing), and metabolic acidosis. Without prompt recognition and intervention, MH can progress rapidly, leading to severe complications such as organ failure, cardiac arrest, and death.

Management of MH involves immediate cessation of triggering agents, administration of the antidote dantrolene to block calcium release from muscle cells, and supportive measures to control hyperthermia, acidosis, and other metabolic disturbances. Prompt treatment is essential to prevent serious complications and improve outcomes.

Prevention of MH relies on careful screening of patients for susceptibility, as the condition is often inherited and can run in families. Preoperative testing, such as the caffeine-halothane contracture test or genetic testing, may be recommended for individuals with a family history of MH or other risk factors.

Overall, while malignant hyperthermia is rare, it is a serious condition that requires prompt recognition, immediate intervention, and coordinated management to ensure the best possible outcomes for affected individuals undergoing anesthesia. (Eger, 1963; Eger, 1974; Eger, 1985; Eger, 1993; Eger, 2000).

Summary

- Between 1920 and 1940, ethylene, cyclopropane, and divinyl ether were introduced into use as anesthetics, gaining acceptance over the older inhaled anesthetics (except for nitrous oxide) by producing a faster, more pleasant induction of anesthesia and by allowing faster awakening after surgery.
- Modern inhaled anesthetics are halogenated partly or entirely with fluorine. Fluorination provides greater stability and lesser toxicity.
- Halothane was introduced into clinical practice in 1956 and became widely used. It had several advantages compared with the older anesthetics, including nonflammability, a pleasant odor, lesser organ toxicity, and pharmacokinetic properties allowing a much faster induction of anesthesia and emergence compared with ether.
- Measurable and universal characteristics of all inhaled anesthetics include the production of immobility and amnestic effects. Immobility is measured by the minimum alveolar concentration (MAC) of anesthetic required to suppress movement to a surgical incision in 50% of patients.
- Inhaled anesthetics produce central nervous system depression by their actions on ion channels, which govern the electrical behavior of the nervous system.4 Inhaled anesthetics probably produce anesthesia by enhancing the function of inhibitory ion channels and by blocking the function of excitatory ion channels.
- Nitrous oxide exists as a gas at ambient temperature, although it becomes a liquid at higher pressures. The remaining inhaled anesthetics are liquids at ambient temperatures.
- Fresh gas flow rate directly impacts the quantity of volatile liquid used, and consequently the cost of the anesthetic delivery. Higher fresh gas flows (at or above minute ventilation) minimize rebreathing and allow faster equilibration between inspired and central nervous system (CNS) partial pressures.
- Anesthetic degradation by metabolism or by an interaction with carbon dioxide absorbents (especially when desiccated) produces several potentially toxic compounds.
- Pharmacokinetics of inhaled anesthetics describe their uptake (absorption) from alveoli into the systemic circulation, distribution in the body, and eventual elimination by the lungs or metabolism principally in the liver.
- A high P_i is necessary during the initial administration of an inhaled anesthetic. This initial high P_i (i.e., input) offsets the impact of uptake into the blood and accelerates induction of anesthesia as reflected by the rate of increase in the P_A.
- Characteristics of the anesthetic breathing system that influence the rate of increase of the P_A include the volume of the system, solubility of inhaled anesthetics in the rubber or plastic components of the system, and gas inflow from the anesthetic machine.
- Nitrous oxide is unique among anesthetics because of its inactivation of methionine synthase, the enzyme regulating vitamin B12 and folate metabolism.
- The blood-gas partition coefficient of nitrous oxide (0.46) is 34 times greater than that of nitrogen (0.014). This differential solubility means that nitrous oxide can leave the

blood to enter an air-filled cavity 34 times more rapidly than nitrogen can leave the cavity to enter the blood.

- An important difference between induction of anesthesia and recovery from anesthesia is the potential impact of metabolism on the rate of decrease in the P_A after anesthesia.
- Diffusion hypoxia may occur after nitrous oxide administration if patients are allowed to inhale room air. The initial high-volume outpouring of nitrous oxide from the blood into the alveoli when inhalation of this gas is discontinued can so dilute the Pao_2 that the Pao_2 decreases.
- Equipotent concentrations of inhaled anesthetics have similar circulatory effects, especially during the maintenance of anesthesia in human volunteers. However, patients undergoing surgery may respond differently from healthy volunteers.
- The cardiac index is minimally influenced by the administration of desflurane, sevoflurane, or isoflurane over a wide range of concentrations in healthy young adults.
- Inhaled anesthetics increase the frequency of breathing and decrease tidal volume as anesthetic concentration increases. Although minute ventilation is relatively preserved, the decreased tidal volume leads to a relatively greater proportion of dead space ventilation relative to alveolar ventilation.
- In the absence of bronchoconstriction, the bronchodilating effects of inhaled anesthetics are small. In volunteers, isoflurane, halothane, and sevoflurane, but not nitrous oxide and thiopental, decrease respiratory systemic resistance after tracheal intubation.
- Volatile anesthetics produce dose-related skeletal muscle relaxation and enhance the activity of neuromuscular blocking drugs. Enhancement of the relaxant effect of rocuronium is more intense with anesthesia from desflurane than with sevoflurane or isoflurane, although all volatile anesthetics enhance skeletal muscle relaxation compared with intravenous anesthetics (e.g., propofol plus fentanyl).

References

1. Akeson, J., & Didricksson, I. (2004). Convulsions on anaesthetic induction with sevoflurane in young children. *Acta Anaesthesiologica Scandinavica, 48*, 405–407.
2. Aronow, W. S., & Ahn, C. (2000). Increased plasma homocysteine is an independent predictor of new coronary events in older persons. *American Journal of Cardiology, 86*(3), 346–347.
3. Badner, N. H., Beattie, W. S., Freeman, D., et al. (2000). Nitrous oxide-induced increased homocysteine concentrations are associated with increased postoperative myocardial ischemia in patients undergoing carotid endarterectomy. *Anesthesia & Analgesia, 91*(5), 1073–1079.
4. Bailey, J. M. (1997). Context-sensitive half-times and other decrement times of inhaled anesthetics. *Anesthesia & Analgesia, 85*, 681–686.
5. Beck, D. H., Doepfmer, U. R., Sinemus, C., et al. (2001). Effects of sevoflurane and propofol on pulmonary shunt fraction during one-lung ventilation for thoracic surgery. *British Journal of Anaesthesia, 86*, 38–43.

6. Bellgardt, M., Bomberg, H., Herzog-Niescery, J., et al. (2016). Survival after long-term isoflurane sedation as opposed to intravenous sedation in critically ill surgical patients: Retrospective analysis. *European Journal of Anaesthesiology, 33*(1), 6–13.
7. Booker, P. D., Whyte, S. D., & Ladusans, E. J. (2003). Long QT syndrome and anaesthesia. *British Journal of Anaesthesia, 90*, 349–366.
8. Brady, J. E., Sun, L. S., Rosenberg, H., et al. (2009). Prevalence of malignant hyperthermia due to anesthesia in New York State, 2001–2005. *Anesthesia & Analgesia, 109*, 1162–1166.
9. Brockwell, R. C., & Andrews, J. J. (2009). Vaporizers (in delivery systems for inhaled anesthetics). In P. G. Barash, B. F. Cullen, R. K. Stoelting, & M. Cahallan (Eds.), *Clinical Anesthesia* (6th ed., pp. 667–669). Philadelphia: Lippincott Williams & Wilkins.
10. Cahalan, M. K. (1996). Hemodynamic effects of inhaled anesthetics. Review Courses. Cleveland: International Anesthesia Research Society.
11. Cahalan, M. K., Weiskopf, R. B., Eger, E. I. II, et al. (1991). Hemodynamic effects of desflurane/nitrous oxide anesthesia in volunteers. *Anesthesia & Analgesia, 73*, 157–164.
12. Carpenter, R. L., Eger, E. I. II, Johnson, B. H., et al. (1986). The extent of metabolism of inhaled anesthetics in humans. *Anesthesiology, 65*, 201–205.
13. Chortkoff, B. S., Bennett, H. L., & Eger, E. I. II. (1993). Subanesthetic concentrations of isoflurane suppress learning as defined by the category-example task. *Anesthesiology, 79*(1), 16–22.
14. Dahan, A., & Teppema, L. J. (2003). Influence of anaesthesia and analgesia on the control of breathing. *British Journal of Anaesthesia, 91*, 40–49.
15. De Hert, S. G., Cromheecke, S., ten Broecke, P. W., et al. (2003). Effects of propofol, desflurane, and sevoflurane on recovery of myocardial function after coronary surgery in elderly high-risk patients. *Anesthesiology, 99*, 314–323.
16. De Hert, S. G., Van der Linden, P. J., Cromheecke, S., et al. (2004). Cardioprotective properties of sevoflurane in patients undergoing coronary surgery and cardiopulmonary bypass are related to the modalities of its administration. *Anesthesiology, 101*, 299–310.
17. Dwyer, R., Bennett, H. L., Eger, E. I. II, et al. (1992). Effects of isoflurane and nitrous oxide in subanesthetic concentrations on memory and responsiveness in volunteers. *Anesthesiology, 77*(5), 888–898.
18. Ebert, T. J., Muzi, M., & Lopatka, C. W. (1995). Neurocirculatory responses to sevoflurane in humans: A comparison to desflurane. *Anesthesiology, 83*, 88–95.
19. Ebert, T. J., Perez, F., Uhrich, T. D., et al. (1998). Desflurane-mediated sympathetic activation occurs in humans despite preventing hypotension and baroreceptor unloading. *Anesthesiology, 88*, 1227–1232.
20. Eger, E. I. (1963). Effect of inspired anesthetic concentration on the rate of rise of alveolar concentration. *Anesthesiology, 24*, 153–157.
21. Eger, E. I. (1985). *Isoflurane (Forane): A Compendium and Reference.* Madison, WI: Ohio Medical Products.
22. Eger, E. I. (1993). *Desflurane (Suprane): A Compendium and Reference.* Nutley, NJ: Anaquest.
23. Eger, E. I. II, & Saidman, L. J. (1965). Hazards of nitrous oxide anesthesia in bowel obstruction and pneumothorax. *Anesthesiology, 26*, 61–66.

24. Eger, E. I. II, Koblin, D. D., Harris, R. A., et al. (1997). Hypothesis: Inhaled anesthetics produce immobility and amnesia by different mechanisms at different sites. *Anesthesia & Analgesia, 84*, 915–918.
25. Eger, E. I. II. (1974). Uptake of inhaled anesthetics: The alveolar to inspired anesthetic difference. In E. I. II Eger (Ed.), *Anesthetic Uptake and Action* (pp. 77–96). Baltimore: Williams & Wilkins.
26. Eger, E. I. II. (1994). New inhaled anesthetics. *Anesthesiology, 80*, 906–922.
27. Eger, E. I. II. (2000). *History of Modern Inhaled Anesthetics: The Pharmacology of Inhaled Anesthetics*. San Antonio, TX: Dannemiller Memorial Educational Foundation.
28. Eshima, R., Maurer, A., King, T., et al. (2003). A comparison of upper airway responses during desflurane and sevoflurane administration via a laryngeal mask airway. *Anesthesia & Analgesia, 96*, 701–705.
29. Fraga, M., Rama-Maceiras, P., Rodino, S., et al. (2003). The effects of isoflurane and desflurane on intracranial pressure, cerebral perfusion pressure, and cerebral arteriovenous oxygen content difference in normocapnic patients with supratentorial brain tumors. *Anesthesiology, 98*, 1085–1090.
30. Frink, E. J., Ghantous, H., Malan, T. P., et al. (1992). Plasma inorganic fluoride with sevoflurane anesthesia: Correlation with indices of hepatic and renal function. *Anesthesia & Analgesia, 74*, 231–235.
31. Goff, M. J., Arain, S. R., Ficke, D. J., et al. (2000). Absence of bronchodilation during desflurane anesthesia: A comparison to sevoflurane and thiopental. *Anesthesiology, 93*, 404–408.
32. Grundmann, U., Muler, M., Kleinschmidt, S., et al. (1996). Cardiovascular effects of desflurane and isoflurane in patients with coronary artery disease. *Acta Anaesthesiologica Scandinavica, 40*, 1101–1107.
33. Guo, T. Z., Poree, L., Golden, W., et al. (1996). Antinociceptive response to nitrous oxide is mediated by supraspinal opiate and spinal alpha 2 adrenergic receptors in the rat. *Anesthesiology, 85*(4), 846–852.
34. Kharasch, E. D. (2008). Adverse drug reactions with halogenated anesthetics. *Clinical Pharmacology & Therapeutics, 84*, 158–162.
35. Laster, M. J., Roth, P., & Eger, E. I. II. (2004). Fires from the interaction of anesthetics with desiccated absorbent. *Anesthesia & Analgesia, 99*, 769–774.
36. Lotto, M. L., Banoub, M., & Schubert, A. (2004). Effects of anesthetic agents and physiologic changes on intraoperative motor evoked potentials. *Journal of Neurosurgical Anesthesiology, 16*, 32–42.
37. Malan, T. P. Jr, DiNardo, J. A., Isner, R. J., et al. (1995). Cardiovascular effects of sevoflurane compared with those of isoflurane in volunteers. *Anesthesiology, 83*, 918–928.
38. Martin, J. L. (2005). Volatile anesthetics and liver injury: A clinical update or what every anesthesiologist should know. *Canadian Journal of Anesthesia, 52*, 125–129.
39. McKay, R. E., Malhotra, A., Cakmakkaya, O. S., et al. (2010). Effect of increased body mass index and anesthetic duration on recovery of protective airway reflexes after sevoflurane vs desflurane. *British Journal of Anaesthesia, 104*, 175–182.

40. Mielck, F., Stephen, H., Buhre, W., et al. (1998). Effects of 1 MAC desflurane on cerebral metabolism, blood flow, and carbon dioxide reactivity in humans. *British Journal of Anaesthesia, 81*, 155–160.

41. Navarro, R., Weiskopf, R. B., Moore, M. A., et al. (1994). Humans anesthetized with sevoflurane or isoflurane have similar arrhythmic response to epinephrine. *Anesthesiology, 80*, 545–549.

42. Njoku, D., Laster, M. J., Gong, D. H., et al. (1997). Biotransformation of halothane, enflurane, isoflurane, and desflurane to trifluoro acetylated liver proteins: Association between protein acetylation and hepatic injury. *Anesthesia & Analgesia, 84*, 173–178.

43. Petersen, K. D., Landsfeldt, U., Cold, G. E., et al. (2003). Intracranial pressure and cerebral hemodynamics in patients with cerebral tumors: A randomized prospective study of patients subjected to craniotomy in propofol-fentanyl, isoflurane-fentanyl, or sevoflurane-fentanyl anesthesia. *Anesthesiology, 98*, 329–336.

44. Quasha, A. L., Eger, E. I. II, Tinker, J. H., et al. (1980). Determination and application of MAC. *Anesthesiology, 53*(4), 315–334.

45. Rampil, I. J. (1994). Anesthetic potency is not altered after hypothermic spinal cord transection in rats. *Anesthesiology, 80*, 606–610.

46. Rosenberg, H., & Shutack, J. G. (1996). Variants of malignant hyperthermia: Special problems for the paediatric anesthesiologist. *Paediatric Anaesthesia, 6*, 87–93.

47. Rosenberg, H., Davis, M., James, D., et al. (2007). Malignant hyperthermia. *Orphanet Journal of Rare Diseases, 2*, 21.

48. Ryan, S., & Neilsen, C. J. (2010). Global warming potential of inhaled anesthetics: Application to clinical use. *Anesthesia & Analgesia, 111*, 92–98.

49. Sackey, P. V., Martling, C. R., Granath, F., & Radell, P. J. (2004). Prolonged isoflurane sedation of intensive care unit patients with the anesthetic conserving device. *Critical Care Medicine, 32*(11), 2241–2246.

50. Sawamura, S., Kingery, W. S., Davies, M. F., et al. (2000). Antinociceptive action of nitrous oxide is mediated by stimulation of noradrenergic neurons in the brainstem and activation of [alpha]2B adrenoceptors. *Journal of Neuroscience, 20*(24), 9242–9251.

51. Sjögren, D., Lindahl, S. G., & Sollevi, A. (1998). Ventilatory responses to acute and sustained hypoxia during isoflurane anesthesia. *Anesthesia & Analgesia, 86*, 403–409.

52. Sonner, J. M., Gong, D., & Eger, E. I. II. (2000). Naturally occurring variability in anesthetic potency among inbred mouse strains. *Anesthesia & Analgesia, 91*(3), 720–726.

53. Sumitani, M., Uchida, K., Yasunaga, H., et al. (2011). Prevalence of malignant hyperthermia and relationship with anesthetics in Japan: Data from the diagnosis procedure combination database. *Anesthesiology, 114*, 84–90.

54. Sundman, E., Witt, H., Sandin, R., et al. (2001). Pharyngeal function and airway protection during subhypnotic concentrations of propofol, isoflurane, and sevoflurane: Volunteers examined by pharyngeal videoradiography and simultaneous manometry. *Anesthesiology, 95*(5), 1125–1132.

55. Wahrenbrock, E. A., Eger, E. I. II, Laravuso, R. B., et al. (1974). Anesthetic uptake—of mice and men (and whales). *Anesthesiology, 40*(1), 19–23.

56. Weiskopf, R. B., Sampson, D., & Moore, M. A. (1994). The desflurane (Tec 6) vaporizer: Design, design considerations and performance evaluation. *British Journal of Anaesthesia, 72*(4), 474–479.

57. Whyte, S. D., Booker, P. D., & Buckley, D. G. (2005). The effects of propofol and sevoflurane on the QT interval and transmural dispersion of repolarization in children. *Anesthesia & Analgesia, 100*, 71–77.

58. Wissing, H., Kuhn, I., Warnken, U., et al. (2001). Carbon monoxide production from desflurane, enflurane, halothane, isoflurane, and sevoflurane with dry soda lime. *Anesthesiology, 95*, 1205–1212.

59. Wu, J., Previte, J. P., Adler, E., et al. (2004). Spontaneous ignition, explosion, and fire with sevoflurane and barium hydroxide lime. *Anesthesiology, 101*, 534–537.

60. Yasuda, N., Lockhart, S. H., Eger, E. I. II, et al. (1992). Comparison of kinetics of sevoflurane and isoflurane in humans. *Anesthesia & Analgesia, 72*, 316–324.

61. Yli-Hankala, A., Vakkuri, A. P., Sarkela, M., et al. (1999). Epileptiform electroencephalogram during mask induction of anesthesia with sevoflurane. *Anesthesiology, 91*, 1596.

62. Zaugg, M., Lucchinetti, E., Spahn, D., et al. (2002). Volatile anesthetics mimic cardiac preconditioning by priming the activation of the mitoKATP channels via multiple signaling pathways. *Anesthesiology, 97*, 4–14.

Chapter

INTRAVENOUS ANESTHETICS

4

Contents

Introduction

In the practice of anesthesia today, intravenous nonopioid anesthetics play a significant role. They are frequently used for patients in critical care units and to enable a quick induction of general anesthesia and sedation during monitored anesthesia care (MAC). The use of intravenous methods for maintaining anesthesia has increased since the advent of propofol. But just like inhaled anesthetics, not all of the effects of the intravenous medications that are currently on the market are positive (hypnosis, amnesia, analgesia, immobility). As a result, rather than starting with larger doses of one or two drugs, the idea of balanced anesthesia developed by using smaller doses of multiple drugs. Inhaled anesthetics, sedative/hypnotics, opioids, and neuromuscular blocking agents are the main medications used with balanced anesthesia.

The quick onset of action of the intravenous anesthetics used to induce general anesthesia is due to their lipophilicity, which allows them to preferentially partition into highly perfused lipid-rich tissues like the brain and spinal cord. Redistribution of the drug into less perfused and inactive tissues, like fat and skeletal muscles, is what causes the effect of a single bolus dose to end, regardless of the amount and rate of their metabolism. As a result, despite having very different metabolisms, all medications used to induce anesthesia have a similar duration of action when taken as a single dose.

Orientation and Directional Terms

Term	Definition	Illustration
Monitored anesthesia care (MAC)	Monitored anesthesia care (MAC) is a type of anesthesia service in which an anesthesia clinician continually monitors and supports the patient's vital functions; diagnoses and treats clinical problems that occur; administers sedative, anxiolytic, or analgesic medications if needed; and converts to general anesthesia if required.	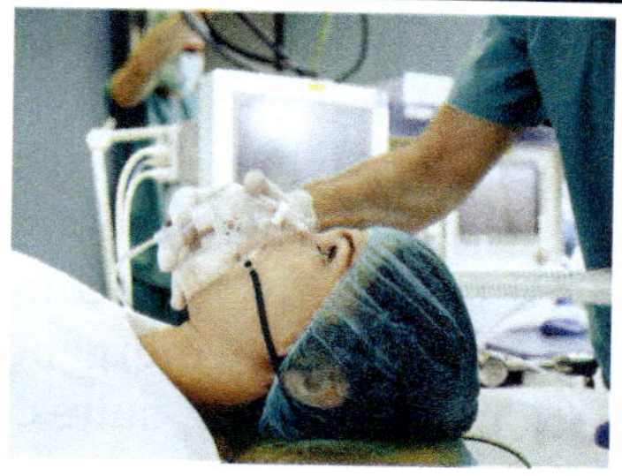
Intensive care unit (ICU)	Intensive care unit (ICU) is a special department of a hospital or health care facility that provides intensive care medicine. An ICU handles severe, potentially life-threatening cases. People who are in a serious accident, undergo major surgery, or have a sudden decline in health may get treatment from an ICU.	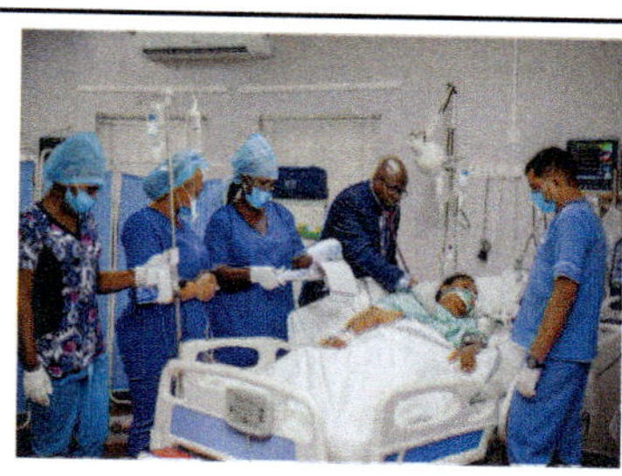
Central nervous system (CNS)	Central nervous system (CNS) is made up of the brain and spinal cord. The CNS is the body's processing center. The brain controls most of the functions of the body, including awareness, movement, thinking, speech, and the 5 senses.	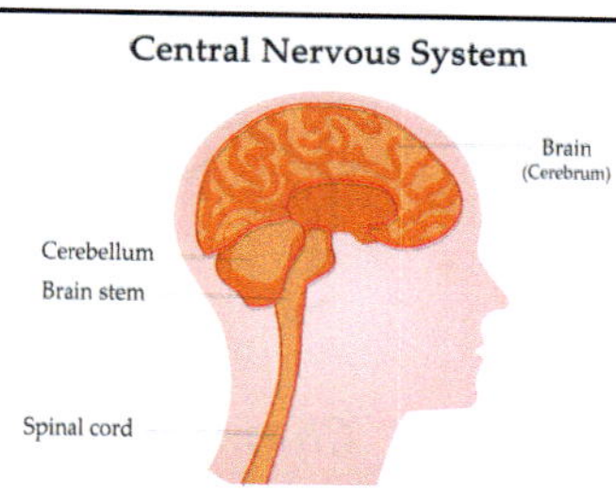
Electroencephalogram (EEG)	Electroencephalogram (EEG) is a test that measures electrical activity in the brain. This test also is called an EEG. The test uses small, metal discs called electrodes that attach to the scalp. Brain cells communicate via electrical impulses, and this activity shows up as wavy lines on an EEG recording. Brain cells are active all the time, even during sleep.	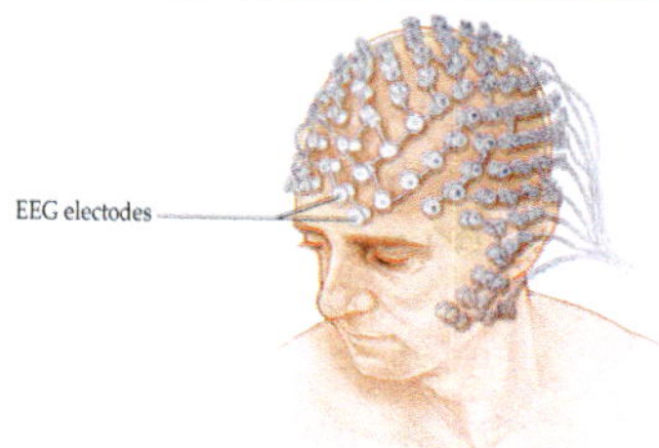
Respiratory System	Respiratory system is the organs and other parts of your body involved in breathing, when you exchange oxygen and carbon dioxide.	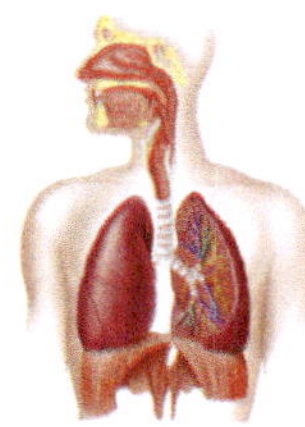

4.1. Propofol

The most commonly used anesthetic medication to induce anesthesia is propofol. Furthermore, propofol is frequently chosen for sedation in both the intensive care unit (ICU) and the operating room, where it is also used for maintaining anesthesia. Propofol is also being used more frequently in settings other than operating rooms, like emergency rooms and interventional radiology suites, for sedation and brief general anesthesia.

4.1.1. Physicochemical Characteristics

The hypnotic alkylphenol propofol (2,6-diisopropylphenol) differs chemically from other classes of intravenous anesthetics (Figure 4.1).

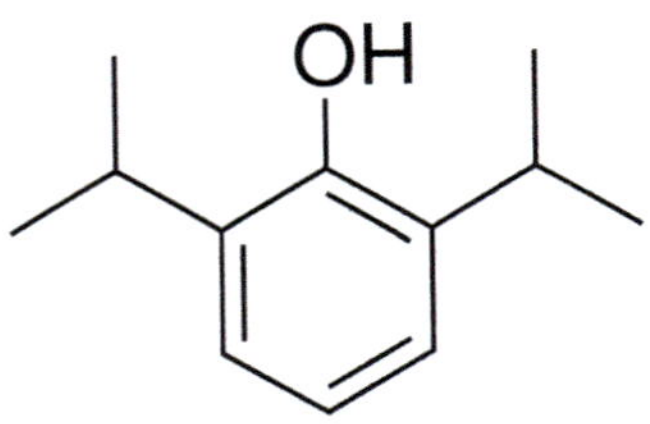

Figure 4.1. *Chemical structure of 2,6-diisopropylphenol (propofol).*

Source: By Harbin - Own work, Public Domain, https://commons.wikimedia.org/w/index.php?curid=5710636.

It is prepared as an emulsion with 10% soybean oil, 2.5% glycerol, and 1.2 percent lecithin (the main ingredient in the egg yolk phosphatide fraction), and it is insoluble in aqueous solutions. The reason the sterile technique is crucial is that the current formulations encourage the growth of bacteria. Although the various manufacturers add ethylenediaminetetraacetic acid (0.05 mg/mL), metabisulfite (0.25 mg/mL), or benzyl alcohol (1 mg/mL) to the emulsions as growth retardants for bacteria, solutions ought to be used right away, or at the very least, within 12 hours of opening the propofol vial. The pH of the solutions is roughly 7, they have a milky white appearance, and the concentration of propofol is 1% (10 mg/mL). There is a 2 percent formulation available in certain nations. Propofol allergies are uncommon, and in patients with immunoglobulin E-confirmed allergies to egg, soy, or peanuts, there is no evidence of cross-reactivity. Patients with sulfite allergies or reactive airways (asthma) should be concerned about the addition of metabisulfite in one of the formulations.

4.1.2. Pharmacokinetics

The water-soluble compounds that are produced when propofol is quickly metabolized in the liver are thought to be inert and eliminated by the kidneys. The anhepatic phase of liver transplantation has confirmed the significance of extrahepatic metabolism, as evidenced by the rapid and greater plasma clearance than hepatic blood flow. Up to 30% of a propofol bolus dose is probably eliminated by the lungs, which are also thought to play a significant role in this extrahepatic metabolism. The more thorough recovery from propofol with less "hangover" than seen with thiopental is explained by the quick plasma clearance. Propofol's effects are terminated, similar to those of other intravenous drugs, by redistribution from the plasma and highly perfused compartments (like the brain) to poorly perfused compartments (like skeletal muscle). Following an induction dose of propofol, a patient typically awakens within 8 to 10 minutes, which is comparable to the time it takes for plasma concentration to drop following a single bolus dose (Table 4.1).

Table 4.1. *Predicted Clearance of Propofol Across Age Groups*

Cardiac Output	Neonates		Infants		Children		Adolescents		Adults	
	Absolute (L/min)	Relative (%)	Absolute (L/min)	Relative (%)	Absolute (L/min)	Relative (%)	Absolute (L/min)	Relative (%)	Absolute (L/min)	Relative (%)
Normal CO	0.05 (0.02)		0.23 (0.11)		0.82 (0.35)		1.58 (0.50)		1.66 (0.45)	
20% ↓CO	0.05 (0.02)	-5.8 (2.3)	0.21 (0.10)	-8.8 (2.4)	0.73 (0.30)	-10.2 (2.2)	1.40 (0.41)	-11.3 (2.2)	1.45 (0.36)	-12.1 (2.3)
30% ↓CO	0.04 (0.018)	-9.4 (3.6)	0.20 (0.09)	-14.0 (3.7)	0.68 (0.27)	-16.2 (3.3)	1.29 (0.37)	-17.7 (3.3)	1.34 (0.32)	-19.0 (3.3)
40% ↓CO	0.04 (0.016)	-13.8 (5.0)	0.18 (0.18)	-20.1 (4.9)	0.62 (0.24)	-23.0 (4.3)	1.17 (0.32)	-25.1 (4.2)	1.21 (0.28)	-26.6 (4.3)
50% ↓CO	0.04 (0.014)	-19.2 (6.4)	0.16 (0.07)	-27.2 (6.1)	0.55 (0.21)	-30.8 (5.3)	1.04 (0.27)	-33.3 (5.0)	1.061 (0.23)	-35.1 (5.1)

CO: cardiac output; relative values were calculated relative to normal CO

Source: Allegaert K, Abbasi MY, Michelet R, Olafuyi O. The Impact of Low Cardiac Output on Propofol Pharmacokinetics across Age Groups—An Investigation Using Physiologically Based Pharmacokinetic Modelling. Pharmaceutics. 2022; 14(9):1957. https://doi.org/10.3390/pharmaceutics14091957.

4.1.2.1. Continuous Intravenous Infusion

Propofol is well suited for continuous intravenous infusion due to its two pharmacokinetic characteristics: (1) quick metabolism and effective plasma clearance; and (2) gradual redistribution from inadequately perfused compartments back into the central compartment. The "context-sensitive half-time," a measure that indicates the amount of time required for a drug's plasma levels to decrease by 50% after the infusion is stopped, can be used to describe an anesthetic infusion. The length of time an infusion has been run determines this time. Even after an extended infusion, propofol's context-sensitive half-life is short, and recovery is still rather quick.

4.1.2.2. Compartmental Model

A three-compartment model provides the best description of the kinetics of propofol (and other intravenous anesthetics) following a single bolus and following continuous infusion. Target-controlled infusion systems have been developed using these mathematical models as their foundation.

4.1.3. Pharmacodynamics

The supposed mode of action involves amplifying the chloride current, which is facilitated by the GABAA receptor complex mediating it.

4.1.3.1. Central Nervous System

Propofol has no analgesic effects and primarily functions as a hypnotic in the central nervous system (CNS). By lowering the cerebral metabolic rate for oxygen (CMRO2), it preserves the flow-metabolism coupling and lowers cerebral blood flow (CBF). Intracranial pressure (ICP), intraocular pressure, and cerebral blood volume all decrease as a result. These alterations are similar in size to those brought about by thiopental. Propofol can lower ICP as desired, but cerebral perfusion may be seriously compromised by the drug's decreased CBF and the peripheral vasodilator's decreased mean arterial pressure. In focal ischemia, propofol most likely provides the same level of neuroprotection as isoflurane or thiopental. Propofol causes burst suppression in the electroencephalogram (EEG), an endpoint that has been utilized to deliver intravenous anesthetics for neuroprotection during neurosurgical procedures, when given in large doses. Occasionally, during the propofol induction of anesthesia, excitatory effects like twitching or spontaneous movement can be seen. Propofol is an anticonvulsant that can be safely given to patients with seizure disorders, despite the fact that these effects may mimic seizure activity. No human study has shown that children who have received propofol anesthesia will experience long-term cognitive or memory problems, despite the fact that propofol may be toxic to growing neurons in animals and cell culture. (Figures 4.2 and 4.3).

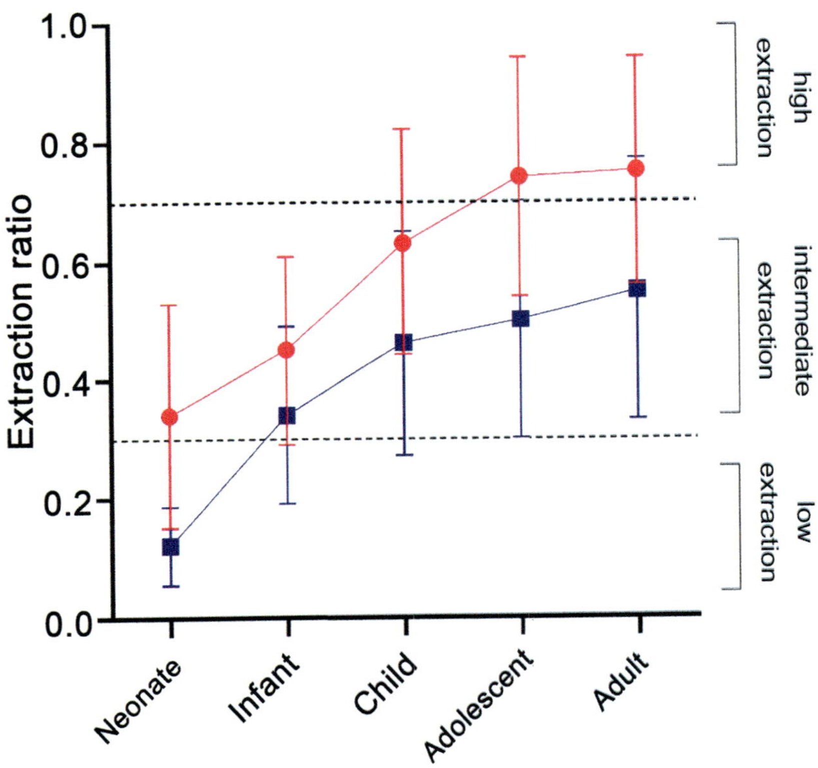

Figure 4.2. *Predicted changes in hepatic extraction ratio (EH) and renal extraction ratio (ER) with age. Red circle and line: EH; blue circle and line: ER; black broken lines: low extraction ratio target (0.3) and high extraction ratio target (0.7). Data points and error bars represent mean and standard deviations of predicted extraction ratios, respectively.*

Source: Allegaert K, Abbasi MY, Michelet R, Olafuyi O. The Impact of Low Cardiac Output on Propofol Pharmacokinetics across Age Groups—An Investigation Using Physiologically Based Pharmacokinetic Modelling. Pharmaceutics. 2022; 14(9):1957. https://doi.org/10.3390/pharmaceutics14091957.

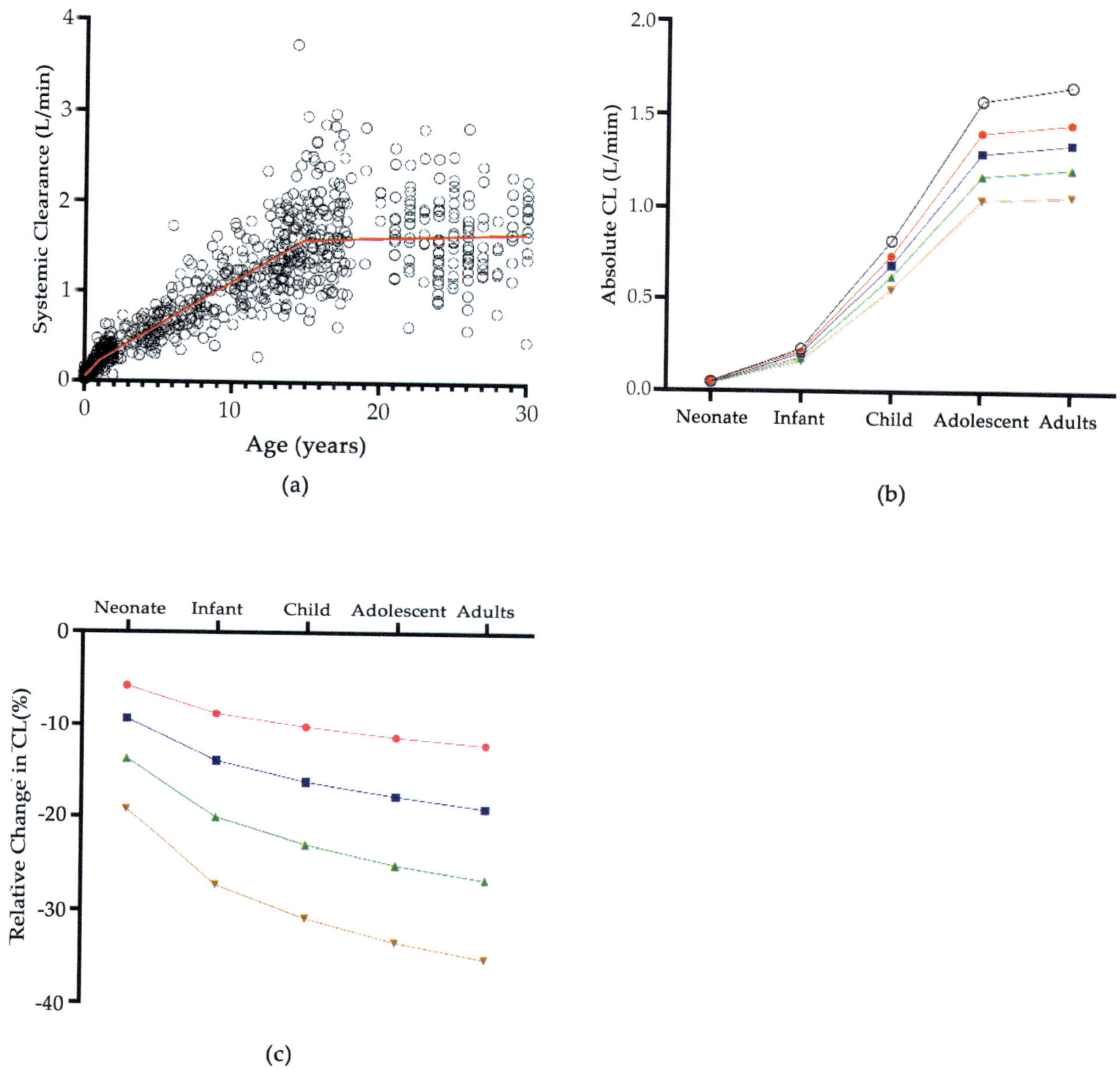

Figure 4.3. *Predicted changes in systemic clearance of propofol under normal or reduced CO conditions. (a) Predicted changes in absolute clearance with age. (b) Predicted changes in absolute clearance with age under reduced CO conditions. (c) Relative percentage changes in systemic clearance under reduced CO conditions with age. Open circles represent individual clearance in virtual subjects. (b) Absolute clearance and (c) relative change in clearance of propofol under reduced cardiac output conditions across age groups. For all Figure 2a–c, black open circle and line, red circles and line, blue squares and line, green triangle and line and brown inverted triangles and line represent clearance under normal, 20%, 30%, 40% and 50%-reduced cardiac reduction, respectively.*

Source: *From Allegaert K, Abbasi MY, Michelet R, Olafuyi O. The Impact of Low Cardiac Output on Propofol Pharmacokinetics across Age Groups—An Investigation Using Physiologically Based Pharmacokinetic Modelling. Pharmaceutics. 2022; 14(9):1957. https://doi.org/10.3390/pharmaceutics14091957.*

4.1.3.2. Cardiovascular System

When used to induce anesthesia, propofol causes the greatest decrease in systemic arterial blood pressure of any other medication. While propofol is known to cause significant vasodilation, its exact mechanism of direct myocardial depression is unknown. Preload and afterload are decreased as a result of vasodilation, which affects both the venous and arterial circulations. Rapid injection exacerbates the effect, which is more noticeable in older patients, particularly those with lower intravascular fluid volumes. Additionally, patients with diabetes, hypertension, or obesity may exhibit altered vasodilation. Propofol exacerbates hypotension by significantly suppressing the typical baroreflex response and causing little to no rise in heart rate. Even in healthy adults, the administration of prophylactic anticholinergic drugs may not prevent profound bradycardia and asystole following propofol administration.

4.1.3.3. Respiratory System

As a respiratory depressant, propofol frequently causes apnea after a dosage that is intended to induce unconsciousness. By lowering both tidal volume and respiratory rate, with a greater impact on tidal volume, a maintenance infusion of propofol reduces minute ventilation. Additionally, there is a decreased ventilatory response to hypercapnia and hypoxia. Propofol is a good choice for airway instrumentation, such as the insertion of a laryngeal mask airway, because it significantly reduces upper airway reflexes more than thiopental does. Propofol inhibits the genioglossus and other muscles, which makes the upper airway more collapsible. Airway obstruction can also happen when waking up from propofol anesthesia or at higher doses of the drug. Propofol reduces the incidence of wheezing in both healthy and asthmatic patients following tracheal intubation and induction of anesthesia when compared to thiopental.

4.1.3.4. Other Effects

Propofol exhibits antiemetic properties, in contrast to many other anesthetics. Contrary to volatile anesthetics and similar to thiopental, propofol most likely does not increase the neuromuscular blockade caused by neuromuscular blocking medications. Propofol, however, frequently offers good clinical circumstances for endotracheal intubation without the need for medications that block neuromuscular pathways. Propofol anesthesia-induced unexpected arrhythmias or changes in the electrocardiogram should be investigated in the laboratory for potential metabolic acidosis, rhabdomyolysis, or hyperkalemia (propofol infusion syndrome).

4.1.4. Clinical Uses

One common complaint that can cause patients to become distressed or dissatisfied is pain from the propofol injection. Choosing an antecubital vein for injection—a vein with a larger, faster venous flow rate—is the most efficient and quick way to lessen injection pain. As an alternative, if a hand vein is selected, it is equally effective to inject a small amount of lidocaine (20 to 40 mg IV) and apply proximal venous occlusion for 15 to 60 seconds before injecting propofol. Premedication with a small dose of opioid, pretreatment with larger doses of lidocaine (40 to 100 mg IV) without venous occlusion, and coadministration of an admixture of propofol and lidocaine are other useful and efficient methods.

4.1.4.1. Induction and Maintenance of General Anesthesia

The most often used medication to induce general anesthesia is propofol (IV, 1 to 2.5 mg/kg). The elderly, particularly those with lowered cardiovascular reserve, or those taking opioids or benzodiazepines as premedication should take less of the medication. Doses between 2.5 and 3 milligrams per kilogram IV are typically higher for children. Patients with obesity need a higher total dose than non-obese patients of comparable height and age; however, to prevent excessive hypotension, boluses for morbidly obese patients should be calculated per kilogram of lean body weight rather than total body weight. Severe hemodynamic alterations are typically avoided by titrating the propofol induction dose, as opposed to administering an arbitrary bolus dose. Additionally, propofol is frequently used in a balanced regimen in conjunction with opioids, nitrous oxide, volatile anesthetics, or sedative-hypnotics to maintain anesthesia. It is also frequently used in total intravenous anesthesia (TIVA) techniques, typically in conjunction with opioids. A small trial size and substantial patient heterogeneity make it difficult to draw firm conclusions, but some clinical trials indicate a decrease in postoperative pain scores and opioid consumption for patients receiving propofol-based TIVA as compared with volatile anesthesia. Combining therapeutic plasma concentrations with nitrous oxide or opioids, the usual range for maintaining anesthesia is 3 to 8 μg/mL, which usually requires a continuous infusion rate of 100 to 200 μg/kg/min.

4.1.4.2. Sedation

When sedating patients in the intensive care unit (ICU) or during procedures conducted within or outside of the operating room, propofol is a commonly used option. A continuous infusion rate of 25 to 75 μg/kg/min is typically necessary to achieve the required plasma concentration of 1 to 2 μg/mL. Propofol should only be given by those with training in airway management due to its strong respiratory depressant effect and limited therapeutic range. For pediatric procedures like magnetic resonance imaging scans, spontaneous ventilation is a good option because it is typically maintained in children at relatively fast propofol infusion rates (200 to 250 μg/kg/min).

4.1.4.3. Antiemetic

Postoperative nausea and vomiting (PONV) can be treated with subanesthetic bolus doses of propofol (10 to 20 mg IV, or 10 to 20 μg/kg/min as an infusion). When compared to volatile anesthetics, propofol TIVA lowers PONV but may not lower the cost of anesthesia in the ambulatory setting, post-discharge nausea and vomiting, or unplanned admissions. (Stoelting and Hillier, 2006)

4.2. Fospropofol

The most often used intravenous anesthetic for conscious sedation and MAC is propofol. It is also frequently used for anesthesia induction and maintenance. As was previously mentioned, there are some drawbacks to the lipid emulsion formulation of propofol, such as injection pain, a potential for bacterial contamination, and the possibility of hypertriglyceridemia with extended infusion. Therefore, a great deal of research has gone into developing related medications or different formulations to deal with some of these issues. An alternative called fospropofol, a water-soluble prodrug of propofol, was created, and the Food and Drug Administration (FDA) licensed it in 2008 as a sedative anesthetic for use during MAC.

4.2.1. Physicochemical Characteristics

Fospropofol, chemically described as 2,6-diisopropylphenoxymethyl phosphate disodium salt, is a water-soluble phosphate ester prodrug of propofol that was first marketed under the name GPI 15715. Propofol, phosphate, and formaldehyde are the products of alkaline phosphatase's metabolism of it. Formaldehyde is quickly metabolized by aldehyde dehydrogenase in the liver and erythrocytes to produce formate, which is then further broken down by 10-formyltetrahydrofolate dehydrogenase. Under the brand name Lusedra, a sterile, aqueous, colorless, and transparent solution containing 35 mg/mL of fospropofol is supplied in a single-dose vial.

4.2.2. Pharmacokinetics

The pharmacokinetics of fospropofol are complicated because it is a prodrug that needs to be metabolized in order to become the active ingredient, propofol. In contrast to propofol, onset and recovery are prolonged. The kinetics have been described using multicompartment models with three compartments for propofol and two for fospropofol. When compared to propofol, a fospropofol bolus should, in theory, result in lower peak plasma levels and a delayed time-to-peak. However, trustworthy data on the kinetics are lacking because earlier research on the pharmacokinetics/pharmacodynamics and tolerability of fospropofol was based on an unreliable analytical assay (Figure 4.4).

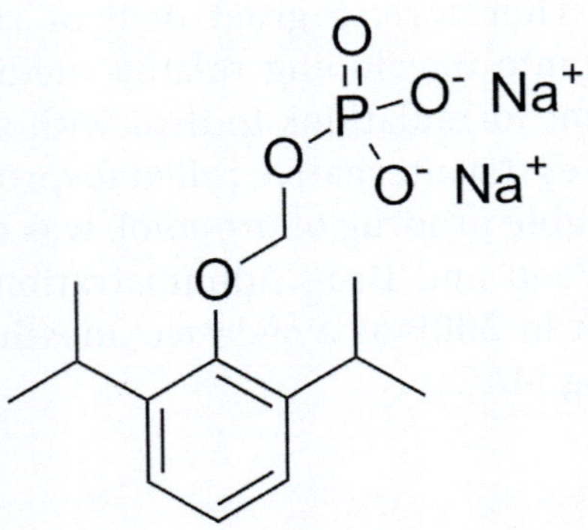

Figure 4.4. *Structure of fospropofol.*

Source: By Ed (Edgar181) - Own work, Public Domain, https://commons.wikimedia.org/w/index.php?curid=16043823.

4.2.3. Pharmacodynamics

Propofol and its effect profile are comparable. According to the previously mentioned kinetics, fospropofol ought to theoretically result in less hypotension and respiratory depression than propofol. Nevertheless, research on humans has not yet proven these advantages.

4.2.4. Clinical Uses

Currently, fospropofol is authorized for use in MAC sedation. When administered as a bolus (6.5% mg/kg IV), the duration of action is extended (5–18 min) compared to an equivalent dose of propofol, and the onset of sedation occurs more slowly (4–8 min). If necessary, repeat the dosage at a rate of 25% of the initial bolus to sustain sedation. Only patients weighing 60 to 90 kg are advised to follow these dosage guidelines, and elderly patients (age > 65) or those with physical classification III or IV according to the American Society of Anesthesiologists (ASA) are advised to reduce their dosage by 25%. Fospropofol frequently causes pruritus and a burning sensation in the perineum. Fospropofol has been shown in small trials to be safe and effective for sedation during bronchoscopies, colonoscopies, and minor surgeries. ICU sedation of patients on mechanical ventilation and fospropofol for TIVA during coronary artery bypass grafting have both been the subject of single studies. As with propofol, airway compromise is still a serious risk. Folicofol should therefore only be given by individuals who have received training in airway management. (Stoelting and Hillier, 2006).

4.3. Barbiturates

Before the development of propofol, barbiturates (thiopental and methohexital) were the most often used intravenous anesthetics for inducing anesthesia.

4.3.1. Physicochemical Characteristics

Barbiturates are produced by substituting barbituric acid (which has no hypnotic qualities) at the N1, C2, and C5 positions (Figure 4.5).

Barbiturates can be classified into thiobarbiturates, containing sulfur substitution at position 2 (such as thiopental), or oxybarbiturates, containing oxygen substitution at position 2 (such as methohexital). The effects of these drugs, including hypnotic, sedative, and anticonvulsant effects, as well as lipid solubility and onset time, are determined by the type and position of substitution.

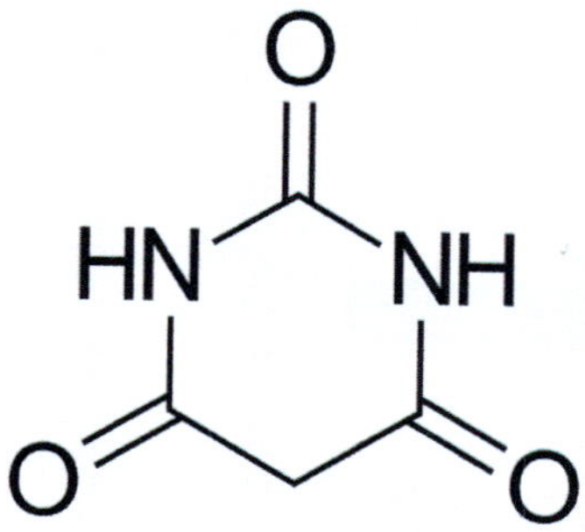

Figure 4.5. *Structure of barbiturates.*

Source: By Manuel Almagro Rivas - Own work, Public Domain, https://commons.wikimedia.org/w/index.php?curid=47183119.

Thiopental and methohexital are commonly formulated as sodium salts combined with anhydrous sodium carbonate. Once reconstituted with water or normal saline, the resulting solutions (with 2.5% thiopental and 1% methohexital) are alkaline with a pH above 10. While this alkalinity helps prevent bacterial growth and extend the shelf life of the solution after reconstitution, it can cause precipitation when mixed with acidic drugs like neuromuscular blockers. This precipitation can lead to blockages in intravenous delivery lines if mixing occurs during administration. In addition, accidental injection into an artery or infiltration into surrounding tissue can result in severe pain and tissue damage. Some barbiturates, like thiopental and methohexital, have different potency levels due to their optical isomers. However, the available formulations are racemic mixtures that reflect the combined potencies of the individual isomers.

4.3.2. Pharmacokinetics

Except for phenobarbital, barbiturates are metabolized in the liver primarily by oxidation, although they can also be metabolized by N-dealkylation, desulfuration, and breaking down the barbituric acid ring structure. Following conjugation, the inactive metabolites are eliminated through bile and urine. Phenobarbital, on the other hand, is mostly excreted unchanged by the kidneys. Barbiturate metabolism is improved by long-term barbiturate administration or by administering other medications that cause oxidative microsomal enzymes (enzyme induction). Porphyrin synthesis is enhanced by stimulating aminolevulinic acid synthetase. Barbiturates should therefore not be given to individuals who have acute intermittent porphyria.

Methohexital has a shorter half-life of elimination than thiopental because it is metabolized by the liver more quickly. This helps to explain why recovery from methohexital administration is quicker and more thorough. Recovery following a single bolus administration of thiopental is similar to that of methohexital and propofol despite the drug's slow metabolism and lengthy elimination half-life. This is because thiopental's mechanism of action is redistribution to inactive tissue sites rather than metabolism. Nevertheless, thiopental induction dosages as low as one bolus may occasionally cause psychomotor impairment that lasts for several hours. Thiopental's long context-sensitive half-time means that recovery from its effects will be significantly prolonged if given as repeated boluses or as a continuous infusion, particularly when using larger doses to produce burst suppression on the EEG.

4.3.3. Pharmacodynamics

Barbiturates are thought to work by enhancing inhibitory neurotransmission and inhibiting excitatory transmission in the central nervous system. The effects on excitatory transmission are less clear, but the effects on inhibitory transmission most likely stem from the activation of the $GABA_A$ receptor complex. Pentameric $GABA_A$ receptors can be found at synapses and extrasynaptic sites. They can consist of various subunit combinations (refer to the Benzodiazepines section for more information). The presence of multiple distinct $GABA_A$-mediated current types in the central nervous system (CNS) could be explained by the variation in their location and composition (fast versus slow, phasic versus tonic). Certain types of $GABA_A$ receptors may be selectively targeted by different intravenous anesthetics (Figure 4.6).

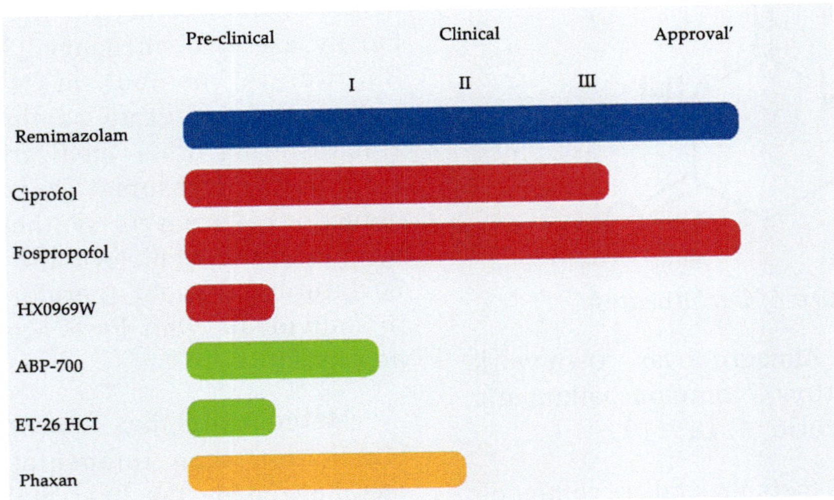

Figure 4.6. *Overview of novel hypnotics and their current status in drug development. 1 By the food and drug administration. blue: benzodiazepine derivative. red: propofol derivatives. green: etomidate derivatives. orange: steroid.*

Source: Vellinga R, Valk BI, Absalom AR, Struys MMRF, Barends CRM. What's New in Intravenous Anaesthesia? New Hypnotics, New Models and New Applications. Journal of Clinical Medicine. 2022; 11(12):3493. https://doi.org/10.3390/jcm11123493.

4.3.3.1. Central Nervous System

If barbiturates are used in induction doses, the CNS is lowered in a dose-dependent manner resulting in sedation or general anesthesia. They may even lower the pain threshold and lack analgesic qualities, so they might be categorized as anti-analgesics. As strong cerebral vasoconstrictors, barbiturates cause consistent drops in cerebral blood volume, ICP, and CBF. Therefore, they reduce CMRO2 until the EEG exhibits a flat line in a dose-dependent manner. Barbiturates can be used to treat patients with space-occupying intracranial lesions because of their capacity to lower ICP and CMRO2. Moreover, they might offer neuroprotection against localized cerebral ischemia (heart attack, surgical retraction, temporary clips during aneurysm surgery), but most likely not against generalized cerebral ischemia (heart attack). Barbiturates can reduce ICP after traumatic brain injury, but doing so is not warranted because the resulting hypotension may worsen outcomes and jeopardize cerebral perfusion pressure. While intravenous infusions may be helpful in the critical care setting to treat refractory status epilepticus (usually third-line therapy after midazolam and propofol have failed), most barbiturates also decrease electrical activity on the EE.G.Methohexital is an exception to this rule since it allows epileptic foci to be identified during surgery intended to ablate these sites by activating them. Methohexital is a common anesthetic option for electroconvulsive therapy for the same reason.

4.3.3.2. Cardiovascular System

When barbiturates are used to induce anesthesia, systemic arterial blood pressure usually drops somewhat, but not as much as when propofol is used. This decrease in systemic arterial blood pressure is primarily caused by peripheral vasodilation, which is a reflection of decreased sympathetic nervous system outflow from the central nervous system and barbiturate-induced depression of the medullary vasomotor center. Barbiturates suppress the baroreceptor reflex, but the amount and duration of hypotension are limited by compensatory heart rate increases. Furthermore, blood pooling and a decrease in venous return are caused by dilation of peripheral capacitance vessels, which lowers systemic arterial blood pressure and cardiac output. In fact, because these patients are less able to compensate for the effects of peripheral vasodilation, exaggerated drops in blood pressure are likely to occur after barbiturates are administered to patients with hypovolemia, cardiac tamponade, cardiomyopathy, coronary artery disease, or cardiac valvular disease. Larger doses and quicker injection times also have more noticeable hemodynamic effects. Barbiturates have detrimental inotropic effects that are easily shown in isolated heart preparations but are typically obscured in vivo by responses mediated by baroreceptor reflexes.

4.3.3.3. Respiratory System

Because barbiturates are respiratory depressants, their smaller tidal volumes and respiratory rates result in decreased minute ventilation. Thiopental and methohexital anesthetic induction doses usually cause transient apnea, which is more noticeable when other respiratory depressants are present. Barbiturates also lessen the response of the ventilator to hypoxia and hypercapnia. A sluggish breathing rate and a reduced tidal volume indicate the return of spontaneous breathing following a barbiturate anesthetic induction dose. Barbiturates are not as effective as propofol in suppressing cough and laryngeal reflexes, which makes them a poor option for airway instrumentation when neuromuscular blocking medications are not available. Moreover, laryngospasm or bronchospasm may arise from stimulation of the upper airway or trachea (secretions, laryngeal mask airway, direct laryngoscopy, tracheal intubation) when airway reflexes are not sufficiently depressed. This phenomenon occurs generally when the anesthetic dose is insufficient to suppress the airway reflexes; it is not specific to barbiturates.

4.3.4. Side Effects

An accidental intra-arterial injection of barbiturates causes severe pain and severe vasoconstriction, which frequently results in gangrene or other severe tissue damage. To preserve perfusion and lower the drug concentration through dilution, aggressive therapy aims to reverse vasoconstriction. Stellate ganglion block is one method of treating the affected extremity by blocking the sympathetic nervous system. Small-diameter arterioles that are distal are likely to become occluded as a result of barbiturate crystal formation. The growing diameter of veins makes crystal formation in veins less dangerous. It is important to use diluted concentrations of barbiturates (2 percent thiopental and 1 percent methohexital) because accidental subcutaneous injection (extravasation) of these drugs can cause local tissue irritation. Some advise injecting 0.5 percent lidocaine (5 to 10 mL) locally into the tissues in the event of extravasation to lessen the concentration of barbiturates. Life-threatening allergic reactions to barbiturates are rare, with an estimated occurrence of 1 in 30,000 patients. However, barbiturate-induced histamine release is occasionally seen.

4.3.5. Clinical Uses

Barbiturates are primarily used in medicine to treat elevated intracranial pressure, induce anesthesia quickly intravenously, and protect against focal cerebral ischemia. Because of its lengthy context-sensitive half-life and drawn-out recovery period, a continuous intravenous infusion of a barbiturate, like thiopental, is rarely used to maintain anesthesia. Extended infusions used to induce a "barbiturate coma" for neuroprotection may lead to hypo- and hyperkalemia, hypothermia, and immunological suppression.

4.3.5.1. Induction of Anesthesia

In less than 30 seconds, thiopental (3 to 5 mg/kg IV) or methohexital (1 to 1.5 mg/kg IV) administration results in unconsciousness. When anesthesia is induced, patients may taste garlic or onions. Compared to propofol, methohexital may allow for longer seizure durations when used as an anesthetic for electroconvulsive therapy. Sugammadex, a medication that reverses rocuronium neuromuscular blockade, may make methohexital and rocuronium a more popular combination of anesthetics for electroconvulsive therapy. Several methods of inducing anesthesia can be used to demonstrate the usefulness of barbiturates.

After a barbiturate, succinylcholine or a nondepolarizing neuromuscular blocking medication is frequently given to induce skeletal muscle relaxation and aid in tracheal intubation. When a patient is more likely to aspirate stomach contents, the anesthesia provider may decide to perform a "rapid-sequence induction" of anesthesia. A barbiturate, typically thiopental, is administered first for rapid-sequence induction, and then succinylcholine is given in quick succession. The avoidance of bag-mask ventilation and the early tracheal intubation with a cuffed tube are significant benefits of this technique. Propofol is now the medication of choice for rapid-sequence induction, though thiopental was once the standard medication.

For patients not at risk of aspiration, intravenous barbiturates can be used to start a gradual induction of anesthesia. Thiopental in small doses (0.5 to 1.0 mg/kg IV) can help patients accept a face mask and avoid unpleasant memories of strong-smelling anesthetics. The induction can be completed with inhaled sevoflurane. This slow induction method allows for careful adjustment of anesthesia levels and prevents extreme changes in blood pressure. Alternatively, a gradual induction can be achieved using intravenous anesthetics alone, with propofol being a better choice due to its shorter half-life. In mentally challenged or uncooperative pediatric patients, rectal administration of methohexital (20 to 30 mg/kg) can aid in anesthesia induction.

4.3.5.2. Neuroprotection

Barbiturates have historically been titrated to produce an isoelectric EEG, an end point that denotes the maximum reduction of $CMRO_2$, when used for neuroprotection. Recent evidence that shows the same level of protection at lower doses has called into question this approach. One risk associated with using high-dose barbiturate therapy to lower intracranial pressure (ICP) or protect against focal cerebral ischemia (carotid endarterectomy, thoracic aneurysm resection, cardiopulmonary bypass) is the associated hypotension, which can critically lower cerebral perfusion pressure and necessitate the use of vasoconstrictors to keep systemic arterial blood pressure stable.

Barbiturates did not prevent permanent neurologic dysfunction in a large registry of patients undergoing repair for acute type A aortic dissection, and it is unlikely that these medications will be helpful during cardiac surgery. (Stoelting and Hillier, 2006)

4.4. Benzodiazepines

Flumazenil is a selective benzodiazepine antagonist that is frequently used in conjunction with diazepam, midazolam, and lorazepam during the perioperative period. Among intravenous anesthetics, benzodiazepines are distinct in that their action can be easily stopped by administering flumazenil, a selective antagonist. Anxiolysis and anterograde amnesia are their most sought-after effects, and they are very helpful for premedication.

4.4.1. Physicochemical Characteristics

Benzodiazepines are compounds that consist of a benzene ring fused to a seven-member diazepine ring, which gives them their name. The three benzodiazepines commonly used in the perioperative setting are highly lipophilic, with midazolam being the most lipid-soluble. These drugs are primarily bound to serum albumin in the body. While they are often given through injections, they can also be taken orally and through other routes such as intramuscular, intranasal, and sublingual administration. When the acidic midazolam formula comes into contact with the blood's pH level, its structure changes to become more lipid-soluble, allowing it to cross the blood-brain barrier quickly and take effect faster.

4.4.2. Pharmacokinetics

The quick onset of action of the highly lipid-soluble benzodiazepines can be attributed to their quick entry into the central nervous system (CNS), which is also responsible for their redistribution to inactive tissue sites and eventual cessation of the drug effect. In the liver, benzodiazepines are metabolized by glucuronide conjugation and microsomal oxidation (N-dealkylation and aliphatic hydroxylation). The main metabolic route for midazolam and diazepam, known as microsomal oxidation, is more vulnerable to outside influences like aging, illnesses (such as hepatic cirrhosis), and the use of other medications that alter the function of the enzyme systems. One of the rare benzodiazepines that is eliminated by a single-step conjugation to glucuronic acid rather than going through oxidative metabolism is lorazepam. Diazepam is metabolized by the liver to produce the active metabolites desmethyldiazepam and oxazepam, which may help explain why the drug's effects last longer. On the other hand, hepatic cytochrome P450 3A4 selectively breaks down midazolam into a single, dominant metabolite called 1-hydroxymidazolam. 1-hydroxymidazolam is quickly glucuronidated and cleared from the body, but it retains the same sedative properties as the parent compound. Patients with normal hepatic and renal function do not experience significant sedation from this metabolite unless they receive a prolonged infusion of midazolam. Moreover, as previously mentioned, midazolam's lipid solubility and quick redistribution account for its brief duration of action after a single dose. Midazolam is thought to have a slower effect-site equilibration time than propofol and thiopental, despite its rapid onset of action in the brain. In this sense, midazolam intravenous doses ought to be spaced sufficiently apart to allow for the identification of the peak clinical effect before considering a repeat dose (Figure 4.7).

The effects of Diazepam on the CNS effects are prolonged, especially in elderly patients, which can be explained by the fact that its elimination half-time is significantly longer than that of midazolam. With the shortest context-sensitive halftime among the three frequently used intravenous benzodiazepines, midazolam is the most appropriate drug for continuous infusion. Remimazolam (CNS-7056), a novel ultrashort-acting benzodiazepine, has just started clinical trials. Similar to remifentanil, remimazolam has a carboxylic ester group that tissue esterases quickly hydrolyze. Remimazolam exhibits a lower volume of distribution, faster clearance, and clearance that is not dependent on body weight when compared to midazolam. Remimazolam's metabolite has a GABAA affinity that is more than 400 times lower than CNS-7056, meaning that it is unlikely to produce sedation that is clinically meaningful. Remimazolam is a potentially less prolonged sedative than midazolam due to its kinetic characteristics; this is especially true for patients with liver disease or those on cytochrome P450-inhibiting medications.

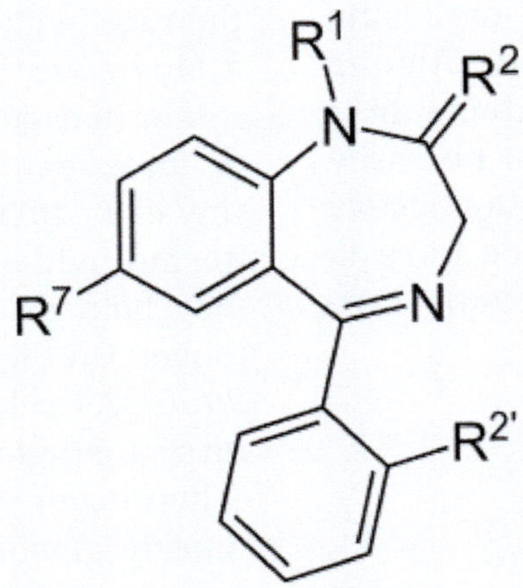

Figure 4.7. *Chemical structure of benzodiazepine.*

Source: https://en.wikipedia.org/wiki/File:Benzodiazepine.svg.

4.4.3. Pharmacodynamics

Benzodiazepines cause neurons to become hyperpolarized and less excitable by activating the $GABA_A$ receptor complex and increasing GABA-mediated chloride currents. $GABA_A$ receptors have particular binding sites for benzodiazepines, which explains why these receptors were first referred to as "benzodiazepine receptors." Midazolam has about twice the affinity of diazepam for $GABA_A$ receptors, which is consistent with its higher potency. Almost all postsynaptic nerve endings in the central nervous system (CNS) have $GABA_A$ receptors that are sensitive to benzodiazepines; the cerebral cortex has the highest density of these receptors. The minimal effects of benzodiazepines outside of the central nervous system are consistent with the anatomic distribution of $GABA_A$ receptors, which are restricted to the CNS. In fact, when benzodiazepines are administered, there is less of a decrease in ventilation depression and the development of hypotension than when barbiturates are used to induce anesthesia.

4.4.3.1. Spectrum of Effects

While the specific potencies of each drug in this class may differ, all benzodiazepines share a similar wide range of effects. The two main effects of benzodiazepines are amnestic (anterograde, but not retrograde) amnesia and their sedative-hypnotic action. Benzodiazepines are also used to treat seizures and have an anticonvulsant effect. While anxiolysis and muscle relaxation are mediated by the γ-subunits of the GABA receptor, these effects are mediated by the α-subunits.

The spinal cord is the site of action for muscle relaxation, and much higher doses are needed to achieve this effect (Figure 4.8).

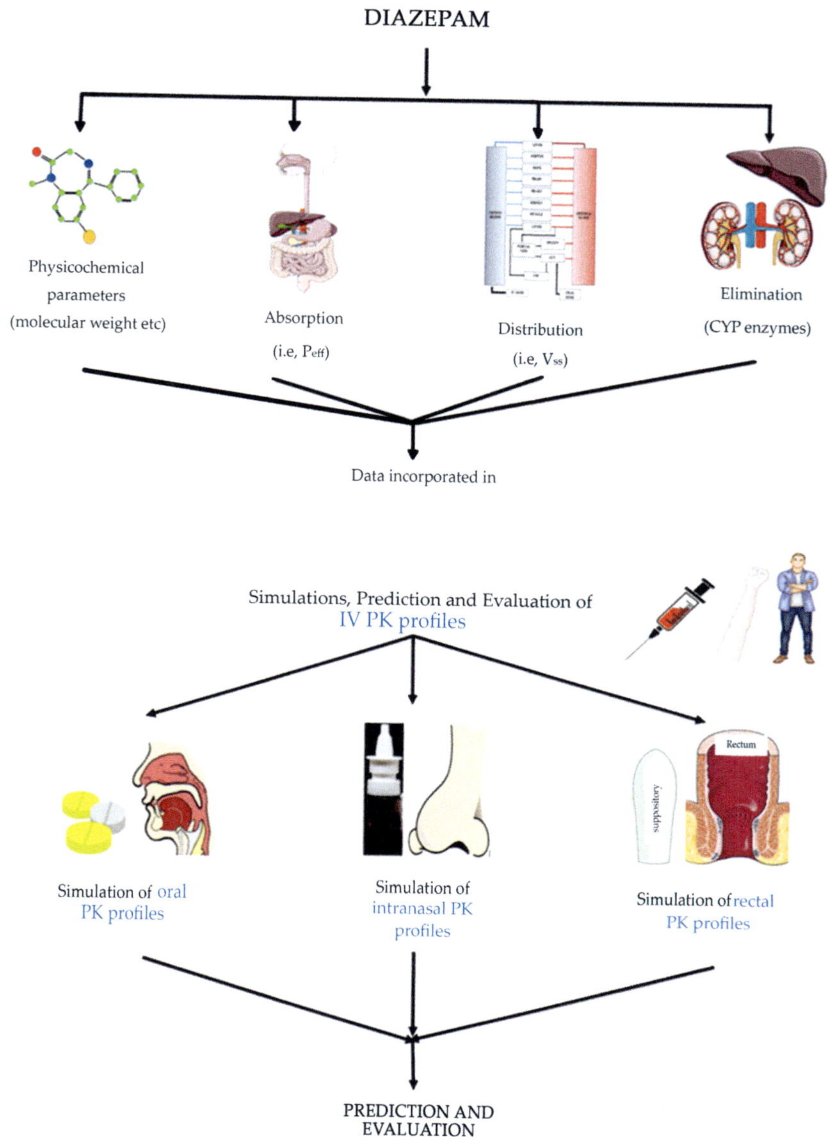

Figure 4.8. *Diazepam pharmacokinetics.*

Source: Khalid S, Rasool MF, Imran I, Majeed A, Saeed H, Rehman Au, Ashraf W, Ahmad T, Bin Jardan YA, Alqahtani F. A Physiologically Based Pharmacokinetic Model for Predicting Diazepam Pharmacokinetics after Intravenous, Oral, Intranasal, and Rectal Applications. Pharmaceutics. 2021; 13(9):1480. https://doi.org/10.3390/pharmaceutics13091480.

4.4.3.2. Safety Profile

The profile of the side effects is remarkably favorable. Even at higher dosages, these medications are generally safe because they only slightly impair breathing and the cardiovascular system when taken by themselves. Moreover, flumazenil, a selective benzodiazepine antagonist, can counteract the central nervous system effects, increasing the margin of safety.

4.4.3.3. Central Nervous System

Benzodiazepines decrease $CMRO_2$ and CBF, albeit less so than barbiturates and propofol. Midazolam does not cause an isoelectric EEG, in contrast to propofol and thiopental, highlighting the fact that benzodiazepines have a ceiling effect on the reduction of $CMRO_2$. After midazolam is administered, patients with reduced intracranial compliance show little to no change in ICP. It has not been demonstrated that benzodiazepines have neuroprotective qualities. They are effective anticonvulsants used to treat alcohol withdrawal, seizures brought on by local anesthetics, and status epilepticus.

4.4.3.4. Cardiovascular System

Midazolam causes a greater drop in arterial blood pressure than diazepam when used to induce anesthesia. Given that cardiac output is unaffected, these alterations are most likely the result of peripheral vasodilation. Hypovolemic patients are more susceptible to midazolam-induced hypotension.

4.4.3.5. Respiratory System

Although transient apnea may occur after fast intravenous midazolam induction of anesthesia, particularly in the presence of opioid premedication, benzodiazepines cause minimal depression of ventilation. When taken by themselves, benzodiazepines typically have little effect on the ventilatory response to carbon dioxide. When given with opioids, benzodiazepines can cause more severe respiratory depression.

4.4.4. Side Effects

Benzodiazepine allergies are extremely rare or nonexistent. Diazepam's poor water solubility is reflected in its most pronounced pain during intravenous injection and subsequent thrombophlebitis. Most likely, the cause of pain during intramuscular or intravenous administration of diazepam, as well as the irregular absorption following intramuscular injection, is the organic solvent propylene glycol, which is needed to dissolve the medication. The higher water solubility of midazolam (but only at low pH) eliminates the need for an organic solvent and lowers the risk of excessive pain or irregular absorption following intramuscular injection or pain during intravenous administration (Table 4.2).

Table 4.2. *Pharmacokinetic and Pharmacodynamic Parameters of Established Hypnotic Agents and New Hypnotic Agents in the Clinical Phase of Drug Development. PONV = Postoperative Nausea and Vomiting. Data after an Established Induction Bolus Dose. Values are Represented as Ranges or Mean ± SD. o is no Effect, -- Strong Negative, - Less Negative, ++ Strong Positive, + Positive, ? is Unknown*

	Mechanism of Action	Elimination Half-Life (min)	Clearance ($mLkg^{-1}min^{-1}$)	Vdss ($L\ kg^{-1}$)	Time to Onset (s)	Effect on							Reversal with Flumazenil	Significant Side Effects
						Heart Rate	Blood Pressure	Respiration	Amnesia	PONV	Analgesia	Pain on Injection		
Propofol [2]	$GABA_A$ receptor	116–834	25.4–32.6	2.27–11	<30	o	--	--	++	--	o	++	o	Propofol infusion syndrome
Etomidate [3]	$GABA_A$ receptor	174–330	9.9–25.0	0.15–4.7	<30	o	o	o		+	o	+	o	Adrenal suppression; Excitation
Ketamine [4]	NMDA receptor	120–240	14.3–35.0	2.28–7.86	<60	++	++	o	+	-	++	o	o	Psychedelic effects, Elevated Intracranial pressure
Midazolam [5]	$GABA_A$ receptor	102–156	6.4–11	1.1–1.7	120–180	+	-	+	++	+	o	o	+	
Remimazolam [6,7]	$GABA_A$ receptor	70 ± 10	1.15 ± 0.12	35.4 ± 4.2	60–90	+	-	+	++	+	o	o	+	
Ciprofol [8]	$GABA_A$ receptor	105.6–125.3	21.7–24.6	3.6–4.3	60–120	-	-	?	?	o	?	o	o	
ABP-700 [3,9]	$GABA_A$ receptor	13.1–16.2	27.8	?	<30	+	+	+	?	+	o	o	o	
Phaxan [10,11]	$GABA_A$ receptor	?	15.4	0.38	<60	o	-	o	?	o	?	o	o	

Source: *Vellinga R, Valk BI, Absalom AR, Struys MMRF, Barends CRM. What's New in Intravenous Anaesthesia? New Hypnotics, New Models and New Applications. Journal of Clinical Medicine. 2022; 11(12):3493. https://doi.org/10.3390/jcm11123493.*

4.4.5. Clinical Uses

Preoperative medicine, intravenous sedation, intravenous induction of anesthesia, and seizure activity suppression are the four uses of benzodiazepines. Lorazepam's slow onset and prolonged duration of action make it less effective for preoperative medication or inducing anesthesia, particularly when it's preferable to awaken slowly and steadily after surgery. Flumazenil (8 to 15 µg/kg IV) may help patients who are having trouble waking up slowly, but it takes about 20 minutes to start working and can make you drowsy.

4.4.5.1. Preoperative Medication and Sedation

Benzodiazepines are used as preoperative medication because of their sedative, anxiolytic, and amnestic properties. For premedication, sedation during regional anesthesia, and short therapeutic procedures, midazolam (1 to 2 mg IV) works well. When combined with propofol sedation for a colonoscopy, midazolam may enhance operating conditions without delaying recovery or exacerbating post-discharge cognitive impairment. Midazolam causes less postoperative sedation, more intense amnesia, and a quicker onset than diazepam. When given midazolam before surgery, many patients have trouble remembering the operating room, and some even forget about the preoperative holding area. When educating patients and their families before surgery, anesthesiologists and surgeons alike should be cognizant of this fact. Barbiturates and ketamine appear to be inferior to benzodiazepines in preventing recall, even though awareness during anesthesia is uncommon. Children are frequently given oral premedication with midazolam. For instance, giving children 0.5 mg/kg orally 30 minutes before the induction of anesthesia reliably induces sedation and anxiolysis without causing delayed awakening. Additionally, midazolam reduces the frequency of PONV. The routine use of benzodiazepines as premedication for elective surgery may not improve patient experience, despite these potential advantages.

The combination of benzodiazepines with other medications, particularly opioids and propofol, has a synergistic effect that improves sedation and acute pain relief. However, taking these medications together also makes respiratory depression worse and increases the risk of apnea or airway blockage. Due to their adverse effects on pharyngeal function and the synchronization of breathing and swallowing, these medications may also raise the risk of aspiration of stomach contents. Smaller dosages and cautious titration may be required for benzodiazepines due to their more pronounced effects and synergistic effects with other respiratory depressants in the elderly. When giving benzodiazepines to critically ill patients who are on mechanical ventilation for sedation, care should be taken because these drugs have been associated with increased delirium and longer ICU stays than other regimens (propofol or dexmedetomidine).

4.4.5.2. Induction of Anesthesia

Although it is rarely used for this purpose, midazolam (0.1 to 0.3 mg/kg IV) can be used to induce general anesthesia. On the other hand, compared to when thiopental, propofol, or etomidate are administered, the onset of unconsciousness is delayed. A small dose of opioid (fentanyl, 50 to 100 µg IV) injected one to three minutes prior to midazolam administration facilitates the onset of unconsciousness. It is unlikely that using midazolam or diazepam to induce anesthesia has any advantages over barbiturates or propofol, even though they might have less circulatory effects. One potential drawback following a benzodiazepine induction dose is delayed awakening.

4.4.5.3. Suppression of Seizure Activity

Benzodiazepines are effective anticonvulsants because they can increase GABA's inhibitory effects, especially in the limbic system. In fact, the effects of local anesthetics or alcohol withdrawal on seizure activity are frequently eliminated by administering 0.1 mg/kg IV diazepam. The preferred intravenous benzodiazepine for status epilepticus is lorazepam (0.01 mg/kg IV). You may also use 0.5 mg/kg IV of diazepam. Intramuscular (IM) administration of midazolam (10 mg IM for patients > 40 kg; 5 mg IM for patients 13 to 40 kg) is a useful and faster method for treating status epilepticus before hospitalization, as it can potentially reduce the need for hospital stays. (Stoelting and Hillier, 2006).

4.5. Ketamine

Ketamine is an intravenous anesthetic that differs from most others in that it produces a significant analgesic effect. It is a derivative of phencyclidine and was approved by the FDA for clinical use in 1970. "Dissociative anesthesia" refers to the distinct cataleptic state that results from a ketamine induction dosage, during which the patient's eyes stay open and they gaze slowly in a nystagmic manner (Figure 4.9).

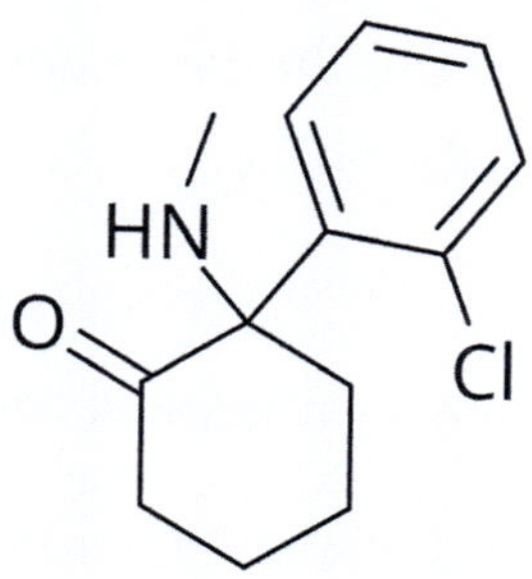

Figure 4.9. *Chemical structure of ketamine.*

Source: By Brenton (talk) - Own work, Public Domain, https://commons.wikimedia.org/w/index.php?curid=61854564.

4.5.1. Physicochemical Characteristics

Ketamine is a derivative of phencyclidine that is highly lipidsoluble and partially water-soluble. Its lipid solubility is five to ten times greater than that of thiopental. The S(+) isomer of the two stereoisomers has greater potency than the R(−) isomer. In the US, there is only one ketamine racemic mixture (10, 50, and 100 mg/mL) available. Ketamine was initially recognized as a safe anesthetic and was used for a while. Ketamine's use in anesthesia has been restricted due to its unpleasant psychomimetic side effects, and its popularity has since declined. However, ketamine's special qualities (strong analgesia with little respiratory depression) make it a very useful substitute in some situations. In recent times, it has gained popularity as an adjuvant for treating major depression and limiting or reversing opioid tolerance when given at subanalgesic doses.

4.5.2. Pharmacokinetics

The high lipid solubility guarantees an immediate onset of action. The effect of a single bolus injection is terminated by redistribution to inactive tissue sites, similar to other intravenous induction drugs. The cytochrome P-450 system is involved in N-demethylation during metabolism, which mostly takes place in the liver. The main active metabolite, norketamine, is conjugated into water-soluble inactive metabolites that are eliminated in urine after being hydroxylated. Norketamine has a potency that is one-third to one-fifth that of ketamine. The only intravenous anesthetic with a low protein binding percentage (12%) is ketamine.

4.5.3. Pharmacodynamics

Although the mode of action is multifaceted, its primary anesthetic effect stems from blocking the N-methyl-d-aspartate (NMDA) receptor complex. Amnesia is not as complete when ketamine is used as the only anesthetic as it is when benzodiazepines are used. Although reflexes are frequently maintained, it is not a given that patients can keep their upper airway safe. The pupils are slightly dilated with a nystagmic gaze, and the eyes stay open. Premedication with an anticholinergic medication may be indicated to limit the frequently increased lacrimation and salivation.

4.5.3.1. Emergence Reactions

The primary factor restricting ketamine use is the unpleasant emergence reactions following administration. These reactions can include increased and distorted visual, tactile, and auditory sensitivity, vivid colorful dreams, hallucinations, and out-of-body experiences. These responses may be linked to feelings of uncertainty and terror. The drug's potential for abuse is explained by the possibility of inducing a euphoric state. The occurrence of severe emergence reactions is generally lower in children. Combining ketamine with benzodiazepines may help reduce unpleasant emergence reactions while simultaneously enhancing amnesia.

4.5.3.2. Central Nervous System

Ketamine is a cerebral vasodilator that raises both CBF and $CMRO_2$, in contrast to other intravenous anesthetics. As a result, patients with intracranial diseases—especially those with elevated ICP—usually avoid ketamine. However, maintaining normocapnia and implementing controlled ventilation may mitigate the negative effects on CBF. Although ketamine has the potential to cause myoclonic activity, it is regarded as an anticonvulsant and may be used to treat status epilepticus in cases where more traditional medications are not working.

4.5.3.3. Cardiovascular System

Ketamine can raise heart rate, cardiac output, and systemic arterial blood pressure significantly but momentarily; this effect is likely the result of centrally mediated sympathetic stimulation. The coadministration of benzodiazepines, opioids, or inhaled anesthetics can mitigate these undesirable effects, which are linked to increased cardiac work and myocardial oxygen consumption. Ketamine is a direct myocardial depressant, despite being more debatable about it. Its stimulation of the sympathetic nervous system usually masks this property, but in critically ill patients, where the ability to increase sympathetic nervous system activity is limited, it may become noticeable.

4.5.3.4. Respiratory System

There is no discernible respiratory depression caused by ketamine. When taken by itself, the medication preserves the respiratory response to hypercapnia and keeps arterial blood gases steady. Rapid intravenous administration of large doses for the induction of anesthesia may result in transient hypoventilation and, in rare cases, a brief period of apnea. Even though there are active airway reflexes, it is not always possible to protect the upper airway when ketamine is present. Anticholinergic medication given ahead of time can lessen the risk of laryngospasm in children, as a result of increased salivation. Ketamine relaxes the smooth muscles in the bronchi, which makes it useful for treating bronchoconstriction and reactive airway patients.

4.5.4. Clinical Uses

Ketamine's usage as a general anesthetic has been limited due to the unpleasant emergence reactions that follow its administration. Nevertheless, ketamine is a valuable substitute for other intravenous anesthetics and a preferred adjunct in many situations due to its special qualities, which include strong analgesia, sympathetic nervous system stimulation, bronchodilation, and minimal respiratory depression. Additionally, ketamine can be given intravenously, intramuscularly, orally, rectally, or epidurally, which makes it a practical choice for premedication in children who are mentally challenged and uncooperative.

4.5.4.1. Induction and Maintenance of Anesthesia

Ketamine can be used to induce anesthesia at a dose of 1 to 2 mg/kg IV or 4 to 6 mg/kg IM. Although it is not frequently used, ketamine should be taken into consideration for the context-sensitive short half-life of anesthesia maintenance. For instance, ketamine alone (30 to 90 μg/kg/min) or in combination with 50–70% nitrous oxide (15 to 45 μg/kg/min) can be used to induce general anesthesia.

4.5.4.2. Analgesia

When additional analgesia is required during regional anesthesia (such as during a cesarean section under neuraxial anesthesia with an inadequate regional block), small bolus doses of ketamine (0.02 to 0.08 mg/kg IV) may be helpful. Effective analgesia is achieved with ketamine without compromising airway integrity. While not all studies investigating the use of ketamine as an adjunct show the desired improvement in pain scores and recovery, an infusion of a subanalgesic dose of ketamine (3 to 5 μg/kg/min) during general anesthesia and in the early postoperative period may be useful to produce analgesia or reduce opioid tolerance and opioid-induced hyperalgesia. The topical and local administration of ketamine seems like a sensible strategy that could enable the achievement of higher local tissue concentrations to prevent undesirable CNS effects because peripheral nociceptors have NMDA receptors. Nevertheless, compelling data from controlled trials is scarce, and case reports are the primary source of current support for this modality.

4.5.4.3. Treatment of Major Depression

As a treatment option for major depression that is resistant to conventional methods, ketamine has gained more and more attention lately. For the reduction of depressive symptoms in less than 24 hours, a single intravenous infusion of ketamine (0.05 mg/kg over 40 minutes) was found to be superior to midazolam. For treatment-resistant patients, the dose, timing, and frequency of treatments are optimized, ketamine may help maintain the antidepressant effects. (Stoelting and Hillier, 2006)

4.6. Etomidate

Etomidate is an intravenous anesthetic that has minimal hemodynamic effects and hypnotic but not analgesic effects. Etomidate is not commonly used due to its endocrine side effects, despite its pharmacokinetics making it suitable for continuous infusion use.

4.6.1. Physicochemical Characteristics

Etomidate is a derivative of carboxylated imidazole with two optical isomers. The only active D(+) isomer in the preparation that is currently available has hypnotic qualities. Due to the medication's low water solubility, it is supplied as a 2 mg/mL solution in 35% propylene glycol. Because of its pH of 6:9, the solution does not lead to precipitation issues like thiopental does.

4.6.2. Pharmacokinetics

Redistribution to inactive tissue sites is necessary for recovery after an etomidate induction dose, which results in a fast onset of anesthesia (similar to thiopental and propofol). The majority of metabolism occurs in the liver via ester hydrolysis, producing inactive metabolites that are subsequently eliminated as bile (22 percent) and urine (78 percent). The amount of etomidate that is eliminated unaltered from the urine is less than 3% of the dose that is given. A shorter elimination half-time indicates that etomidate is cleared roughly five times faster than thiopental. The duration of action is directly proportional to the dose, with approximately 100 seconds of unconsciousness being provided by every 0.1 mg/kg. Larger doses, repeated boluses, or continuous infusions can be safely administered due to its short context-sensitive half-time and negligible effects on hemodynamics. Etomidate exhibits high protein binding (77 percent), mainly to albumin, similar to the majority of other intravenous anesthetics. The goal of creating an analog with minimal adverse effects on the adrenal gland is being pursued through the development of novel short-acting etomidate derivatives, such as ABP-700 (Figure 4.10).

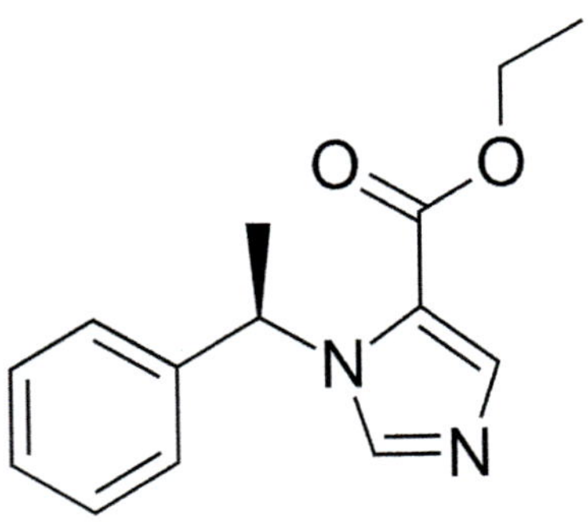

Figure 4.10. *Chemical structure of etomidate.*

Source: Public Domain, https://commons.wikimedia.org/w/index.php?curid=1543631.

4.6.3. Pharmacodynamics

Etomidate, like the majority of other intravenous anesthetics, has GABA-like effects and appears to primarily act through potentiation of $GABA_A$-mediated chloride currents.

4.6.3.1. Central Nervous System

Potent cerebral vasoconstrictor etomidate is demonstrated by reductions in CBF and ICP. Etomidate's effects are comparable to those of thiopental at similar dosages. Despite its reduction of CMRO2, etomidate failed to show neuroprotective properties in animal studies, and human studies are lacking. Compared to thiopental, etomidate causes more frequent excitatory spikes on the EE.G.Etomidate, like methohexital, has the potential to trigger seizure foci, which show up as rapid activity on the EE.G. Furthermore, over 50% of patients on etomidate experience spontaneous movements known as myoclonus. This myoclonic activity may be connected to seizure-like activity on the EEG.

4.6.3.2. Cardiovascular System

Cardiovascular stability following bolus injection is a desirable and characteristic aspect of etomidate-induced anesthesia induction. Reduces in systemic vascular resistance are the main cause of the slight or nonexistent drops in arterial blood pressure. Etomidate's hypotensive effects are likely overstated when hypovolemia is present. Heart rate and cardiac output are barely affected by etomidate. At the dosages required to induce anesthesia, etomidate has negligible depressive effects on cardiac contractility.

4.6.3.3. Respiratory System

A fast intravenous injection of etomidate can occasionally cause apnea, but its depressant effects on ventilation are not as severe as those of barbiturates. When inhaled opioids or anesthetics are combined with etomidate, the depression of ventilation may be exacerbated.

4.6.3.4. Endocrine System

Etomidate suppresses adrenocortical function by inhibiting 11β-hydroxylase, an enzyme required to convert cholesterol to cortisol, in a dose-dependent manner. After a single etomidate induction dose, this suppression lasts for at least 4 to 8 hours, and relative adrenal insufficiency can linger for up to 24 or 48 hours. The safety of etomidate as an induction drug for general anesthesia and for the intubation of critically ill patients has been hotly debated due to this property.

4.6.4. Clinical Uses

When it comes to a quick intravenous induction of anesthesia, etomidate is a better option than propofol and barbiturates, particularly for patients with severe aortic stenosis, coronary artery disease, or compromised myocardial contractility. The onset of unconsciousness following a standard induction dose of 0.2 to 0.3 mg/kg IV is similar to that caused by propofol and thiopental. Intravenous injection of etomidate is often associated with pain, which may be followed by venous irritation. While involuntary myoclonic movements are common, they can be concealed by concurrent neuromuscular blocking medication administration. Following a single intravenous dose of etomidate, awakening occurs quickly and there is minimal indication of any lingering depressant effects. Etomidate does not cause analgesia, and PONV might occur more frequently than it would following the use of propofol or thiopental. Due to its temporary suppression of adrenocortical function, etomidate's clinical use for inducing anesthesia is primarily limited. In theory, this suppression could be advantageous if it lessens the neurohormonal stresses associated with surgery and anesthesia, or harmful if it inhibits helpful defensive reactions against perioperative stressors. The earlier findings that etomidate increases mortality after a single dose for intubating septic patients have been contested by recent meta-analyses. Compared to propofol or methohexital, ethosomalate offers a longer duration of seizure, making it a valuable hypnotic for ECT (Figure 4.11).

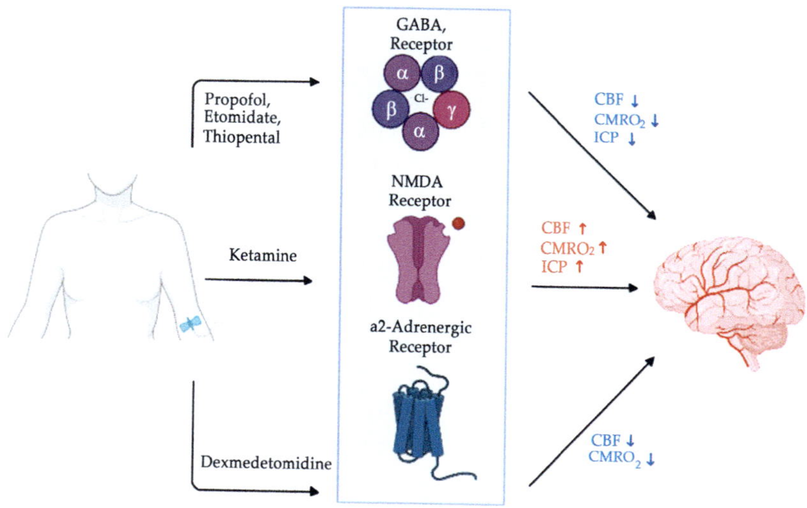

Figure 4.11. *Etomidate, but not thiopental, is associated with decreases in the plasma concentrations of cortisol.*

Source: Nguyen A, Mandavalli A, Diaz MJ, Root KT, Patel A, Casauay J, Perisetla P, Lucke-Wold B. Neurosurgical Anesthesia: Optimizing Outcomes with Agent Selection. Biomedicines. 2023; 11(2):372. https://doi.org/10.3390/biomedicines11020372.

4.7. Dexmedetomidine

A very selective α_2-adrenergic agonist is dexmedetomidine. The observation that patients on chronic clonidine therapy require less anesthesia led to the recognition of the value of α_2-agonists. With α_2-antagonist medications, the effects of dexmedetomidine can be counteracted. (Stoelting and Hillier, 2006)

4.7.1. Physicochemical Characteristics

Medetomidine, an imidazole derivative and highly selective α_2-adrenergic agonist, has an active S-enantiomer called dexmedetomidine, which is utilized in veterinary care. There is a parenteral formulation of dexmedetomidine that is soluble in water.

4.7.2. Pharmacokinetics

The hepatic metabolism of dexmedetomidine proceeds quickly and involves conjugation, N-methylation, and hydroxylation. Urine and bile are the excretion routes for metabolites. There is little half-time for elimination and a high clearance rate. The context-sensitive half-time, on the other hand, significantly increases from 4 minutes following a 10-minute infusion to 250 minutes following an 8-hour infusion.

4.7.3. Pharmacodynamics

Dexmedetomidine produces its effects through the activation of CNS α_2-receptors.

4.7.3.1. Central Nervous System

The analgesic effect starts at the spinal cord level, and hypnosis is most likely caused by activation of α_2- receptors in the locus coeruleus. Because dexmedetomidine activates endogenous sleep pathways, its sedative effect is distinct from that of other intravenous anesthetics in that it more closely resembles a physiologic sleep state (Figure 4.12).

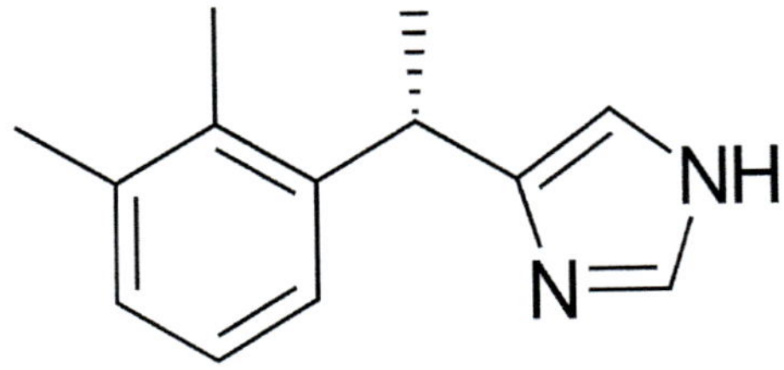

Figure 4.12. *Chemical structure of dexmedetomidine.*

Source: By Icey - Own work, created in Inkscape, Public Domain, https://commons.wikimedia.org/w/index.php?curid=1069540.

Dexmedetomidine lowers CBF without appreciably altering $CMRO_2$ or ICP. Dependency and tolerance can grow. While there are EEG changes, spikes from seizure foci are not suppressed, which makes dexmedetomidine a valuable medication for epilepsy surgery. At standard infusion dosages, evoked potentials observed during spine surgery are not suppressed.

4.7.3.2. Cardiovascular System

The infusion of dexmedetomidine causes moderate reductions in heart rate and systemic vascular resistance, leading to a decrease in systemic arterial blood pressure. A single bolus injection can temporarily increase systemic arterial blood pressure and significantly lower heart rate, likely due to vasoconstriction through peripheral α_2-adrenergic receptors. Initial doses of 0.5 to 1 μg/kg IV over 10 minutes can increase systemic vascular resistance and mean arterial pressure without a significant effect on pulmonary vascular resistance. If bradycardia or hypotension occurs during dexmedetomidine infusion, treatment may be necessary. Older age and low baseline arterial blood pressure (<70 mm Hg) are risk factors for hemodynamic instability with dexmedetomidine. Vagal stimulation can lead to heart block, severe bradycardia, or asystole. Anticholinergic medications have no effect on this response. As an adjunct to general anesthesia, dexmedetomidine can lower plasma catecholamine levels and reduce heart rate elevation during emergence.

4.7.3.3. Respiratory System

Dexmedetomidine causes a minor to moderate reduction in tidal volume and a negligible shift in the respiratory rate in the respiratory system. While there is a slight impairment in the ventilatory response to carbon dioxide, there appears to be a reduction in the response to hypoxia comparable to that of propofol. Sedation may cause upper airway obstruction, even though the respiratory effects are minimal. Furthermore, when combined with other sedative-hypnotics, dexmedetomidine has a synergistic sedative effect.

4.7.4. Clinical Uses

In an intensive care unit, patients who are mechanically ventilated and are tracheally intubated are primarily given dexmedetomidine for brief periods of sedation. While there is no proof that dexmedetomidine lowers the risk of death, it can shorten the time spent in the intensive care unit, minimize the need for mechanical ventilation, and enhance sleep. In the operating room, dexmedetomidine can be used as a sedative during awake fiberoptic tracheal intubation, as a supplement to general anesthesia, or both. Dexmedetomidine (0.5–1 μg/kg IV initial dose over 10–15 minutes, followed by an infusion of 0.2–0.7 μg/ kg/h) reduces the dose requirements for both intravenous and inhaled anesthetics when given during general anesthesia. The sedative and analgesic effects of dexmedetomidine without respiratory depression may be helpful during awakening and the transition to the postoperative setting. Although analgesic benefits have not been demonstrated in all settings, dexmedetomidine appears to reduce perioperative opioid consumption and improve pain scores. Children have benefited greatly from the widespread use of dexmedetomidine, which has been shown to be effective in this demographic. It might be especially helpful in preventing emergent delirium following pediatric anesthesia. When it comes to elderly patients who need sedation after cardiac or noncardiac surgery, dexmedetomidine may be a better option than propofol in terms of minimizing delirium. (Stoelting and Hillier, 2006)

A Closer Look

Remifentanil Viatris

Remifentanil Viatris represents a significant advancement in pain management and anesthesia, particularly in surgical settings. Manufactured by Viatris, a reputable pharmaceutical company known for its commitment to quality healthcare solutions, Remifentanil Viatris is a formulation of the potent opioid analgesic remifentanil. This medication is characterized by its unique pharmacokinetic profile, featuring rapid onset and offset of action, making it an invaluable asset for anesthesiologists and surgeons alike.

The swift onset of action of Remifentanil Viatris allows for rapid pain relief, which is especially crucial during the induction phase of anesthesia. This feature is particularly advantageous in scenarios where immediate control of pain is necessary, such as during rapid sequence inductions or procedures requiring fastidious hemodynamic control. Furthermore, Remifentanil Viatris offers unparalleled titratability, enabling clinicians to adjust the dosage promptly and precisely to meet the individualized needs of each patient throughout the surgical procedure. This capability ensures optimal pain management while minimizing the risk of under- or over-sedation, a challenge often encountered with other opioids.

Another distinguishing feature of Remifentanil Viatris is its ultra-short duration of action, largely due to its rapid metabolism by non-specific tissue and plasma esterases. This characteristic makes it an attractive choice for procedures of varying lengths, as its effects dissipate quickly upon discontinuation, allowing for smooth emergence from anesthesia without prolonged sedation or respiratory depression. Moreover, the short duration of action reduces the risk of accumulation and residual effects, mitigating concerns regarding postoperative respiratory depression and delayed recovery.

Despite its numerous benefits, Remifentanil Viatris, like all opioids, is not without risks. Respiratory depression, hypotension, and bradycardia are potential adverse effects associated with its use, particularly when administered rapidly or in high doses. Additionally, like other opioids, remifentanil has the potential for abuse and addiction if used improperly or for extended periods.

Remifentanil Viatris represents a valuable addition to the armamentarium of anesthetic agents available to healthcare providers. Its rapid onset, titratability, and ultra-short duration of action make it a versatile and effective option for pain management and anesthesia in a variety of surgical settings. However, prudent clinical judgment and careful patient monitoring are essential to maximize the benefits of Remifentanil Viatris while minimizing the risks associated with its use. (Stoelting and Hillier, 2006)

Summary

- Intravenous nonopioid anesthetics have an important role in modern anesthesia practice. They are widely used to facilitate a rapid induction of general anesthesia and provide sedation during monitored anesthesia care (MAC) and for patients in intensive care settings.
- Propofol is the most frequently administered anesthetic drug for induction of anesthesia. In addition, propofol is used during the maintenance of anesthesia and is a common selection for sedation in the operating room as well as in the intensive care unit (ICU).
- Plasma clearance is rapid and exceeds hepatic blood flow, thus indicating the importance of extrahepatic metabolism, which has been confirmed during the anhepatic phase of liver transplantation.
- In the central nervous system (CNS), propofol primarily acts as a hypnotic and does not have any analgesic properties. It reduces the cerebral metabolic rate for oxygen (CMRO2), which leads to decreased cerebral blood flow (CBF) through preserved flow-metabolism coupling.
- Propofol is a respiratory depressant and often produces apnea following a dose used to induce anesthesia. A maintenance infusion of propofol decreases minute ventilation via reductions in tidal volume and respiratory rate, with the effect on tidal volume being more pronounced.
- Barbiturates, except for phenobarbital, undergo hepatic metabolism most importantly by oxidation, but also by N-dealkylation, desulfuration, and destruction of the barbituric acid ring structure. The resulting metabolites are inactive and excreted through urine and, after conjugation, through bile.
- The mechanism of action for the effect of barbiturates in the CNS presumably involves both enhancement of inhibitory neurotransmission and inhibition of excitatory transmission. Although the effects on inhibitory transmission probably result from activation of the $GABA_A$ receptor complex, the effects on excitatory transmission are less well understood.
- Barbiturates are respiratory depressants and lead to decreased minute ventilation via smaller tidal volumes and respiratory rates. Anesthetic induction doses of thiopental and methohexital typically induce transient apnea, which is more pronounced in the presence of other respiratory depressants.
- Benzodiazepines commonly used in the perioperative period include diazepam, midazolam, and lorazepam, as well as the selective benzodiazepine antagonist flumazenil.
- Benzodiazepines work through activation of the $GABA_A$ receptor complex and enhancement of GABA-mediated chloride currents, thereby leading to hyperpolarization of neurons and reduced excitability.
- Ketamine is a partially water-soluble and highly lipid-soluble derivative of phencyclidine. It is between 5 and 10 times more lipid soluble than thiopental. Of the two stereoisomers the S(+) form is more potent than the R(−) isomer.
- Etomidate is a carboxylated imidazole derivative that has two optical isomers. The available preparation contains only the active D(+) isomer, which has hypnotic properties.

The drug is poorly soluble in water and is therefore supplied as a 2 mg/mL solution in 35% propylene glycol.

- Hypnosis presumably results from stimulation of α_2- receptors in the locus ceruleus, and the analgesic effect originates at the level of the spinal cord.

References

1. Albanese, J., Arnaud, S., Rey, M., et al. (1997). Ketamine decreases intracranial pressure and electroencephalographic activity in traumatic brain injury patients during propofol sedation. *Anesthesiology, 87*(6), 1328–1334.
2. Alexopoulou, C., Kondili, E., Diamantaki, E., et al. (2014). Effects of dexmedetomidine on sleep quality in critically ill patients: A pilot study. *Anesthesiology, 121*(4), 801–807.
3. Antonik, L. J., Goldwater, D. R., Kilpatrick, G. J., et al. (2012). A placebo- and midazolam-controlled phase I single ascending-dose study evaluating the safety, pharmacokinetics, and pharmacodynamics of remimazolam (CNS 7056): Part I. Safety, efficacy, and basic pharmacokinetics. *Anesthesia & Analgesia, 115*(2), 274–283.
4. Apfel, C. C., Korttila, K., Abdalla, M., et al. (2004). A factorial trial of six interventions for the prevention of postoperative nausea and vomiting. *New England Journal of Medicine, 350*(24), 2441–2451.
5. Asserhøj, L. L., Mosbech, H., Krøigaard, M., et al. (2016). No evidence for contraindications to the use of propofol in adults allergic to egg, soy or peanut. *British Journal of Anaesthesia, 116*(1), 77–82.
6. Avramov, M. N., Husain, M. M., & White, P. F. (1995). The comparative effects of methohexital, propofol, and etomidate for electroconvulsive therapy. *Anesthesia & Analgesia, 81*(3), 596–602.
7. Bailey, P. L., Pace, N. L., Ashburn, M. A., et al. (1990). Frequent hypoxemia and apnea after sedation with midazolam and fentanyl. *Anesthesiology, 73*(5), 826–830.
8. Bendel, S., Ruokonen, E., Pölönen, P., & Uusaro, A. (2007). Propofol causes more hypotension than etomidate in patients with severe aortic stenosis: A double-blind, randomized study comparing propofol and etomidate. *Acta Anesthesiologic Scandinavica, 51*(3), 284–289.
9. Blaudszun, G., Lysakowski, C., Elia, N., & Tramer, M. R. (2012). Effect of perioperative systemic alpha 2 agonists on postoperative morphine consumption and pain intensity: Systematic review and meta-analysis of randomized controlled trials. *Anesthesiology, 116*(6), 1312–1322.
10. Borgeat, A., Wilder-Smith, O. H., Saiah, M., & Rifat, K. (1992). Subhypnotic doses of propofol possess direct antiemetic properties. *Anesthesia & Analgesia, 74*(4), 539–541.
11. Bosnjak, Z. J., Logan, S., Liu, Y., & Bai, X. (2016). Recent insights into molecular mechanisms of propofol-induced developmental neurotoxicity. *Anesthesia & Analgesia, 123*(5), 1286–1296.
12. Bruder, E. A., Ball, I. M., Ridi, S., et al. (2015). Single induction dose of etomidate versus other induction agents for endotracheal intubation in critically ill patients. *Cochrane Database of Systematic Reviews, 2015*(1), CD010225.
13. Bulach, R., Myles, P. S., & Russnak, M. (2005). Double-blind randomized controlled trial to determine extent of amnesia with midazolam given immediately before general anesthesia. *British Journal of Anaesthesia, 94*(3), 300–305.

14. Campagna, J. A., Pojasek, K., Grayzel, D., et al. (2014). Advancing novel anesthetics: Pharmacodynamic and pharmacokinetic studies of cyclopropyl-methoxycarbonyl metomidate in dogs. *Anesthesiology, 121*(6), 1203–1216.
15. Candiotti, K. A., Gan, T. J., Young, C., et al. (2011). A randomized, open-label study of the safety and tolerability of fospropofol for patients requiring intubation and mechanical ventilation in the intensive care unit. *Anesthesia & Analgesia, 113*(3), 550–556.
16. Cedborg, A. I., Sundman, E., Boden, K., et al. (2015). Effects of morphine and midazolam on pharyngeal function, airway protection, and coordination of breathing and swallowing in healthy adults. *Anesthesiology, 122*(6), 1253–1267.
17. Chan, C. M., Mitchell, A. L., & Shorr, A. F. (2012). Etomidate is associated with mortality and adrenal insufficiency in sepsis: A meta-analysis. *Critical Care Medicine, 40*(11), 2945–2953.
18. Chen, K., Lu, Z., Xin, Y. C., et al. (2015). Alpha-2 agonists for long-term sedation during mechanical ventilation in critically ill patients. *Cochrane Database of Systematic Reviews, 2015*(1), CD010269.
19. Chen, Y., Cai, A., Dexter, F., et al. (2016). Amnesia of the operating room in the B-Unaware and BAG-RECALL Clinical Trials. *Anesthesia & Analgesia, 122*(4), 1158–1168.
20. Cote, C. J., Cohen, I. T., Suresh, S., et al. (2002). A comparison of three doses of a commercially prepared oral midazolam syrup in children. *Anesthesia & Analgesia, 94*(1), 37–43.
21. Dahmani, S., Delivet, H., & Hilly, J. (2014). Emergence delirium in children. *Current Opinion in Anaesthesiology, 27*(3), 309–315.
22. Djaiani, G., Silverton, N., Fedorko, L., et al. (2016). Dexmedetomidine versus propofol sedation reduces delirium after cardiac surgery: A randomized controlled trial. *Anesthesiology, 124*(2), 362–368.
23. Eames, W. O., Rooke, G. A., Wu, R. S., et al. (1996). Comparison of the effects of etomidate, propofol, and thiopental on respiratory resistance after tracheal intubation. *Anesthesiology, 84*(6), 1307–1311.
24. Ellens, N., Figueroa, B., & Clark, J. (2015). The use of barbiturate-induced coma during cerebrovascular neurosurgery procedures: A review of the literature. *Brain Circulation, 1*(2), 140–146.
25. Erdoes, G., Basciani, R. M., & Eberle, B. (2014). Etomidate—A review of robust evidence for its use in various clinical scenarios. *Acta Anaesthesiologica Scandinavica, 58*(4), 380–389.
26. Euasobhon, P., Dej-arkom, S., Siriussawakul, A., et al. (2016). Lidocaine for reducing propofol-induced pain on induction of anesthesia in adults. *Cochrane Database of Systematic Reviews, 2016*(2), CD007874.
27. Farrant, M., & Nusser, Z. (2005). Variations on an inhibitory theme: Phasic and tonic activation of GABAA receptors. *Nature Reviews Neuroscience, 6*(3), 215–229.
28. Fechner, J., Ihmsen, H., Jeleazcov, C., & Schüttler, J. (2009). Fospropofol disodium, a water-soluble prodrug of the intravenous anesthetic propofol (2,6-diisopropylphenol). *Expert Opinion on Investigational Drugs, 18*(10), 1565–1571.
29. Fechner, J., Ihmsen, H., Schüttler, J., & Jeleazcov, C. (2013). A randomized open-label phase I pilot study of the safety and efficacy of total intravenous anesthesia with fospropofol for

coronary artery bypass graft surgery. *Journal of Cardiothoracic and Vascular Anesthesia, 27*(5), 908–915.

30. Fragen, R. J., Shanks, C. A., Molteni, A., et al. (1984). Effects of etomidate on hormonal responses to surgical stress. *Anesthesiology, 61*(6), 652–656.

31. Franks, N. P. (2008). General anesthesia: From molecular targets to neuronal pathways of sleep and arousal. *Nature Reviews Neuroscience, 9*, 370–386.

32. Franks, N. P. (2006). Molecular targets underlying general anesthesia. *British Journal of Pharmacology, 147*(Suppl 1), S72–S81.

33. Fraser, G. L., Devlin, J. W., Worby, C. P., et al. (2013). Benzodiazepine versus nonbenzodiazepine-based sedation for mechanically ventilated, critically ill adults: A systematic review and meta-analysis of randomized trials. *Critical Care Medicine, 41*(9 Suppl 1), S30–S38.

34. Friesen, R. H., Nichols, C. S., Twite, M. D., et al. (2013). The hemodynamic response to dexmedetomidine loading dose in children with and without pulmonary hypertension. *Anesthesia & Analgesia, 117*(4), 953–959.

35. Glass, P. S. (2010). Half-time or half-life: What matters for recovery from intravenous anesthesia? *Anesthesiology, 112*(6), 1266–1269.

36. Gorlin, A. W., Rosenfeld, D. M., & Ramakrishna, H. (2016). Intravenous sub-anesthetic ketamine for perioperative analgesia. *Journal of Anesthesiology Clinical Pharmacology, 32*(2), 160.

37. Grady, M. V., Mascha, E., Sessler, D. I., & Kurz, A. (2012). The effect of perioperative intravenous lidocaine and ketamine on recovery after abdominal hysterectomy. *Anesthesia & Analgesia, 115*(5), 1078–1084.

38. Grant, M. C., Kim, J., Page, A. J., et al. (2016). The effect of intravenous midazolam on postoperative nausea and vomiting. *Anesthesia & Analgesia, 122*(3), 656–663.

39. Gu, W. J., Wang, F., Tang, L., & Liu, J. C. (2015). Single-dose etomidate does not increase mortality in patients with sepsis: A systematic review and meta-analysis of randomized controlled trials and observational studies. *Chest, 147*(2), 335–346.

40. Haessler, R., Madler, C., Klasing, S., et al. (1992). Propofol/fentanyl versus etomidate/fentanyl for the induction of anesthesia in patients with aortic insufficiency and coronary artery disease. *Journal of Cardiothoracic and Vascular Anesthesia, 6*(2), 173–180.

41. He, X. Y., Cao, J. P., He, Q., & Shi, X. Y. (2014). Dexmedetomidine for the management of awake fiberoptic intubation. *Cochrane Database of Systematic Reviews, 2014*(1), CD009798.

42. Heard, C., Harutunians, M., Houck, J., et al. (2015). Propofol anesthesia for children undergoing magnetic resonance imaging. *Anesthesia & Analgesia, 120*(1), 157–164.

43. Hughes, M. A., Glass, P. S., & Jacobs, J. R. (1992). Context-sensitive half-time in multicompartment pharmacokinetic models for intravenous anesthetic drugs. *Anesthesiology, 76*(3), 334–341.

44. Ice, C. J., Personett, H. A., Frazee, E. N., et al. (2016). Risk factors for dexmedetomidine associated hemodynamic instability in noncardiac intensive care unit patients. *Anesthesia & Analgesia, 122*(2), 462–469.

45. Ilic, R. G. (2015). Fospropofol and remimazolam. *International Anesthesiology Clinics, 53*(2), 76–90.

46. Ingrande, J., Brodsky, J. B., & Lemmens, H. J. (2011). Lean body weight scalar for the anesthetic induction dose of propofol in morbidly obese subjects. *Anesthesia & Analgesia, 113*(1), 57–62.
47. Jalota, L., Kalira, V., George, E., et al. (2011). Prevention of pain on injection of propofol: Systematic review and meta-analysis. *BMJ, 342*, d1110.
48. Kamibayashi, T., & Maze, M. (2000). Clinical uses of alpha2-adrenergic agonists. *Anesthesiology, 93*(5), 1345–1349.
49. Kassam, S. I., Lu, C., Buckley, N., et al. (2011). The mechanisms of propofol-induced vascular relaxation and modulation by perivascular adipose tissue and endothelium. *Anesthesia & Analgesia, 112*(6), 1339–1345.
50. Kohrs, R., & Durieux, M. E. (1998). Ketamine: Teaching an old drug new trick. *Anesthesia & Analgesia, 87*(6), 1186–1193.
51. Krajčová, A., Waldauf, P., Anděl, M., & Duška, F. (2015). Propofol infusion syndrome: A structured review of experimental studies and 153 published case reports. *Critical Care, 19*, 398.
52. Krüger, T., Hoffmann, I., Blettner, M., et al. (2013). GERAADA Investigators. Intraoperative neuroprotective drugs without beneficial effects? Results of the German Registry for Acute Aortic Dissection Type A (GERAADA). *European Journal of Cardiothoracic Surgery, 44*(5), 939–946.
53. Kumar, G., Stendall, C., Mistry, R., et al. (2014). A comparison of total intravenous anaesthesia using propofol with sevoflurane or desflurane in ambulatory surgery: Systematic review and meta-analysis. *Anesthesia, 69*(10), 1138–1150.
54. Li, Y., Wang, B., Zhang, L. L., et al. (2016). Dexmedetomidine combined with general anesthesia provides similar intraoperative stress response reduction when compared with a combined general and epidural anesthetic technique. *Anesthesia & Analgesia, 122*(4), 1202–1210.
55. Lihua, P., Su, M., Ke, W., & Ziemann-Gimmel, P. (2014). Different regimens of intravenous sedatives or hypnotics for electroconvulsive therapy (ECT) in adult patients with depression. *Cochrane Database of Systematic Reviews, 2014*(4), CD009763.
56. Lodenius, Å., Ebberyd, A., Hårdemark-Cedborg, A., et al. (2016). Sedation with dexmedetomidine or propofol impairs hypoxic control of breathing in healthy male volunteers: A nonblinded, randomized crossover study. *Anesthesiology, 125*(4), 700–715.
57. MacIver, M. B. (2014). Anesthetic agent-specific effects on synaptic inhibition. *Anesthesia & Analgesia, 119*(3), 558–569.
58. Mason, K. P., & Lerman, J. (2011). Dexmedetomidine in children. *Anesthesia & Analgesia, 113*(5), 1129–1142.
59. Maurice-Szamburski, A., Auquier, P., Viarre-Oreal, V., et al. (2015). PremedX Study Investigators. Effect of sedative premedication on patient experience after general anesthesia: A randomized clinical trial. *JAMA, 313*(9), 916–925.
60. Mcintosh, M. P., Iwasawa, K., Rajewski, R. A., et al. (2012). Hemodynamic profile in rabbits of fospropofol disodium injection relative to propofol emulsion following rapid bolus injection. *Journal of Pharmaceutical Sciences, 101*(9), 3518–3525.
61. Messina, A. G., Wang, M., Ward, M. J., et al. (2016). Anesthetic interventions for prevention of awareness during surgery. *Cochrane Database of Systematic Reviews, 2016*(10), CD007272.

62. Mohler, H., & Richards, J. G. (1988). The benzodiazepine receptor: A pharmacological control element of brain function. *European Journal of Anaesthesiology, 2*, 15–24.

63. Morel, J., Salard, M., Castelain, C., et al. (2011). Hemodynamic consequences of etomidate administration in elective cardiac surgery: A randomized double-blinded study. *British Journal of Anaesthesia, 107*(4), 503–509.

64. Murrough, J. W., Iosifescu, D. V., Chang, L. C., et al. (2013). Antidepressant efficacy of ketamine in treatment-resistant major depression: A two-site randomized controlled trial. *American Journal of Psychiatry, 170*(10), 1134–1142.

65. Naik, B. I., Nemergut, E. C., Kazemi, A., et al. (2016). The effect of dexmedetomidine on postoperative opioid consumption and pain after major spine surgery. *Anesthesia & Analgesia, 122*(5), 1646–1653.

66. Oda, Y., Toriyama, S., Tanaka, K., et al. (2007). The effect of dexmedetomidine on electrocorticography in patients with temporal lobe epilepsy under sevoflurane anesthesia. *Anesthesia & Analgesia, 105*(5), 1272–1277.

67. Olkkola, K. T., & Ahonen, J. (2008). Midazolam and other benzodiazepines. In *Handbook of Experimental Pharmacology* (Vol. 182, pp. 335–360). Springer.

68. Padmanabhan, U., Leslie, K., Eer, A. S., et al. (2009). Early cognitive impairment after sedation for colonoscopy: The effect of adding midazolam and/or fentanyl to propofol. *Anesthesia & Analgesia, 109*(5), 1448–1455.

69. Peltoniemi, M. A., Hagelberg, N. M., Olkkola, K. T., & Saari, T. I. (2016). Ketamine: A review of clinical pharmacokinetics and pharmacodynamics in anesthesia and pain therapy. *Clinical Pharmacokinetics, 55*, 1059–1077.

70. Peng, K., Liu, H. Y., Wu, S. R., et al. (2016). Does propofol anesthesia lead to less postoperative pain compared with inhalational anesthesia? *Anesthesia & Analgesia, 123*(4), 846–858.

71. Prasad, M., Krishnan, P. R., Sequeira, R., & AlRoomi, K. (2014). Anticonvulsant therapy for status epilepticus. *Cochrane Database of Systematic Reviews, 2014*(9), CD003723.

72. Purdon, P. L., Sampson, A., Pavone, K. J., & Brown, E. N. (2015). Clinical electroencephalography for anesthesiologists: Part I: Background and basic signatures. *Anesthesiology, 123*(4), 937–960.

73. Reves, J. G., Fragen, R. J., Vinik, H. R., et al. (1985). Midazolam: Pharmacology and uses. *Anesthesiology, 62*(3), 310–324.

74. Reznik, M. E., Berger, K., & Claassen, J. (2016). Comparison of intravenous anesthetic agents for the treatment of refractory status epilepticus. *Journal of Clinical Medicine, 5*(5), E54.

75. Roberts, I., & Sydenham, E. (2012). Barbiturates for acute traumatic brain injury. *Cochrane Database of Systematic Reviews, 2012*(12), CD000033.

76. Rozet, I., Metzner, J., Brown, M., et al. (2015). Dexmedetomidine does not affect evoked potentials during spine surgery. *Anesthesia & Analgesia, 121*(2), 492–501.

77. Saidman, L. J. (1974). Uptake, distribution, and elimination of barbiturates. In Eger, E. I. (Ed.), *Anesthetic Uptake and Action* (pp. 264–284). Williams & Wilkins.

78. Sawynok, J. (2014). Topical and peripheral ketamine as an analgesic. *Anesthesia & Analgesia, 119*(1), 170–178.

79. Schulman, S. R., Rockett, C. B., Canada, A. T., & Glass, P. (1995). Long-term propofol infusion for refractory postoperative nausea—A case-report with quantitative propofol analysis. *Anesthesia & Analgesia, 80*(3), 636–637.

80. Short, T. G., Hannam, J. A., Laurent, S., et al. (2016). Refining target-controlled infusion. *Anesthesia & Analgesia, 122*(1), 90–97.

81. Simons, J. C., Pierce, E., Diaz-Gil, D., et al. (2016). Effects of depth of propofol and sevoflurane anesthesia on upper airway collapsibility, respiratory genioglossus activation, and breathing in healthy volunteers. *Anesthesiology, 125*(3), 525–534.

82. Singh, J. B., Fedgchin, M., Daly, E. J., et al. (2016). A double-blind, randomized, placebo controlled, dose-frequency study of intravenous ketamine in patients with treatment-resistant depression. *American Journal of Psychiatry, 173*(8), 816–826.

83. Stoelting, R. K., & Hillier, S. C. (2006). Barbiturates. In R. K. Stoelting & S. C. Hillier (Eds.), *Pharmacology and Physiology in Anesthetic Practice* (4th ed., pp. 127–139). Lippincott Williams & Wilkins.

84. Stoelting, R. K., & Hillier, S. C. (2006). Benzodiazepines. In R. K. Stoelting & S. C. Hillier (Eds.), *Pharmacology and Physiology in Anesthetic Practice* (4th ed., pp. 140–154). Lippincott Williams & Wilkins.

85. Stoelting, R. K., & Hillier, S. C. (2006). Nonbarbiturate intravenous anesthetic drugs. In R. K. Stoelting & S. C. Hillier (Eds.), *Pharmacology and Physiology in Anesthetic Practice* (4th ed., pp. 155–178). Lippincott Williams & Wilkins.

86. Struys, M. M., Fechner, J., Schüttler, J., & Schwilden, H. (2010). Erroneously published fospropofol pharmacokinetic-pharmacodynamic data and retraction of the affected publications. *Anesthesiology, 112*(4), 1056–1057.

87. Su, X., Meng, Z. T., Wu, X. H., et al. (2016). Dexmedetomidine for prevention of delirium in elderly patients after noncardiac surgery: A randomized, double-blind, placebo-controlled trial. *The Lancet, 388*(10054), 1893–1902.

88. Talke, P., Chen, R., Thomas, B., et al. (2000). The hemodynamic and adrenergic effects of perioperative dexmedetomidine infusion after vascular surgery. *Anesthesia & Analgesia, 90*(4), 834–839.

89. Tramer, M. R., Moore, R. A., & McQuay, H. J. (1997). Propofol and bradycardia: Causation, frequency and severity. *British Journal of Anesthesia, 78*, 642–651.

90. Vanlersberghe, C., & Camu, F. (2008). Etomidate and other non-barbiturates. In *Handbook of Experimental Pharmacology* (Vol. 182, pp. 267–282). Springer.

91. Vanlersberghe, C., & Camu, F. (2008). Propofol. In *Handbook of Experimental Pharmacology* (Vol. 182, pp. 227–252). Springer.

92. Vuyk, J., Sitsen, E., & Reekers, M. (2015). Intravenous anesthetics. In R. D. Miller (Ed.), *Miller's Anesthesia* (8th ed., pp. 821–863). Elsevier.

93. Zaal, I. J., Devlin, J. W., Hazelbag, M., et al. (2015). Benzodiazepine-associated delirium in critically ill adults. *Intensive Care Medicine, 41*(12), 2130–2137.

Chapter 5

LOCAL ANESTHETICS

Contents

Introduction

Local anesthetics have revolutionized pain management and made a wide range of medical procedures possible with minimal discomfort, making them essential tools in modern medicine. By blocking the transmission of pain signals, these agents can be applied locally to particular nerve pathways or tissues. This results in a significant reduction or elimination of pain perception during surgical procedures, dental work, and diagnostic tests. Through their interaction with sodium channels in nerve cell membranes, local anesthetics block the generation and propagation of action potentials along nerve fibers. A key benefit of local anesthetics over general anesthesia in many clinical situations is their ability to selectively target sensory neurons, resulting in a reversible loss of sensation in the targeted area while maintaining motor function and consciousness. Because there are formulations for topical application, infiltration, nerve block, and spinal or epidural injection, among other routes of administration, local anesthetics are highly versatile. This adaptability enables healthcare providers to customize the selection and approach.

Local anesthetics exhibit a favorable safety profile when used appropriately, with adverse effects typically limited to the site of administration and transient in nature. However, systemic toxicity can occur, particularly with inadvertent intravascular injection or excessive dosing, underscoring the importance of meticulous technique and vigilant monitoring during administration.

Continuous research and development efforts seek to enhance the efficacy, duration, and safety of local anesthetics, with ongoing exploration of novel formulations, delivery methods, and adjuvants. Additionally, advancements in understanding the pharmacokinetics and pharmacodynamics of these agents contribute to improved dosing strategies and patient outcomes.

Local anesthetics play a vital role in modern healthcare, facilitating a wide range of medical procedures with minimal pain and discomfort. With ongoing innovation and refinement, these agents continue to evolve, promising further improvements in pain management and patient care.

Loss of sensation in a specific area of the body brought on by interference with impulse generation or propagation is known as local anesthesia. Numerous chemical and physical processes can be used to create local anesthesia. In contrast, many substances with similar mechanisms of action but varying action durations are used in routine clinical practice to produce local anesthesia, from which recovery is typically spontaneous, predictable, and total (American Society of Regional Anesthesia and Pain Medicine; Covino and Vassallo, 1976; Covino, Scott, Lambert, 1994).

Orientation and Directional Terms

<table>
<tr><th>Term</th><th>Definition</th><th>Illustration</th></tr>
<tr><td>Pain management</td><td>Pain management is an aspect of medicine and health care involving relief of pain in various dimensions, from acute and simple to chronic and challenging.</td><td>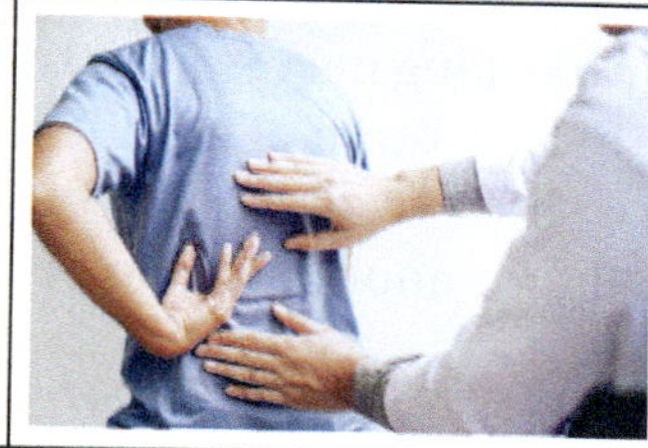</td></tr>
<tr><td>Neuronal membrane</td><td>Neuronal membrane is the site where most processes involved in neuronal preservation and functioning are triggered. These actions require the participation of membrane-related molecular agents, which associate in protein/lipid clusters to initiate molecular processing and signal transduction.</td><td>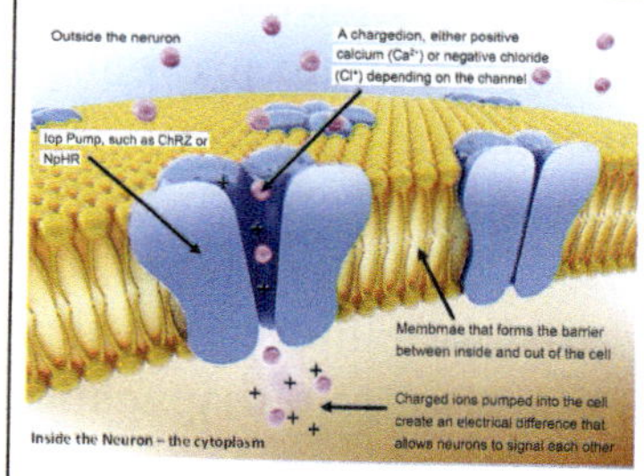
</td></tr>
<tr><td>Vasodilation</td><td>Vasodilation is the widening of blood vessels as a result of the relaxation of the blood vessel's muscular walls. Vasodilation is a mechanism to enhance blood flow to areas of the body that are lacking oxygen and/or nutrients.</td><td>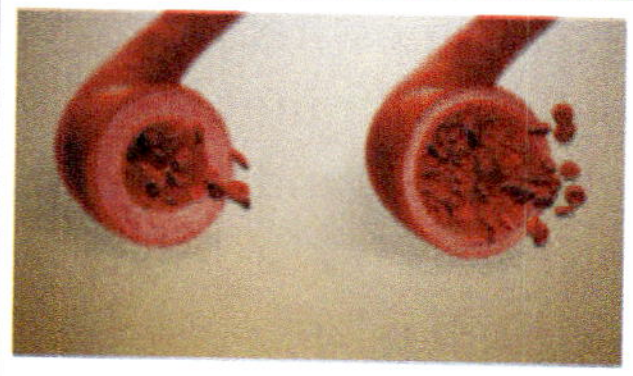</td></tr>
<tr><td>Epinephrine</td><td>Epinephrine is both a neurotransmitter and a hormone, but it acts mainly as a hormone. Epinephrine, also known as adrenaline, plays an important role in your body's fight-or-flight response. It's also used as a medication to treat many life-threatening conditions.</td><td>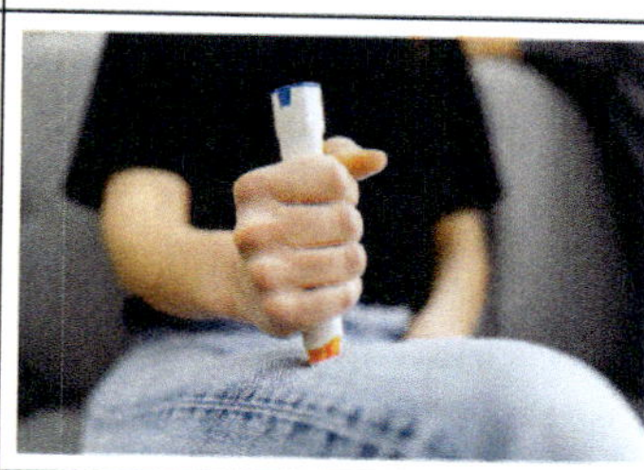</td></tr>
<tr><td>Cardiovascular system</td><td>Cardiovascular system provides blood supply throughout the body. Responding to various stimuli can control the velocity and amount of blood carried through the vessels. The cardiovascular system comprises the heart, arteries, veins, and capillaries.</td><td>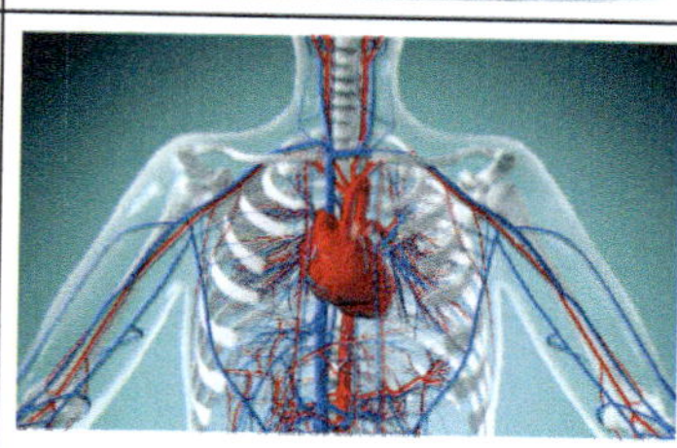</td></tr>
</table>

5.1. Overview of Local Anesthesia

Local anesthesia prevents pain during procedures by blocking nerves from transmitting pain signals to the brain. The effects of local anesthetic are short-lived, so healthcare teams primarily use it for minor outpatient procedures.

Local anesthesia is a type of anesthesia that numbs a specific part of the body, typically a small area or region, to prevent pain during medical procedures. It works by blocking the nerves in the targeted area from sending pain signals to the brain. Local anesthesia is commonly used for minor surgical procedures, dental work, and certain diagnostic tests.

There are different forms of local anesthesia, including topical anesthetics applied to the skin or mucous membranes, local anesthetics injected into the tissue, and regional anesthesia which involves blocking a larger area of the body, such as a limb or an entire section of the body, using nerve blocks.

Unlike general anesthesia, which renders a person unconscious and affects the entire body, local anesthesia allows the individual to remain conscious and aware during the procedure. It's generally considered safer and associated with fewer risks and side effects compared to general anesthesia. However, the administering healthcare provider needs to consider factors such as allergies, potential drug interactions, and the patient's medical history before administering local anesthesia.

5.1.1. History

In the 1880s, cocaine was the first local anesthetic to be used clinically. The local anesthetic benzocaine, which is applied topically, and the injectable medications procaine, tetracaine, and chloroprocaine were subsequently created by modifying the structure of cocaine, which is an amino ester. 1948 saw the introduction of lidocaine as the first medication in a brand-new class of local anesthetics known as amino amides. More stability and a lower incidence of allergic reactions were two benefits of the amino amides over the previous amino esters. Due to these advantageous characteristics, lidocaine was used as a model to create a number of amino-amide anesthetics. The aromatic amine xylidine is the source of lidocaine as well as the majority of amino-amide local anesthetics, such as levobupivacaine, ropivacaine, mepivacaine, and bupivacaine. Another unique feature that sets levobupivacaine and ropivacaine apart is that they are single enantiomers as opposed to racemic mixtures. They are the result of a developmental strategy that aims to lessen the possibility of cardiac toxicity by utilizing the different stereoselectivity of cardiac and neuronal sodium ion channels. In the liver, almost all amides go through biotransformation, while the esters go through hydrolysis in the plasma (Figure 5.1).

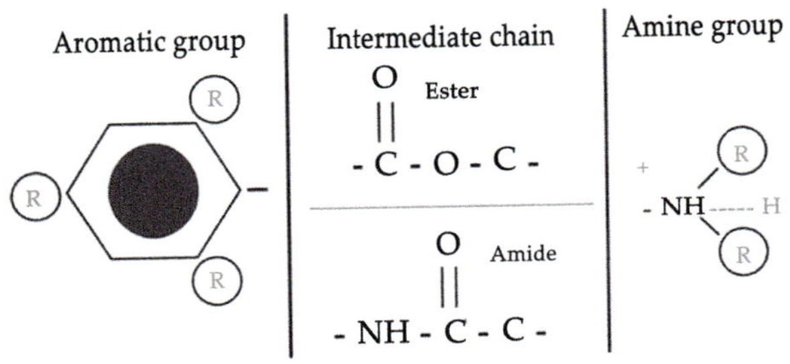

Figure 5.1. *Typical structural formula of a local anesthetic.*

Source: M. Whizar-Lugo, V., L. Íñiguez-López, K., C. Cárdenas-Maytorena, A., & D. Ramírez-Puerta, C. (2020). Local Anesthetics. IntechOpen. doi: 10.5772/intechopen.93643.

5.2. Nerve Conduction

The neural membrane has a negative potential of about −90 mV when it is at rest or in a normal state (the potential inside the nerve fiber is negative relative to the extracellular fluid). Together with increased membrane permeability to potassium ions in comparison to sodium ions, energy-dependent outward and inward transport of sodium and potassium ions produce this negative potential. The transmembrane potential decreases when the nerve is stimulated because of an increase in the membrane's permeability to sodium ions. A fast and self-sustaining influx of sodium ions causes a propagating wave of depolarization, known as the action potential, if a critical potential, also known as the threshold potential, is reached. The resting membrane potential then returns. The function, fiber diameter, and myelin type (type C) or absence (type A and B) can all be used to categorize nerve fibers. Conduction velocity is dependent on the diameter of the nerve fiber; a wider diameter corresponds to faster nerve conduction. Conduction velocity is also accelerated by myelin. The axolemma's insulation from the environment around it causes this effect (American Society of Regional Anesthesia and Pain Medicine; Covino and Vassallo, 1976; Covino, Scott, Lambert, 1994).

5.3. Local Anesthetic Actions on Sodium Channels

Although local anesthetics have a broad range of molecular targets, voltage-gated sodium channels are the primary mechanism by which they achieve their intended clinical effects. Complex transmembrane proteins with large alpha subunits and much smaller beta subunits make up voltage-gated sodium channels. The pore is located in the middle of the four homologous domains (four square-shaped domains made up of six transmembrane helices) that make up the alpha subunits. In addition to controlling the channel's electrophysiologic characteristics, beta subunits play a significant part in the channel's localization, adhesion molecule binding, and intracellular cytoskeleton attachment. In mammalian tissues, sodium channel alpha subunits have nine major subtypes, while beta subunits have four major subtypes.

Diverse tissues, developmental stages, and disease states exhibit the expression of distinct sodium channel subtypes. Subtypes of sodium channels are being actively studied in relation to human diseases involving spontaneous pain and pain insensitivity, as potential targets for novel analgesics, and in other medical domains such as neurology and cardiology. From an electrophysiological perspective, local anesthetics prevent the threshold potential from being reached by slowing down the rate at which the body depolarizes in response to stimulation. They barely affect the threshold potential and do not change the transmembrane potential at rest. Sodium channels alternate between their open, inactive, and resting states. Excitation causes the sodium channel to change from its closed, resting state to an open, activated state, increasing the inward flow of sodium ions and causing depolarization as a result. The channel changes from a resting state to an inactive state and needs more conformational changes to return to that state (Table 5.1). (Figures 5.2 and 5.3).

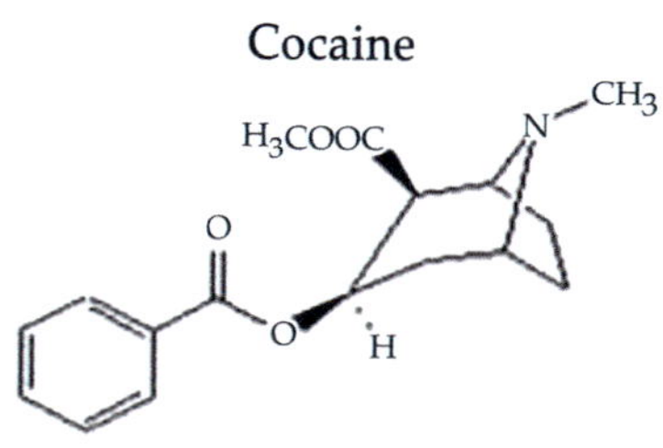

Figure 5.2. *Chemical structures of ester local anesthetics.*

Source: M. Whizar-Lugo, V., L. Íñiguez-López, K., C. Cárdenas-Maytorena, A., & D. Ramírez-Puerta, C. (2020). Local Anesthetics. IntechOpen. doi: 10.5772/intechopen.93643.

Table 5.1. *Nerve Fibers: Details*

Fiber Type	Function	Myelinated	Diameter (mm)	Conduction Velocity (m/s)	Spike Duration (ms)
Aα	Proprioception, somatic motor	Yes	12–20	70–120	0.4–0.5
Aβ	Touch, pressure	Yes	5–12	30–70	0.4–0.5
Aγ	Motor to muscle spindle	Yes	3–6	15–30	0.4–0.5
Aδ	Pain, cold, touch	Yes	2–5	12–30	0.4–0.5
C	Pain, temperature (dr) mechanoreception, reflex responses	No	0.4–1.2	0.5–2	2
B	Preganglionic autonomic	Yes	<3	3–15	1.2
C	Postganglionic sympathetic	No	0.3–1.3	0.7–2.3	2

Source: Marcos Michel-Levy, J. (2020). Pharmacokinetics and Pharmacodynamics of Local Anesthetics. IntechOpen. doi: 10.5772/intechopen.91700.

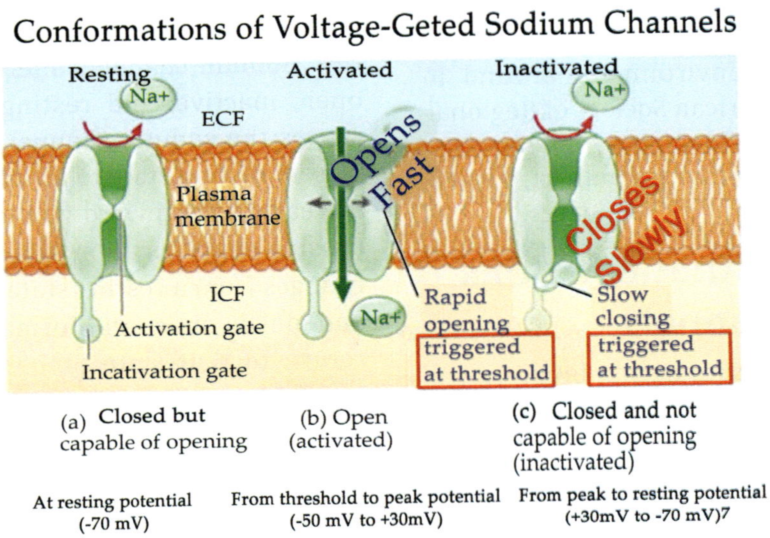

Figure 5.3. *During the propagation of impulses, from left to right, the current entering the axon at the initial rising phase of the impulse (large vertical arrows) passes through the axoplasm (local circuit current) and depolarizes the adjacent membrane. Plus, and minus signs adjacent to the axon membrane indicate the polarization state of the axon membrane: negative inside at rest, positive inside during active depolarization under the action potential, and less negative in regions where local circuit currents flow. This ionic current passes relatively uniformly across the nonmyelinated axon, but in the myelinated axon, it is restricted to entry at the nodes of Ranvier, several of which are simultaneously depolarized during a single action potential.*

Source: Marcos Michel-Levy, J. (2020). Pharmacokinetics and Pharmacodynamics of Local Anesthetics. IntechOpen. doi: 10.5772/intechopen.91700.

The modulated receptor model states that local anesthetics work through an allosteric mechanism, which alters the relative stability and kinetics of the channel's cycling through resting, open, and inactive conformations, rather than by physically "plugging the pore" of the channel. By doing this, the proportion of channels that are open and able to conduct inward sodium currents in reaction to a depolarization wave is decreased. This mechanism produces "use-dependent" or "frequency-dependent" nerve blocks, meaning that the intensity of the block increases with increased nerve firing frequency.

5.3.1 PH, Net Charge, and Lipid Solubility

Local anesthetics primarily bind to sodium channels close to the cytoplasmic side of the plasma membrane. Sufficient solubility and quick diffusion in both the hydrophobic environment of the lipid bilayers in plasma membranes and the hydrophilic environments of extracellular fluid, cytosol, and the headgroup region of membrane phospholipids are essential structural requirements for a molecule to be an effective local anesthetic. Because each of the commonly used clinical amino-amide and amino-ester local anesthetics contains a tertiary amine group that can quickly transition between an unprotonated base form (uncharged, hydrophobic) and a protonated hydrochloride form (charged, hydrophilic), they can achieve the goal of good solubility in both water and fat. At sodium channel binding sites, the most common active species is the charged, protonated form.

The relative proportion of charged and uncharged local anesthetic molecules is a function of the dissociation constant of the drug and the environmental pH. Recalling the Henderson-Hasselbalch equation, the dissociation constant (Ka) can be expressed as follows:

$$pKa = pH - \log([base]/[conjugate\ acid])$$

The conjugate acid component of the equation cancels out if the base and conjugate acid concentrations are equal (log 1 = 0). Therefore, the pKa offers a helpful means of characterizing a local anesthetic's tendency to exist in either a charged or uncharged state. At a particular pH, the percentage of un-ionized fraction increases with decreasing pKa. Conversely, less than half of the molecules of the widely used injectable anesthetics are un-ionized at physiological pH because their pKa values fall between 7 and 8 points. Since the base forms of local anesthetics are less stable and poorly soluble in water, they are typically sold as slightly acidic hydrochloride salts that are soluble in water. In an attempt to speed up the onset of anesthesia, bicarbonate is occasionally added to local anesthetic solutions right before injection to raise the un-ionized fraction. The onset and effectiveness of local anesthesia may also be adversely affected by other conditions that lower pH, such as tissue acidosis brought on by an infection, inflammation, or ischemia.

A local anesthetic's lipid solubility has an impact on its tissue penetration, potency, time course of uptake, and duration of action. Protein binding is also correlated with the duration of the local anesthetic action, which probably helps to keep the anesthetic in the nerve. The system used to measure these effects, whether in vitro or in vivo, may change the degree of anesthetic potency. For instance, when measured in isolated nerve, tetracaine is about 20 times more potent than bupivacaine; however, when measured in vivo, these medications are almost equally potent. Comparisons between local anesthetics, even when evaluated in vivo, may differ depending on the precise application site (spinal versus peripheral block) due to secondary effects like the anesthetic's intrinsic vasoactive qualities (American Society of Regional Anesthesia and Pain Medicine; Covino and Vassallo, 1976; Covino, Scott, Lambert, 1994).

5.4. Differential Local Anesthetic Blockade

Clinical observations and electrophysiologic measurements demonstrate that local anesthesia is not a binary state: after receiving injections of local anesthetic, patients experience varying degrees of sensory and motor blockade that change over time (Figure 5.4).

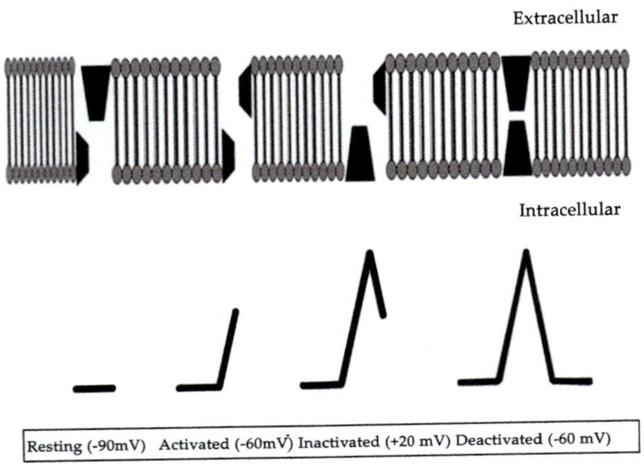

Figure 5.4. *Structural features of the Na+ channel that determine local anesthetic (LA) interactions.*

Source: *M. Whizar-Lugo, V., L. Íñiguez-López, K., C. Cárdenas-Maytorena, A., & D. Ramírez-Puerta, C. (2020). Local Anesthetics. IntechOpen. doi: 10.5772/intechopen.93643.*

Intraneural concentrations of local anesthetics are typically correlated with clinically apparent "numbness," but complex integration and processing of inputs at supraspinal sites in the somatosensory pathway as well as in the spinal dorsal horn also contribute to this phenomenon. Conduction blockade is facilitated by either increasing the concentration of local anesthetic or increasing the length of the nerve exposed to more diluted concentrations when compound action potentials are recorded in peripheral nerves exposed to local anesthetics in varying concentrations and lengths of nerve exposed (Figure 5.5).

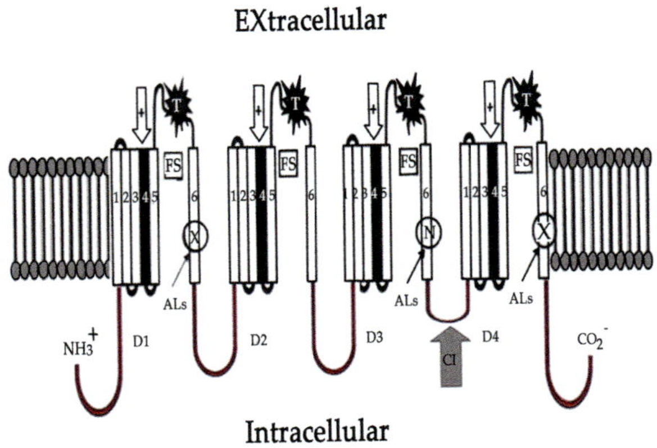

Figure 5.5. *Diagram of the voltage-dependent sodium channel with its 4 domains. Each domain has 6 helices that cross the cell membrane. The black stars located at the junctions of the helices 5 and 6 of each domain (pore handle) are the sites where cellular toxins (TTX) act. The sodium channel inactivation gate (IC) is located on the intracellular face between domains 3 and 4. The effector site of local anesthetics is located on helix 6 (or segment 6) of domains 3 and 4, although some schemes also draw it in domain 1.*

Source: *M. Whizar-Lugo, V., L. Íñiguez-López, K., C. Cárdenas-Maytorena, A., & D. Ramírez-Puerta, C. (2020). Local Anesthetics. IntechOpen. doi: 10.5772/intechopen.93643.*

Conduction blockade prevents the action potential from "skipping over" the region of local anesthetic exposure at the limit of short lengths of nerve exposed to the anesthetic by requiring exposure of at least three successive Ranvier nodes. In clinical textbooks, the term "differential blockade" originally described the finding that analgesia and autonomic blockade signs could be produced by infusions of diluted local anesthetic concentrations while comparatively sparing motor strength. The electrophysiologic findings of action potential blockade in large and small fibers perfused to a steady state do not easily account for this clinical trend. Although the mechanisms underlying this discrepancy between experimental and clinical data are not well understood, they could be associated with intrinsic impulse activity, variations in the longitudinal spread necessary for neural blockade, the anatomic and geographic arrangement of nerve fibers, and effects on other ion channels (American Society of Regional Anesthesia and Pain Medicine; Covino and Vassallo, 1976; Covino, Scott, Lambert, 1994).

5.5. Spread of Local Anesthesia After Injection

Local anesthetics applied around a peripheral nerve have to get past several diffusion barriers to enter the sodium channels found in the axons of the nerves. They diffuse along a concentration gradient from the nerve's outer surface (mantle) to its core (core) in large nerve trunks. As a result, the mantle's nerve fibers of a mixed nerve are blocked first. While fibers close to the core innervate distal structures, these mantle fibers are typically found in closer proximity to more proximal anatomic structures. This anatomical configuration explains why proximal anesthesia develops first, and then distal involvement occurs when the local anesthetic diffuses to reach more central core nerve fibers. If there are more superficial motor nerve fibers, skeletal muscle weakness may occur before sensory blockade. The anatomical location of the sympathetic, sensory, and motor nerve fibers within a mixed peripheral nerve plays a significant role in determining the sequence of events that occur during and after conduction blockade, in addition to their inherent sensitivity to local anesthetics (American Society of Regional Anesthesia and Pain Medicine; Covino and Vassallo, 1976; Covino, Scott, Lambert, 1994).

5.6. Pharmacokinetics

Systemic uptake transports the majority of oral and intravenous medications from the site of administration to the site of effect. Local anesthetics work differently because systemic absorption competes with drug entry into nerve effect sites when the drug is applied close to the intended location. As a result, effective and quick systemic absorption from an injection site reduces rather than boosts the effectiveness of nerve blockade. Unwanted intravascular injection or high plasma concentrations of local anesthetics following absorption from injection sites are the source of their potential toxicity. The rate of systemic absorption and, to a lesser extent, the rate of local anesthetic clearance determine the peak plasma concentrations that are reached. Numerous elements pertaining to the local anesthetic's physiochemical characteristics and the blood flow within the tissue have an impact on uptake. Local anesthetics with high lipophilicity and protein binding tend to have delayed uptake.

5.6.1. Local Anesthetic Vasoactivity

The tendency of anesthetics to cause vasodilation or constriction of blood vessels varies. The location of the injection, its concentration, and the ratio of local direct actions on vascular smooth muscle to indirect actions through blocking sympathetic efferent fibers all affect these outcomes. It could be clinically significant for these variations. For instance, S (−) ropivacaine has less frequent incidence of systemic toxicity in comparison to the R (+) enantiomer may be partially attributed to its vasoconstrictive activity (. Another illustration is the erratic result of adding vasoconstrictors to local anesthetic solutions used for spinal anesthesia. There is evidence that tetracaine causes a notable increase in spinal cord blood flow, which is different from what happens with lidocaine or bupivacaine. As a result, tetracaine exhibits a more marked prolongation of spinal anesthesia by epinephrine or other vasoconstrictors than other widely used spinal anesthetics (Table 5.2). (Figures 5.6, 5.7 and 5.8).

Table 5.2. *Comparative Pharmacology of Local Anesthetics*

Physico-chemical Characteristics				**Relative Potency in Different Blocks**			
Anesthetic	**pKa**	**Ionized % at pH 7.4**	**Partition Coefficient**	**% Protein Binding**	**Epidural**	**Spinal**	**Peripheral Nerve**
• Bupivacaine	8.1	83	3420	95	4	9.6	3.6
• Levobupiva-caine	8.1	83	3420	97	4	9.6	3.6
• Etidocaine	7.7	66	7317	94	2	6.7	0.7
• Lidocaine	7.9	76	366	64	1	1	1
• Mepivacaine	7.6	61	130	77	1	1	2.6
• Prilocaine	7.9	76	129	55	1	¿	0.8
• Ropivacaine	8.1	83	775	94	4	4.8	3.6
• Chloroprocaine	8.7	95	810	—	0.5	—	—
• Procaine	8.9	97	100	6	—	—	—
• Tetracaine	8.5	93	5822	94	—	—	—

Source: M. Whizar-Lugo, V., L. Íñiguez-López, K., C. Cárdenas-Maytorena, A., & D. Ramírez-Puerta, C. (2020). Local Anesthetics. IntechOpen. doi: 10.5772/intechopen.93643.

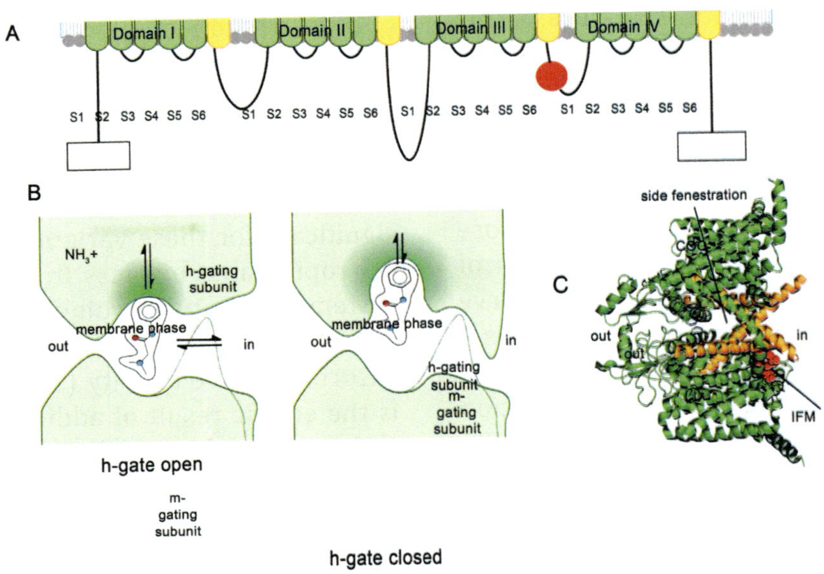

Figure 5.6. *Voltage-gated Navs as targets of LAs.* ***(A)****: 2D representation of Nav. Inactivation motif is indicated by red circle labelled with IFM (isoleucine, phenylalanine, methionine).* ***(B)****: View of 1977: Diagram of a LA molecule binding into the pore of a Nav indicating the activation gate (m-gate) and inactivation gate (h-gate) according to an early view and description of Nav modification (Hille, 1977). LAs were assumed to enter via* the membrane phase or passing the m- and h-gate from

the intracellular side. Many assumptions proved to be correct, such as the possibility for LAs to enter into the channel's pore from the membrane phase. The figure was partially readapted from (Hille, 1977). ***(C)**: Cryo-EM structure of hNav1.7 (Shen et al., 2019) (PDB ID: 6J8G) depicting the side fenestrations, which allow LAs to enter the channel from the lipid phase and the inactivation motif (IFM-motif, shown in red), which was previously described as h-gate.*

Source: Körner J, Albani S, Sudha Bhagavath Eswaran V, Roehl AB, Rossetti G and Lampert A (2022) Sodium Channels and Local Anesthetics—Old Friends With New Perspectives. Front. Pharmacol. 13:837088. doi: 10.3389/fphar.2022.837088.

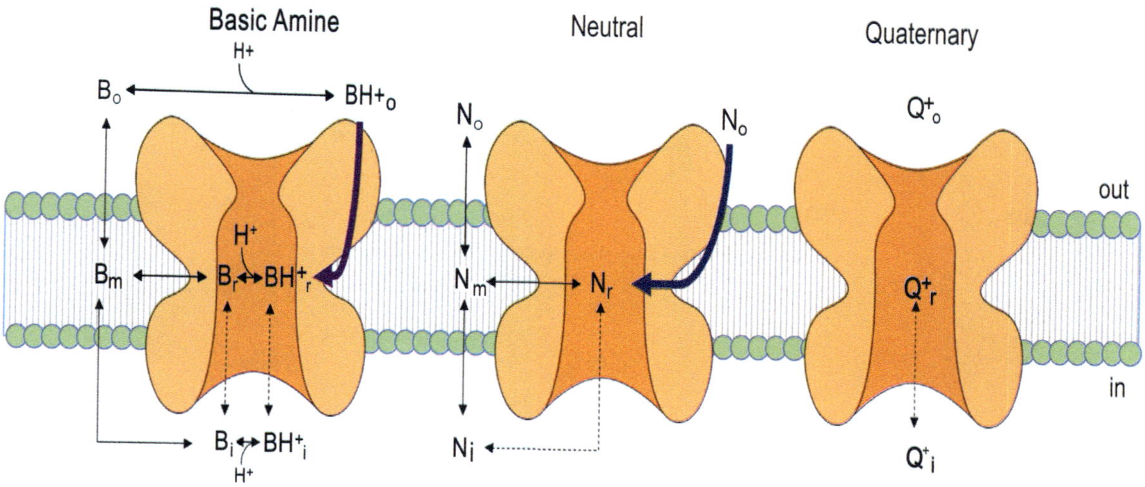

Figure 5.7. *Entry pathways of LAs with different chemical properties. Diagram of the movements of differently charged LA molecules (B, basic amine, N, neutral LA, Q, quaternary charged LA) to and from the channel. Black dashed lines are transitions requiring open activation and fast inactivation gates, as the drug enters from the intracellular side. Black solid lines are transitions probably not strongly depending on the gating state. Violet and blue lines indicate two pathways observed in MD studies for lidocaine and benzocaine, respectively, (Boiteux et al., 2014; Nguyen et al., 2019), where the LA does not pass through the membrane phase but enters a lipophilic pathway within the channel protein towards the side fenestrations. Subscript characters represent membrane phase (m), receptor site (r), extracellular (o) and intracellular (i) space.*

Source: Körner J, Albani S, Sudha Bhagavath Eswaran V, Roehl AB, Rossetti G and Lampert A (2022) Sodium Channels and Local Anesthetics—Old Friends With New Perspectives. Front. Pharmacol. 13:837088. doi: 10.3389/fphar.2022.837088.

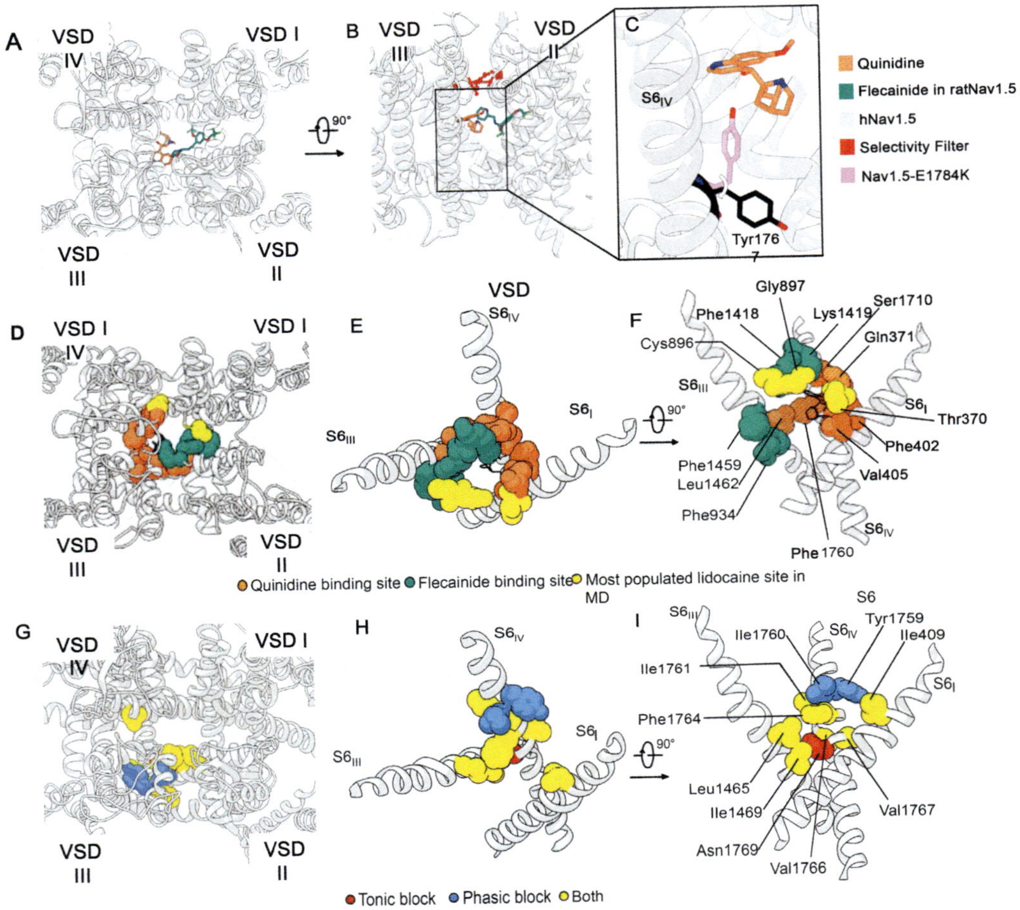

Figure 5.8. *LAs binding sites.* ***(A,B)*** Quinidine in hNav1.5 and *flecainide binding poses in rNav1.5 (PDB IDs: 6LQA and 6UZ0, respectively) and* ***(C)*** quinidine's effect on the rotation Tyr1767, as observed in hNav1.5 (PDB ID: 7DTC). ***(D–F)*** Sphere representation of the residues that appear in the binding site of quinidine (black wires) [in PDB ID: 6LQA (Li et al., 2021a)], and the corresponding hNav1.5 residues that were additionally observed in the binding pose of *flecainide [PDB ID: 6UZ0 (Jiang et al., 2020)], and the lidocaine molecules simulated in (Nguyen et al., 2019). The overlapping residues are colored in stripes in Panel F.* ***(G–I)*** Rat Nav1.2 homology model (https://alphafold.ebi.ac.uk/entry/P04775) and sphere representation of the residues characterized in mutagenesis experiments (Ragsdale et al., 1994; *Yarov-Yarovoy et al., 2002). Panels D-F and G-I show a partial overlapping of the binding regions of quinidine on hNav1.5 and lidocaine on rNav1.2, respectively.*

Source: Körner J, Albani S, Sudha Bhagavath Eswaran V, Roehl AB, Rossetti G and Lampert A (2022) Sodium Channels and Local Anesthetics—Old Friends With New Perspectives. Front. Pharmacol. 13:837088. doi: 10.3389/fphar.2022.837088.

5.6.2. Metabolism

Local anesthetics that are amino-amides are metabolized by hepatic microsomal enzymes, while those that are amino-esters are hydrolyzed by plasma esterases. Additionally, the lungs can draw local anesthetics from the bloodstream, including prilocaine, bupivacaine, and lidocaine. See

"Systemic Toxicity" for information on how this metabolism and first-pass pulmonary extraction may affect toxicity. This is because other local anesthetics, especially the amino amides, are more likely to produce sustained plasma concentrations than the ester local anesthetic chloroprocaine due to its relatively rapid hydrolysis. Yet, because of absent or restricted plasma hydrolysis, patients with atypical plasma cholinesterase levels may be more susceptible to experiencing excessive plasma concentrations of chloroprocaine or other ester local anesthetics. Lidocaine is extensively metabolized by the liver, and the liver's blood flow and the removal of this local anesthetic from plasma coincide. Diseases of the liver or reductions in hepatic blood flow, such as those brought on by congestive heart failure or general anesthesia, can slow down the rate at which lidocaine is metabolized. Less than 5% of local anesthetics injected into the body are expelled.

5.6.3. Additives

The most often used ingredient in solutions for local anesthetics is epinephrine. Epinephrine causes local vasoconstriction at a typical concentration of 5 μg/mL (1:200,000). This slows the rate of tissue absorption, lowering peak systemic concentrations and lowering the risk of systemic toxicity. Epinephrine may cause a temporary prolongation of a sensory or motor block, depending on the injection site and the local anesthetic used. Based on effects on arterial blood pressure, heart rate, or symptoms, epinephrine can also be used as a marker for intravascular injection detection. Still, in susceptible patients, systemic absorption of epinephrine may exacerbate systemic hypertension or contribute to cardiac dysrhythmias. In peripheral nerve blocks, epinephrine should be avoided in areas that might not have collateral flow (e.g., virtual blocks). On the other hand, vasoconstriction induced by epinephrine reduces local bleeding and might be advantageous when combined with local anesthetics used for infiltration anesthesia. A number of additional additives, such as the glucocorticoid dexamethasone and the α2-agonist clonidine, have been investigated to extend the analgesia resulting from peripheral nerve blocks. Meaningful prolongations from certain blocks more than others are caused by both of these additives, along with meaningful prolongations of sensory block and clinical analgesia from both local and systemic perineural administration. Anesthesia providers have historically had a great deal of latitude in creating their own blends and additions. It's becoming increasingly acknowledged that this procedure can lead to mistakes in the administration of drugs. Furthermore, while certain additives have been thoroughly tested in preclinical settings to guarantee that they do not cause local tissue toxicity in nerve and muscle, others have not. Clinical use of novel additives without adequate preclinical safety data and a regulatory review procedure is probably not warranted (American Society of Regional Anesthesia and Pain Medicine; Covino and Vassallo, 1976; Covino, Scott, Lambert, 1994).

5.7. Adverse Effects

Important adverse effects of local anesthetics, although rare, may occur from systemic absorption, local tissue toxicity, allergic reactions, and drug-specific effects.

5.7.1. Systemic Toxicity

Local anesthetics can become toxic to the system due to high plasma concentrations, which are typically caused by an unintentional intravascular injection given during peripheral nerve blocks. Less frequently, the absorption of local anesthetics from tissue injection sites leads to excessive plasma concentrations. A vasoconstrictor's presence in the local anesthetic solution, the injection site, and the dose administered all affect how much of the anesthetic is absorbed systemically. After injection for caudal anesthesia and intercostal nerve blocks, the systemic absorption of local anesthetic is at its highest; it is intermediate following epidural anesthesia, and it is at its lowest following brachial plexus blocks.

Systemic toxicity that is clinically significant is caused by effects on the cardiovascular and central nervous systems. To control plasma concentrations that may arise from these medications' systemic absorption, the maximum permissible local anesthetic doses have been established to perform regional anesthesia. However, standard dosage recommendations lack consideration for the unique injection site and patient-related factors, and they are inconsistent and not fully supported by the available evidence. However, dose recommendations serve as a basis for dose modifications based on changing evidence and clinical circumstances.

5.7.1.1. Central Nervous System Toxicity

Although significant deviation from this pattern is fairly common, increasing plasma concentrations of local anesthetics typically cause circumoral numbness, facial tingling, restlessness, vertigo, tinnitus, and slurred speech, which ultimately culminate in tonic-clonic seizures.

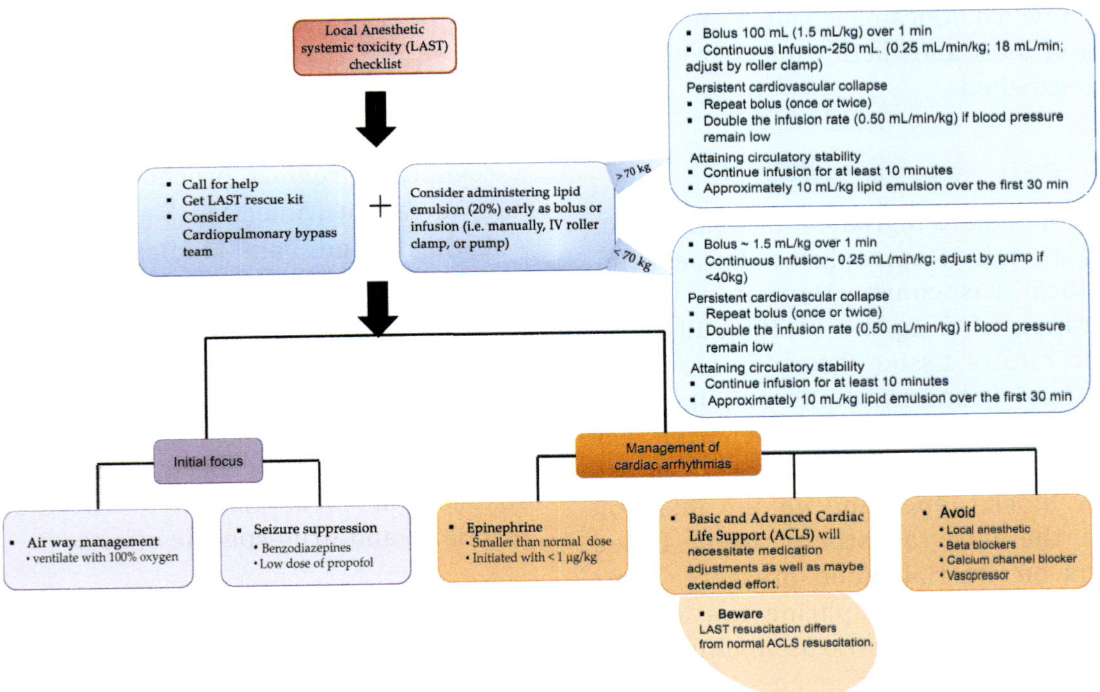

Figure 5.9. *The American Society of Regional Anesthesia and Pain Medicine (ASRAPM) guidelines for the management of local anesthetic systemic toxicity (LAST).*

Source: Bahar E, Yoon H. Lidocaine: A Local Anesthetic, Its Adverse Effects and Management. Medicina. 2021; 57(8):782. https://doi.org/10.3390/medicina57080782.

Since local anesthetics are neural depressants, it is likely that the selective depression of cortical inhibitory neurons that causes seizures first occurs, allowing excitatory pathways to remain unopposed. Larger doses, however, may alter excitatory and inhibitory pathways, depressing the central nervous system and possibly putting a person in a coma. These outcomes typically follow the potency of anesthetics. During seizure activity, arterial hypoxemia and metabolic acidosis can happen quickly. Additionally, both hypoxemia and acidosis can increase the toxicity of local anesthetics on the central nervous system (Figure 5.9).

When treating toxic reactions to the central nervous system, quick action is required to prevent hypoxemia and hypercarbia. This includes giving extra oxygen and supporting ventilation as needed. When benzodiazepines (i.e., due to their effectiveness and relative hemodynamic stability, midazolam, lorazepam, and diazepam) are typically the first-choice medications to stop seizures. Propofol can impair cardiac function, so even though it is more readily available, it should be used cautiously when suppressing seizures.

5.7.1.2. Cardiovascular System Toxicity

In general, the central nervous system is less vulnerable to the harmful effects of local anesthetics than the cardiovascular system. However, significant hypotension can be caused by high plasma concentrations of local anesthetics because they relax the smooth muscle in the arteriolar arteries and cause direct cardiac depression. Part of the cardiac toxicity can be attributed to local anesthetics' capacity to block cardiac sodium ion channels in addition to other ion channels. Cardiac automaticity and cardiac impulse conduction are thereby compromised, resulting in an ECG that shows an elongated PR interval and a widened QRS complex. Myocardial contractility may be significantly and to differing degrees depressed by local anesthetics. For instance, the amount of lidocaine needed to cause cardiovascular collapse is roughly twice that of bupivacaine compared to the dose needed to cause seizures. These results are consistent with the theory that bupivacaine is more likely to result in cardiac toxicity, which has fueled the creation of single-enantiomer anesthetics like levobupivacaine and ropivacaine.

5.7.2. Lipid Resuscitation

Lipid emulsion intravenous infusions are now a routine treatment for systemic toxicity (LAST) associated with local anesthetics. The mechanism of action is unclear, but it probably has to do with the capacity of lipids to extract lipophilic medications like bupivacaine from tissue targets or aqueous plasma, lowering the drugs' effective free concentration (also known as a "lipid sink"). As a result, lipid emulsion solutions ought to be kept on hand and easily accessible in any area where major conduction blockade is carried out, as well as in any area where overdoses from any lipophilic medication may be handled. An extensive publication by the American Society of Regional Anesthesia and Pain Medicine (ASRA) Task Force on Local Anesthetic Systemic Toxicity provides guidelines for the administration of lipid emulsions (20 percent), checklists, and treatment protocols.

The ASRA guidelines state that a lipid emulsion intravenous bolus dose consists of a bolus of 1.5 mL/kg (100 mg in adults) and a continuous infusion at 0.25 mL/kg/min. Lipid rescue is crucial and ought to be utilized, but it is not a 100% foolproof solution. It is not a replacement for adhering to safe practices and dosage guidelines concerning patient monitoring, fractionated dosing, and keeping an eye out for any early warning indicators of systemic toxicity. Additional modifications to standard advanced cardiac life support (ACLS) protocols are recommended by ASRA guidelines. These modifications include refraining from using vasopressin, calcium channel blockers, β-adrenergic blockers, or other local anesthetics such as lidocaine or amiodarone. Reduce the incremental dosage of adrenaline to less than 1 μg/kg.

5.7.3. Local Tissue Toxicity

The effects of local anesthetics on local tissue are generally well tolerated. However, all of the local anesthetics on the market today have inherent toxicities to muscles and nerves that can occasionally manifest clinically. These risks may be made worse by conditions that increase nerve vulnerability and predispose to nerve ischemia, such as preexisting nerve dysfunction, metabolic and inflammatory conditions, increased tissue pressure, and systemic hypotension. These incidences of toxicities increase with local tissue concentration and duration of exposure. Long-term perineural infusions can cause intraneural concentrations to rise gradually. Due to these factors, we advise using relatively diluted local anesthetic concentrations for prolonged perineural infusions—generally, no more than 0–2% for ropivacaine or bupivacaine.

5.7.4. Allergic Reactions

Even though local anesthetics are used frequently, allergic reactions to them are uncommon. Allergy mechanisms account for less than 1% of adverse reactions to local anesthetics. The majority of unfavorable reactions that are mistakenly attributed to allergic reactions are actually the result of additives or systemic toxicity symptoms brought on by high local anesthetic plasma concentrations. Syncope-related hypotension may be vagally mediated, while systemic epinephrine absorption may cause tachycardia and palpitations.

5.7.4.1. Cross-Sensitivity

Hypersensitivity reactions are more common with amino-ester local anesthetics than with amino amides because they generate metabolites linked to para-aminobenzoic acid. Commercial formulations of ester and amide local anesthetics contain methylparaben or similar compounds that resemble para-aminobenzoic acid as preservatives; these compounds can also trigger allergic reactions. It is recommended that patients who are known to be allergic to amino-ester local anesthetics be given amino-amide local anesthetics; however, this recommendation should be regarded with caution as it presumes that the local anesthetic, rather than a common preservative, was the cause of the initial allergic reaction.

5.7.4.2. Documentation

The primary basis for recording an allergy to local anesthetics is the patient's clinical history, which includes symptoms like rash, laryngeal edema, hypotension, and bronchospasm. However, if other medications (such as sedative-hypnotics or opioids) have been taken at the same time as the local anesthetic, intradermal testing may help identify the local anesthetic as the offending antigen. Increases in serum tryptase, a marker of mast cell degranulation, may also be useful for confirmation (American Society of Regional Anesthesia and Pain Medicine; Covino and Vassallo, 1976; Covino, Scott, Lambert, 1994).

5.8. Specific Local Anesthetics

5.8.1. Amino Esters

5.8.1.1. Procaine

Throughout the first half of the 20th century, procaine—the first injectable local anesthetic—was widely used, mostly as a spinal anesthetic. Because of its instability and significant risk of hypersensitivity reactions, lidocaine was introduced, which limited its use. Procaine is once again being considered as a spinal anesthetic due to concerns about transient neurologic symptoms (TNS) linked to spinal lidocaine (see "Lidocaine"). Nevertheless, scant information indicates that procaine provides little benefit in terms of TNS, and spinal procaine is linked to a noticeably higher rate of nausea.

5.8.1.2. Tetracaine

Spinal anesthesia is still frequently achieved with tetracaine. As a result, it acts for a long time, especially when combined with a vasoconstrictor, though doing so carries a surprisingly high risk of TNS. Tetracaine is available as Niphanoid crystals or as a 1% solution; the anesthetic in solution is relatively unstable, so the crystal form is preferred. Tetracaine's profound motor blockade, slow onset, and potential toxicity at high doses make it an uncommon choice for epidural anesthesia and peripheral nerve blocks. Despite being an ester, it has a metabolism that is a tenth that of chloroprocaine and a fourth that of procaine.

5.8.1.3. Chloroprocaine

Because of its quick hydrolysis, chloroprocaine was first widely used as an epidural anesthetic, especially in obstetrics, where worries about systemic toxicity and fetal exposure to the local anesthetic were essentially eliminated. Unfortunately, enthusiasm for neuraxial chloroprocaine administration was tempered by neurotoxic injury, which was thought to result from an accidental intrathecal injection of large doses intended for the epidural space. It was believed that the preservative sodium bisulfite, which was a part of the commercial formulation, was what caused this toxicity. Subsequent research, on the other hand, has shown intrathecal bisulfite to be neither neurotoxic nor neuroprotective, but rather non-toxic. Regardless, a version of chloroprocaine free of antioxidants and preservatives is available.

Epidural anesthesia produced by chloroprocaine lasts for a comparatively short time. Since it reduces the anesthetic or analgesic effect of epidural bupivacaine and opioids used concurrently or sequentially, epidural administration of chloroprocaine is occasionally avoided. Because of clinical concerns about the potential toxicity of lidocaine injected into the subarachnoid space and because toxicity is not expected at the small doses needed for spinal anesthesia, chloroprocaine's status as a spinal anesthetic has been reevaluated. Because of these positive early reports, chloroprocaine is now frequently used off-label for this purpose. Despite the debate, intrathecal doses of chloroprocaine for spinal anesthesia should not exceed 60 mg, and solutions should be bisulfite-free.

A repeat loading dose with the more frequently used amino-amide local anesthetic would cause a stepwise increase in blood concentrations into a toxic range. This is why chloroprocaine is unique in pediatric regional anesthesia because of its rapid plasma clearance. (1) As a continuous epidural infusion in neonates and very young infants. (2) For patients receiving postoperative epidural or peripheral perineural infusions.

5.8.2. Amino Amides

5.8.2.1. Lidocaine

The most widely used local anesthetic is lidocaine. It is applied to peripheral nerve block, spinal and epidural anesthesia, and local, topical, and regional intravenous block. Lidocaine is still widely used for all other local anesthetic uses, such as epidural anesthesia, even though recent problems have limited its use for spinal anesthesia. Possibly neurotoxic (i.e., cauda equina syndrome) when spinal anesthesia is provided with lidocaine has become a concern, particularly when a continuous spinal technique is employed. The majority of the initial injuries were caused by neurotoxic anesthetic concentrations in the caudal region of the subarachnoid space, which was obtained by combining relatively large anesthetic doses with maldistribution via small-gauge spinal catheters. Even the 75–100 mg doses of lidocaine that are frequently used for single-injection spinal anesthesia have been linked to neurotoxicity, though.

When patients receive intrathecal doses of lidocaine, up to one-third of them may experience TNS, a syndrome characterized by pain and dysesthesia (but rarely with bupivacaine). TNS was eventually adopted in place of the original term, transient radicular irritation, due to the uncertainty surrounding the etiology of these symptoms. The lithotomy position, knee arthroscopy positioning, and outpatient status are among the cofactors that increase the risk of TNS in addition to the administration of intrathecal lidocaine. On the other hand, the incidence of TNS with lidocaine remains unchanged regardless of the concentration of local anesthetic, glucose levels, concurrent administration of epinephrine, and technique-related factors like needle size or type. TNS symptoms usually appear 12 to 24 hours after surgery, go away in 3 days, and then rarely come back for more than a week. While self-limiting, the pain can be extremely intense, frequently worse than what the surgery caused, and in rare cases necessitating a return hospital stay in order to manage the pain. As a first line of treatment, nonsteroidal anti-inflammatory drugs (NSAIDs) are frequently quite effective. TNS does not.

5.8.2.2. Mepivacaine

The first of the pipecholyl xylidine series, mepivacaine combined the xylidine ring of lidocaine with the piperidine ring of cocaine. This produced an anesthetic with properties that were almost exactly like lidocaine, but with less vasodilation and a little bit longer half-life. With the exception of being comparatively ineffective as a topical local anesthetic, mepivacaine is used in clinical settings similarly to lidocaine. For short-duration spinal anesthesia, mepivacaine is a desirable substitute for lidocaine due to its decreased incidence of TNS.

5.8.2.3. Prilocaine

When prilocaine was first used in clinical settings, it was thought to be a useful medication due to its quick metabolism and rare acute toxicity (which is roughly 40% less harmful to the central nervous system than lidocaine). Sadly, administering large doses (>600 mg) may cause the metabolite ortho-toluidine, an oxidizing substance that can change hemoglobin into methemoglobin, to accumulate to a clinically significant level. Methemoglobinemia induced by pliolocaine resolves on its own and can be corrected by injecting 1 to 2 mg/kg of methylene blue intravenously over a 5-minute period. However, prilocaine's ability to cause dose-related methemoglobinemia has hindered its clinical acceptability.

Like other anesthetics, prilocaine has gained attention lately as a spinal anesthetic because spinal lidocaine isn't working well enough. Though scarce, the data that is currently available indicates that prilocaine acts similarly to lidocaine for a longer period of time while causing less TNS. Neither the drug nor any formulation that would be suitable for intrathecal delivery is currently authorized for use in the United States.

5.8.2.4. Bupivacaine

Bupivacaine is a derivative of mepivacaine that has a longer duration of action due to a modification on the piperidine ring: a butyl group instead of a methyl group. This feature, along with its superior sensory anesthesia in comparison to motor blockade, has made bupivacaine the most widely used local anesthetic for postoperative pain management and epidural anesthesia during labor. Bupivacaine has a fairly clean record as a spinal anesthetic and is also frequently used for peripheral nerve block.

The use of 0.75 percent bupivacaine, which is no longer advised for epidural anesthesia, has been linked to irreversible cardiac arrest when administered intravenously during an attempted epidural anesthesia. Its interaction with cardiac sodium ion channels is most likely the mechanism responsible for bupivacaine's cardiotoxicity. Comparing the electrophysiologic differences between anesthetics, lidocaine exhibits a rapid entry and exit from the sodium ion channel. Bupivacaine blockade, on the other hand, has a much greater effect on lowering the maximum upstroke velocity of the cardiac action potential (V_{max}) in ventricular cardiac muscle during diastole due to the relatively longer recovery period. Bupivacaine is therefore known as a "fast-in, slowout" local anesthetic. It is possible that this feature facilitates unidirectional block and reentry.

Bupivacaine may also be cardiotoxic due to other mechanisms, such as atrioventricular nodal conduction disruption, myocardial contractility depression, and indirect effects through the central nervous system. This risk of cardiotoxicity significantly restricts the overall amount of bupivacaine and emphasizes the need of fractional dosing and techniques to identify unintentional intravascular injection when large amounts of local anesthetic, particularly bupivacaine, are administered for regional block. The significance of these precautionary measures is not lessened by the discovery that lipid emulsion is a viable therapeutic intervention for bupivacaine cardiotoxicity. When spinal anesthesia is administered in small doses, cardiotoxicity is not a concern.

5.8.3. Single Enantiomers

The stereoisomers of bupivacaine and its homolog, ropivacaine, have come under scrutiny due to worries about bupivacaine's cardiotoxicity.

5.8.3.1. Stereochemistry

Despite having the same molecular formula, isomers are distinct compounds. Stereoisomers are subsets of isomers with different spatial orientations of atoms joined by the same bonding sequence. A specific class of stereoisomers known as enantiomers are those that exist as mirror images. Because the forms are essentially nonsuperimposable mirror images, the term "chiral" comes from the Greek word cheir, which means "hand." With the exception of the direction in which the plane of polarized light rotates, enantiomers are identical in every way. The enantiomer is classified as levorotatory (–) if the rotation is to the left or counterclockwise, and as dextrorotatory (+) if it is to the right or clockwise, based on this property. A mixture of equal parts of enantiomers, known as a racemic mixture, is optically inactive because the opposite rotation of one isomer cancels out the rotation caused by its molecules. On the basis of their absolute configuration, chiral compounds can also be categorized; these are typically denoted as R (rectus) or S (sinister). Regarding a particular biologic activity, enantiomers can vary. For instance, the bupivacaine S (–) enantiomer has l by nature.

5.8.3.2. Ropivacaine

Levopropivacaine, also known as ropivacaine, is the S (–) enantiomer of the piperidine ring-containing homolog of bupivacaine and mepivacaine. Moreover, there is a better connection with cardiac sodium ion channels. Its greater propensity to cause vasoconstriction could be a factor in its lower cardiotoxicity. Ropivacaine may more readily cause a differential block since motor blockade is less severe and electrophysiologic research suggests that C fibers may be blocked preferentially. However, ropivacaine is not as effective as bupivacaine, which makes sense given its decreased lipid solubility. Any comparison of these anesthetics must take potency into account; if more medication is required to produce the desired result, then when more appropriate equipotent dose comparisons are made, the apparent benefits with regard to cardiotoxicity (or differential block) may not exist. In terms of cardiotoxicity, ropivacaine probably has some advantage over bupivacaine; however, in terms of differential block, the difference is, at most, negligible.

5.8.3.3. Levobupivacaine

The single S (–) enantiomer of bu-pivacaine is called levobupivacaine. Cardiotoxicity is decreased similarly to ropivacaine, but differential blockade is not improved over bupivacaine. Similar to ropivacaine, this compound's clinically meaningful advantage over the racemic mixture is limited to circumstances involving the administration of relatively high anesthetic doses.

5.8.4. Topical Local Anesthetics

Local anesthetics are frequently applied to mucosal surfaces, intact skin, especially when performing needle procedures on children, and cut skin to aid in the healing of lacerations. Through mucosal surfaces, systemic absorption occurs fairly quickly and effectively. Overdosing on local anesthetic sprays and gels from the oral, nasal, or tracheobronchial mucosa has been known to cause systemic toxicity, especially in young children and infants.

It is comparatively more difficult to achieve anesthesia of intact skin by topical application because the keratinized layer of the skin acts as an effective barrier to the diffusion of topical anesthetics. This restriction can be addressed by applying local anesthetic in relatively high concentrations (e.g.5% lidocaine (like in LMX) or 4% gel tetracaine (like in Ametop). A mixture consisting of 2.5 percent lidocaine and 2.5 percent prilocaine cream (i.e. On intact skin, eutectic mixture of local anesthetics (EMLA) is frequently used. This mixture exists at room temperature as an oil that can penetrate the skin's barrier, and its melting point is lower than that of either component alone. EMLA cream is especially helpful for preventing or lessening pain related to venipuncture or intravenous catheter insertion in children, though it may take up to an hour to produce sufficient topical anesthesia. An additional product called Synera uses a heating element to hasten the onset of tetracaine-and lidocaine-induced skin analgesia.

5.8.5. Tumescent Local Anesthesia

Tumescent local anesthesia is a common technique used for a range of plastic and cosmetic surgical procedures. It entails the subcutaneous infusion of large volumes of very dilute local anesthetic. This method uses very high total doses of lidocaine—eight times higher than what is advised for infiltration or peripheral nerve blockade. However, this strategy has a pharmacokinetic foundation. Plasma lidocaine concentrations stay within a safe range when suggested dosage guidelines and procedures are followed, however plasma concentrations typically peak more than 12 hours after injection. The general safety of this approach is supported by multiple case series when suggested guidelines are adhered to. On the other hand, bad things have happened when rules weren't followed. Specifically, toxic reactions have occurred when other local anesthetics were dosed more over the course of the following day. Any medical facility employing this method needs to have LAST treatment protocols and resources.

5.8.6. Systemic Local Anesthetics for Acute and Chronic Pain

In addition to being used for local anesthesia,

related sodium channel blockers like mexiletine can also be used as systemic analgesics. Evidence supports the efficacy of these medications as adjuvant analgesics for both postoperative pain and various neuropathic pain conditions. Brief intravenous lidocaine infusions may provide a notable, if not well-understood, prolonged duration of pain relief for certain patients suffering from neuropathic pain (e.g., days or weeks) that significantly surpasses the apparent pharmacologic half-life of lidocaine (American Society of Regional Anesthesia and Pain Medicine; Covino and Vassallo, 1976; Covino, Scott, Lambert, 1994).

5.9. When Local Anesthesia Fails

Enhancing the clinical efficacy of local anesthetic administration should be a goal for anesthesia providers and other healthcare professionals. Technical failure, or the placement of the needle and solution injection not close enough to the intended site of action, has historically been a common cause of failed local anesthesia. The technical success of many forms of regional anesthesia, particularly those involving peripheral nerve and plexus blocks, has undoubtedly improved due to the widespread use of ultrasound guidance. Despite the fact that numerous studies show that ultrasound helps regional anesthesia go more smoothly and with significantly lower amounts of local anesthetics, the median effective dose or volume (i.e., effectiveness for 50% of subjects) is not a useful variable for clinical practice; an ED95 (an effective dose that prevents movement in 95% of subjects) is more pertinent. When "blind" techniques like loss of resistance are used alone, there is a significant technical failure rate for well-established procedures like thoracic epidural anesthesia. More comprehensive roles for more objective approaches to confirm needle and catheter placement for various forms are becoming increasingly appreciated.

There are several other reasons why local anesthesia may not work properly besides a technical issue with the needle's placement. Clinicians may overlook certain nerves that innervate a surgical site because of incorrect assumptions they make about the relevant neuroanatomy of pain resulting from a surgical procedure. Furthermore, biologic sources of variation in local anesthetic responsiveness are not fully appreciated. For instance, a small percentage of individuals with type III Ehlers-Danlos syndrome exhibit a relative resistance to local anesthetics.

Local anesthetics frequently work less well at places where there is inflammation or infection. Both pharmacodynamic factors, such as peripheral and central sensitization, and pharmacokinetic factors, such as local acidosis, edema, and hyperemia, which decrease drug entry into nerves, are likely responsible for inflammation-induced local anesthetic resistance. Certain patients may experience tachyphylaxis, or rapidly developing tolerance, after repeated doses or extended infusions. Clinical observations and animal research link tachyphylaxis to the emergence of hyperalgesia. By concurrently administering antihyperalgesic medications or other analgesics with central actions, tachyphylaxis can be lessened or avoided.

In addition to coadministration of other analgesic or antihyperalgesic medications, patients with chronic pain and hyperalgesia that has persisted over time often seem to require larger volumes or concentrations, or both, of local anesthetics to achieve adequate analgesia. While psychological factors might affect a patient's capacity to withstand surgery under regional anesthesia, physicians shouldn't "blame the patient" for inadequate levels of analgesia or sensory block because there are a number of technical or biologic factors that affect how effective the block is. Peripheral nerves and sodium channels may also be impacted by chronic pain and its treatment. Different sodium channel subtypes express themselves differently in response to inflammation and nerve injury. While the sodium channel's alpha subunit makes up the "pore," beta subunits are also expressed differently in response to inflammation or nerve injury. These beta subunits change the electrophysiology of the channel, which may change how responsive the area is to local anesthetics. According to a 2016 study, the ability of the rat sciatic nerve to respond to local anesthetic was hampered by chronic opioid exposure, but not by acute exposure (American Society of Regional Anesthesia and Pain Medicine; Covino and Vassallo, 1976; Covino, Scott, Lambert, 1994).

5.10. Future Local Anesthetics

In contemporary anesthetic practice, local anesthetics are essential. However, this class of compounds has a relatively narrow therapeutic index with respect to their potential for neurotoxicity and for adverse effects on the cardiovascular and central nervous systems, despite significant advancements in pharmacology and administration techniques over the past century. Site 1 sodium channel blockers are a different class of molecules that block sodium channels through a different site and mechanism. Several early studies suggest they are not neurotoxic or myotoxic. These findings imply that there may not be a shared mechanism between sodium channel blockade and local tissue toxicity to nerve and muscle. Additionally, site 1 blockers seem to have less cardiotoxicity, most likely because of their much lower affinity for Nav1.5, the predominant sodium channel subtype in the myocardium.

The use of regional anesthesia both during surgery and afterward has become more and more common. One acknowledged benefit of employing regional anesthesia and analgesia is opioid sparing. After a single injection, the majority of local anesthetics on the market provide analgesia for less than 12 hours. While continuous catheter approaches can prolong analgesia, there are risks associated with these infusions, including increased risk of dislodgement and increased postoperative care and expenses. As a result, there are various ways to achieve long-lasting local anesthesia with a single injection for peripheral nerve blockade or wound infiltration. It has been possible to release bupivacaine under control using hydrogels, liposomes, microparticles, and other vehicles. Exparel, a liposomal bupivacaine product approved for wound infiltration, is currently available for purchase in the US market. The results of clinical trials have been inconsistent.

The lack of modality selectivity in current local anesthetics is another drawback. For instance, it would be ideal to have strong analgesia, prevent weakness and hypotension, and maintain enough sensation to feel the need to push when using epidural analgesia for labor. Two main approaches to sensory-selective blockade have been used in recent research: (1) developing drugs that bind preferentially to subtypes of sodium channels located predominantly in small sensory fibers, and (2) targeting local anesthetic entry preferentially into small sensory nerve fibers (American Society of Regional Anesthesia and Pain Medicine; Covino and Vassallo, 1976; Covino, Scott, Lambert, 1994).

A Closer Look

Spinal Anesthesia

Spinal anesthesia, also known as spinal block or subarachnoid block, is a form of regional anesthesia commonly used in surgical procedures below the umbilicus (belly button), including cesarean sections, hernia repairs, and orthopedic surgeries. This technique involves injecting a local anesthetic medication into the subarachnoid space surrounding the spinal cord, temporarily blocking the transmission of nerve impulses and effectively numbing the lower half of the body. Unlike epidural anesthesia, which involves placing a catheter into the epidural space outside the spinal cord, spinal anesthesia delivers the medication directly into the cerebrospinal fluid, resulting in a faster onset of action and typically requiring smaller doses of anesthetic. The procedure is performed with the patient positioned either sitting upright or lying on their side, and after sterilizing the area and administering a local anesthetic to numb the skin, a needle is inserted into the lower back between the vertebrae of the lumbar spine. Once the needle is correctly positioned in the subarachnoid space, the anesthetic medication is injected, and its effects are rapidly felt within minutes. Patients may experience sensations of warmth, numbness, and heaviness in the lower body as the anesthesia takes effect, and they are closely monitored throughout the procedure for any signs of complications such as hypotension (low blood pressure) or headache. Spinal anesthesia provides excellent pain relief during surgery while allowing patients to remain awake and alert, making it a preferred choice for many surgical procedures, particularly those involving the lower abdomen, pelvis, or lower extremities. After the surgery is completed, the effects of spinal anesthesia gradually wear off, and sensation and movement return to the lower body over the course of several hours. However, some temporary side effects such as urinary retention, headache, and back pain may occur, and rare complications such as nerve injury or infection are possible but uncommon with proper technique and monitoring. Overall, spinal anesthesia is a safe and effective option for providing localized pain relief and anesthesia for a variety of surgical procedures, contributing to improved patient comfort and outcomes.

Summary

- The mechanism of action of local anesthetics involves their interaction with sodium channels in nerve cell membranes, thereby preventing the generation and propagation of action potentials along nerve fibers.
- Local anesthetics play a vital role in modern healthcare, facilitating a wide range of medical procedures with minimal pain and discomfort. With ongoing innovation and refinement, these agents continue to evolve, promising further improvements in pain management and patient care.
- Local anesthetics act on a wide range of molecular targets, but they exert their predominant desired clinical effects by blocking sodium ion flux through voltage-gated sodium channels. Voltage-gated sodium channels are complex transmembrane proteins comprising large alpha subunits and much smaller beta subunits.
- When local anesthetics are deposited around a peripheral nerve, they must cross a series of diffusion barriers to access sodium channels in nerve axons. With large nerve trunks, they diffuse from the outer surface (mantle) toward the center (core) of the nerve along a concentration gradient.
- Anesthetics differ in their tendencies to cause either vasoconstriction or vasodilation of blood vessels. These effects vary with site of injection, concentration, and balance of local direct actions on vascular smooth muscle versus indirect actions via blockade of sympathetic efferent fibers.
- The amino-ester local anesthetics undergo hydrolysis by plasma esterases, whereas the amino-amide local anesthetics undergo metabolism by hepatic microsomal enzymes. The lungs are also capable of extracting local anesthetics such as lidocaine, bupivacaine, and prilocaine from the circulation.
- Epinephrine is the most common additive in local anesthetic solutions. In a typical concentration of 5 μg/mL (1:200,000), epinephrine produces local vasoconstriction, which slows the rate of tissue absorption and therefore reduces peak systemic concentrations, decreasing the odds of systemic toxicity
- Systemic toxicity of local anesthetics results from excessive plasma concentrations of these drugs, most often from accidental intravascular injection during performance of peripheral nerve blocks.
- Increasing plasma concentrations of local anesthetics classically produce circumoral numbness, facial tingling, restlessness, vertigo, tinnitus, and slurred speech, culminating in tonic-clonic seizures, though marked variation from this pattern is quite common.
- Allergic reactions to local anesthetics are rare, despite the frequent use of these drugs. Less than 1% of all adverse reactions to local anesthetics are caused by allergic mechanisms.
- Chloroprocaine initially gained popularity as an epidural anesthetic, particularly in obstetrics, because its rapid hydrolysis virtually eliminated concern about systemic toxicity and fetal exposure to the local anesthetic.

- Local anesthetics are commonly administered on mucosal surfaces, on cut skin to facilitate laceration repair, and on intact skin, especially for needle procedures in children. Systemic absorption through mucosal surfaces is relatively rapid and efficient (American Society of Regional Anesthesia and Pain Medicine; Covino and Vassallo, 1976; Covino, Scott, Lambert, 1994).

References

1. Albright, G. A. (1979). Cardiac arrest following regional anesthesia with etidocaine or bupivacaine. *Anesthesiology, 51*, 285–287.
2. Araujo, M. C., Sinnott, C. J., & Strichartz, G. R. (2003). Multiple phases of relief from experimental mechanical allodynia by systemic lidocaine: Responses to early and late infusions. *Pain, 103*, 21–29.
3. Arendt-Nielsen, L., Kaalund, S., Bjerring, P., & Hogsaa, B. (1990). Insufficient effect of local analgesics in Ehlers Danlos type III patients (connective tissue disorder). *Acta Anesthesiologic Scandinavica, 34*, 358–361.
4. Bernards, C. M., & Artu, A. A. (1991). Hexamethonium and midazolam terminate dysrhythmias and hypertension caused by intracerebroventricular bupivacaine in rabbits. *Anesthesiology, 74*, 89–96.
5. Binshtok, A. M., Bean, B. P., & Woolf, C. J. (2007). Inhibition of nociceptors by TRPV1-mediated entry of impermeant sodium channel blockers. *Nature, 449*, 607–610.
6. Bromage, P. R., Pettigrew, R. T., & Crowell, D. E. (1969). Tachyphylaxis in epidural analgesia: I. Augmentation and decay of local anesthesia. *Journal of Clinical Pharmacology and New Drugs, 9*, 30–38.
7. Butler-O'Hara, M., LeMoine, C., & Guillet, R. (1998). Analgesia for neonatal circumcision: A randomized controlled trial of EMLA cream versus dorsal penile nerve block. *Pediatrics, 101*, E5.
8. Cairns, B. E., Gambarota, G., Dunning, P. S., et al. (2003). Activation of peripheral excitatory amino acid receptors decreases the duration of local anesthesia. *Anesthesiology, 98*, 521–529.
9. Casati, A., Fanelli, G., Danelli, G., et al. (2007). Spinal anesthesia with lidocaine or preservative-free 2-chlorprocaine for outpatient knee arthroscopy: A prospective, randomized, double-blind comparison. *Anesthesia & Analgesia, 104*, 959–964.
10. Catterall, W. A. (2012). Voltage-gated sodium channels at 60: Structure, function and pathophysiology. *The Journal of Physiology, 590*, 2577–2589.
11. Challapalli, V., Tremont-Lukats, I. W., McNicol, E. D., et al. (2005). Systemic administration of local anesthetic agents to relieve neuropathic pain. *Cochrane Database of Systematic Reviews, 2019*(10), CD003345.
12. Clarkson, C. W., & Hondeghem, L. M. (1985). Mechanism for bupivacaine depression of cardiac conduction: Fast block of sodium channels during the action potential with slow recovery from block during diastole. *Anesthesiology, 62*, 396–405.
13. Covino, B. G., & Vassallo, H. G. (1976). *Local Anesthetics: Mechanisms of Action and Clinical Use.* Grune & Stratton.

14. Covino, B. G., Scott, D. B., & Lambert, D. H. (1994). *Handbook of Spinal Anesthesia and Analgesia*. WB Saunders.

15. de Jong, R. H., Ronfeld, R. A., & DeRosa, R. A. (1982). Cardiovascular effects of convulsant and supraconvulsant doses of amide local anesthetics. *Anesthesia & Analgesia, 61*, 3–9.

16. Dib-Hajj, S. D., Cummins, T. R., Black, J. A., & Waxman, S. G. (2010). Sodium channels in normal and pathological pain. *Annual Review of Neuroscience, 33*, 325–347.

17. Drasner, K. (1997). Lidocaine spinal anesthesia: A vanishing therapeutic index? *Anesthesiology, 87*, 469–472.

18. Drasner, K. (2002). Local anesthetic neurotoxicity: Clinical injury and strategies that may minimize risk. *Regional Anesthesia and Pain Medicine, 27*, 576–580.

19. Drasner, K. (2005). Chloroprocaine spinal anesthesia: Back to the future? *Anesthesia & Analgesia, 100*, 549–552.

20. Drasner, K. (2010). Local anesthetic systemic toxicity: A historical perspective. *Regional Anesthesia and Pain Medicine, 35*, 162–166.

21. Eichenfield, L. F., Funk, A., Fallon-Friedlander, S., & Cunningham, B. B. (2002). A clinical study to evaluate the efficacy of ELAMax (4% liposomal lidocaine) as compared with eutectic mixture of local anesthetics cream for pain reduction of venipuncture in children. *Pediatrics, 109*, 1093–1099.

22. Eisenach, J. C., Schlairet, T. J., Dobson, C. E. II, & Hood, D. H. (1991). Effect of prior anesthetic solution on epidural morphine analgesia. *Anesthesia & Analgesia, 73*, 119–123.

23. Epstein-Barash, H., Shichor, I., Kwon, A. H., et al. (2009). Prolonged duration local anesthesia with minimal toxicity. *Proceedings of the National Academy of Sciences of the United States of America, 106*, 7125–7130.

24. Fisher, D. (2007). What if half of your patients moved (or remembered or did something else bad) at incision? *Anesthesiology, 107*, 1–2.

25. Freedman, J. M., Li, D. K., Drasner, K., et al. (1998). Transient neurologic symptoms after spinal anesthesia: An epidemiologic study of 1,863 patients. *Anesthesiology, 89*, 633–641.

26. Gissen, A. J., Covino, B. G., & Gregus, J. (1980). Differential sensitivities of mammalian nerve fibers to local anesthetic agents. *Anesthesiology, 53*, 467–474.

27. Gissen, A., Datta, S., & Lambert, D. (1984). The chloroprocaine controversy. II. Is chloroprocaine neurotoxic? *Regional Anesthesia, 9*, 135–144.

28. Grazer, F. M., & de Jong, R. H. (2000). Fatal outcomes from liposuction: Census survey of cosmetic surgeons. *Plastic and Reconstructive Surgery, 105*, 436–446. Discussion 447–448.

29. Hadley, R. M., & Dine, A. P. (2014). Where is the evidence? A critical review of bias in the reporting of clinical data for Exparel: A liposomal bupivacaine formulation. *Journal of Clinical Research & Bioethics, 5*, 189.

30. Hampl, K. F., Schneider, M. C., Ummenhofer, W., & Drewe, J. (1995). Transient neurologic symptoms after spinal anesthesia. *Anesthesia & Analgesia, 81*, 1148–1153.

31. Hodgson, P. S., Liu, S. S., Batra, M. S., et al. (2000). Procaine compared with lidocaine for incidence of transient neurologic symptoms. *Regional Anesthesia and Pain Medicine, 25*, 218–222.

32. Housman, T. S., Lawrence, N., Mellen, B. G., et al. (2002). The safety of liposuction: Results of a national survey. *Dermatologic Surgery, 28*, 971–978.

33. Kirksey, M. A., Haskins, S. C., Cheng, J., & Liu, S. S. (2015). Local anesthetic peripheral nerve block adjuvants for prolongation of analgesia: A systematic qualitative review. *PLoS ONE, 10*, e0137312.

34. Kouri, M. E., & Kopacz, D. J. (2004). Spinal 2-chloroprocaine: A comparison with lidocaine in volunteers. *Anesthesia & Analgesia, 98*, 75–80.

35. Kranke, P., Jokinen, J., Pace, N. L., et al. (2015). Continuous intravenous perioperative lidocaine infusion for postoperative pain and recovery. *Cochrane Database of Systematic Reviews, 6*(6), CD009642.

36. Lambert, L. A., Lambert, D. H., & Strichartz, G. R. (1994). Irreversible conduction block in isolated nerve by high concentrations of local anesthetics. *Anesthesiology, 80*, 1082–1093.

37. Lee, K. C., Wilder, R. T., Smith, R. L., & Berde, C. B. (1994). Thermal hyperalgesia accelerates and MK-801 prevents the development of tachyphylaxis to rat sciatic nerve blockade. *Anesthesiology, 81*, 1284–1293.

38. Liu, Q., & Gold, M. S. (2016). Opioid-induced loss of local anesthetic potency in the rat sciatic nerve. *Anesthesiology, 125*(4), 755–764.

39. Lobo, K., Donado, C., Cornelissen, L., et al. (2015). A phase 1, dose-escalation, double-blind, block-randomized, controlled trial of safety and efficacy of neosaxitoxin alone and in combination with 0.2% bupivacaine, with and without epinephrine, for cutaneous anesthesia. *Anesthesiology, 123*, 873–885.

40. Lund, C., Mogensen, T., Hjortso, N. C., & Kehlet, H. (1985). Systemic morphine enhances spread of sensory analgesia during postoperative epidural bupivacaine infusion. *Lancet, 2*, 1156–1157.

41. Neal, J. M., Bernards, C. M., Butterworth, J. F., et al. (2010). ASRA practice advisory on local anesthetic systemic toxicity. *Regional Anesthesia and Pain Medicine, 35*, 152–161.

42. Nordstrom, H., & Stange, K. (2005). Plasma lidocaine levels and risks after liposuction with tumescent anesthesia. *Acta Anesthesiologic Scandinavica, 49*, 1487–1490.

43. Noviasky, J., Pierce, D. P., Whalen, K., et al. (2014). Bupivacaine liposomal versus bupivacaine: Comparative review. *Hospital Pharmacy, 49*, 539–543.

44. Pollock, J. E., Neal, J. M., Stephenson, C. A., & Wiley, C. E. (1996). Prospective study of the incidence of transient radicular irritation in patients undergoing spinal anesthesia. *Anesthesiology, 84*, 1361–1367.

45. Rigler, M. L., & Drasner, K. (1991). Distribution of catheter-injected local anesthetic in a model of the subarachnoid space. *Anesthesiology, 75*, 684–692.

46. Roberts, M. H., & Gildersleve, C. D. (2016). Lignocaine topicalization of the pediatric airway. *Paediatric Anaesthesia, 26*, 337–344.

47. Rosenberg, P. H., Veering, B. T., & Urmey, W. F. (2004). Maximum recommended doses of local anesthetics: A multifactorial concept. *Regional Anesthesia and Pain Medicine, 29*, 564–575. Discussion 524.

48. Rosenblatt, M. A., Abel, M., Fischer, G. W., et al. (2006). Successful use of a 20% lipid emulsion

to resuscitate a patient after a presumed bupivacaine-related cardiac arrest. *Anesthesiology, 105*, 217–218.

49. Sakura, S., Bollen, A. W., Ciriales, R., & Drasner, K. (1995). Local anesthetic neurotoxicity does not result from blockade of voltage-gated sodium channels. *Anesthesia & Analgesia, 81*, 338–346.

50. Smith, G. A., Strausbaugh, S. D., Harbeck-Weber, C., et al. (1997). New non-cocaine-containing topical anesthetics compared with tetracaine-adrenaline-cocaine during repair of lacerations. *Pediatrics, 100*, 825–830.

51. Spence, A. G. (2007). Lipid reversal of central nervous system symptoms of bupivacaine toxicity. *Anesthesiology, 107*, 516–517.

52. Taenzer, A. H., Clark, C. T., & Kovarik, W. D. (2010). Experience with 724 epidurograms for epidural catheter placement in pediatric anesthesia. *Regional Anesthesia and Pain Medicine, 35*, 432–435.

53. Taniguchi, M., Bollen, A. W., & Drasner, K. (2004). Sodium bisulfite: Scapegoat for chloroprocaine neurotoxicity? *Anesthesiology, 100*, 85–91.

54. Templin, J. S., Wylie, M. C., Kim, J. D., et al. (2015). Neosaxitoxin in rat sciatic block: Improved therapeutic index using combinations with bupivacaine, with and without epinephrine. *Anesthesiology, 123*, 886–898.

55. Tsui, B. C., Wagner, A., Cave, D., & Kearney, R. (2004). Thoracic and lumbar epidural analgesia via the caudal approach using electrical stimulation guidance in pediatric patients: A review of 289 patients. *Anesthesiology, 100*, 683–689.

56. Wang, G. K., & Strichartz, G. R. (2012). State-dependent inhibition of sodium channels by local anesthetics: A 40-year evolution. *Biochemistry (Moscow) Supplement Series A: Membrane and Cell Biology, 6*, 120–127.

57. Weinberg, G. (n.d.). LipidRescue Resuscitation. Retrieved from www.lipidrescue.org

58. Weinberg, G., Ripper, R., Feinstein, D. L., & Hoffman, W. (2003). Lipid emulsion infusion rescues dogs from bupivacaine-induced cardiac toxicity. *Regional Anesthesia and Pain Medicine, 28*, 198–202.

59. Winnie, A. P., Tay, C. H., Patel, K. P., et al. (1977). Pharmacokinetics of local anesthetics during plexus blocks. *Anesthesia & Analgesia, 56*, 852–861.

60. Wylie, M. C., Johnson, V. M., Carpino, E., et al. (2012). Respiratory, neuromuscular, and cardiovascular effects of neosaxitoxin in isoflurane-anesthetized sheep. *Regional Anesthesia and Pain Medicine, 37*, 152–158.

Chapter 6

ANESTHETIC NEUROTOXICITY

Contents

Introduction

The effects of general anesthesia and sedative medications on neurodevelopment and cognition throughout life have long been a major concern in the field of anesthesiology. Anesthesia providers should stay up to date on the latest findings regarding the long-term effects of anesthesia on the brain, even though conclusive conclusions are impossible to reach. Unquestionably, laboratory animal models have shown that general anesthesia causes neuronal cell death and neurocognitive impairments. A Drug Safety Communication was released by the Food and Drug Administration in response to a public health concern. It contains a warning that children's brain development may be impacted by the repeated or prolonged use of general anesthetic and sedation drugs during surgeries or procedures in children under three years old or in pregnant women during the third trimester. That being said, this is not a novel worry. Eckenhoff issued a warning in 1953 regarding an unusually high rate of postoperative personality changes in kids. Since then, preclinical studies on young animal models have conclusively shown that general anesthesia causes later neurotoxic and neurocognitive impairment. Additionally, Bedford wrote in 1955 about how general anesthesia causes behavioral changes in the elderly. A number of lab reports have discovered that anesthetic medications cause mature rodents to exhibit histologic, biochemical, and neurocognitive abnormalities.

Anesthetic drugs are powerful agents that affect the central nervous system (CNS) and temporarily make patients unable to feel pain during medical procedures and surgery. While the exact ways in which they work to induce immobility, pain relief, and memory loss are not fully understood, most anesthetic and sedative medications act on the γ-aminobutyric acid (GABA) receptors or N-methyl-d-aspartate (NMDA) glutamate receptors, or a combination of both. General anesthesia and sedation can be achieved through the inhaled or intravenous administration of specific drugs. However, it is important to be aware of the potential risk of anesthetic-induced developmental neurotoxicity (AIDN) associated with these medications. The short-term and long-term neurocognitive effects of general anesthesia should also be taken into consideration.

Orientation and Directional Terms

<table>
<tr><th>Term</th><th>Definition</th><th>Illustration</th></tr>
<tr><td>Neuronal morphogenesis</td><td>The process in which the anatomical structures of a neuron projection are generated and organized. A neuron projection is any process extending from a neural cell, such as axons or dendrites.</td><td>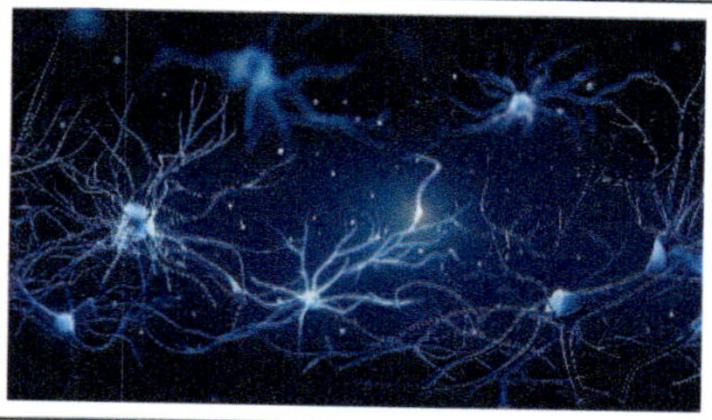</td></tr>
<tr><td>Glucocorticoids</td><td>Glucocorticoids are steroid hormones produced from the cortex of adrenal glands (gluco-corti-coids: glucose-cortex-steroids). Glucocorticoids have a pivotal role in the glucose, protein, and fat metabolism of the body.</td><td>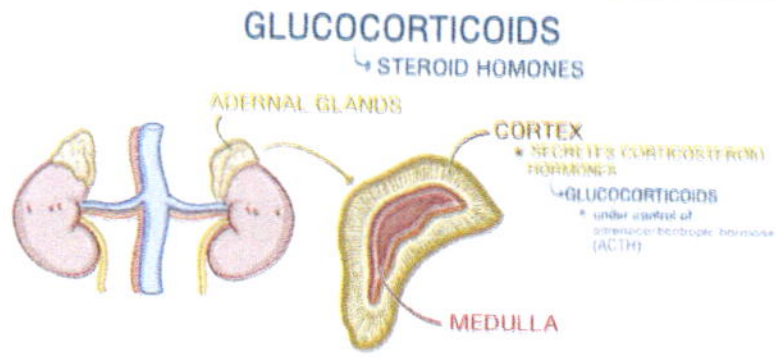
</td></tr>
<tr><td>Reactive oxygen species' (ROS)</td><td>Reactive oxygen species (ROS) is an umbrella term for an array of derivatives of molecular oxygen that occur as a normal attribute of aerobic life. Elevated formation of the different ROS leads to molecular damage, denoted as 'oxidative distress.'</td><td>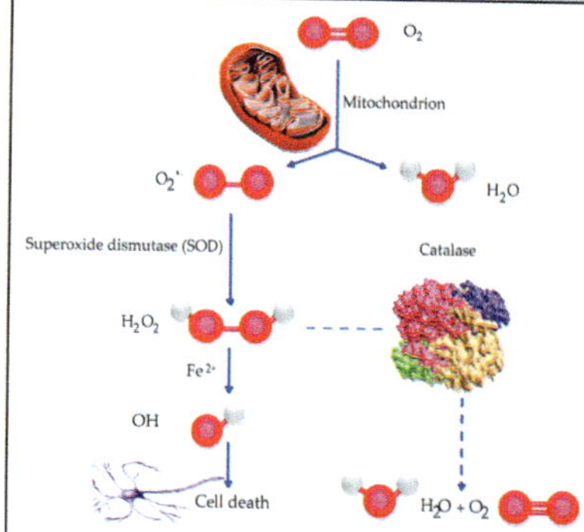
</td></tr>
<tr><td>Dendritic spines</td><td>Dendritic spines are tiny protrusions from dendrites, which form functional contacts with neighboring axons of other neurons. Dendritic spines are very plastic and their size and shape are constantly changing in response to neuronal activity.</td><td>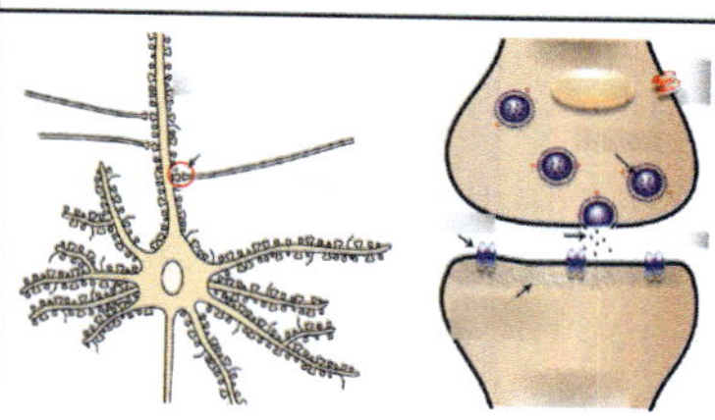</td></tr>
<tr><td>Minimum alveolar concentration (MAC)</td><td>Minimum alveolar concentration (MAC) is the minimum concentration of an inhaled anesthetic at 1 atm of pressure that prevents skeletal muscle movement in response to a surgical incision in 50% of patients. The MAC of a volatile anesthetic changes with the patient's age</td><td>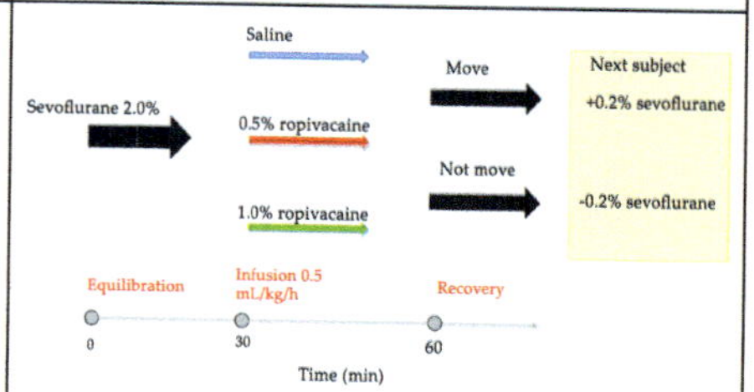
</td></tr>
</table>

6.1. Anesthetic Drugs as a Cause for Neurodegeneration and Long-Term Neurocognitive Deficits

6.1.1. Basic Science of Anesthetic-Induced Developmental Neurotoxicity

There are many different molecular targets for CNS depressant drugs, and the exact mechanism by which they produce general anesthesia is still unknown, making it difficult to pinpoint the underlying cause of their neurotoxic effect on the developing brain. AIDN has been shown in lab models exposed to the majority of anesthetic and sedative medications typically given to pediatric patients, both in vivo and in vitro. Anticonvulsant medications and alcohol given to fetuses have been linked to a similar pattern of neurodegeneration and impaired neurocognitive progress. AIDN was first identified in fetal and postnatal rats exposed to halothane over 40 years ago, but its significance was not fully understood by the scientific or general public until a 1999 report highlighted the increased neurodegeneration in neonatal rat pups caused by ketamine. It was later discovered that the combination of isoflurane, nitrous oxide, and midazolam, three commonly used anesthetic medications, not only caused neuroapoptosis but also impaired hippocampal synaptic function and learning behavior. While ketamine and nitrous oxide, which are NMDA antagonists, and isoflurane, a GABA agonist, have anesthetic mechanisms as well.

The trophic support necessary for neurogenesis and context-dependent neuroplasticity modulation is reduced when anesthesia occurs because it eliminates sensory input and suppresses normal neural activity. Nonetheless, a number of studies have detailed the mechanisms underlying neuronal cell death, including excitotoxicity, mitochondrial malfunction, aberrant cell cycle reentry, dysregulation of trophic factors, and disruption of cytoskeletal assembly. In the mature brain, GABA functions as an inhibitory drug; however, in the early stages of brain development, it acts as an excitatory agent due to the presence of the immature Na/K/2Cl transporter protein NKCC1, which causes a chloride influx that depolarizes neurons. Therefore, until the mature chloride transporter, KCC2, is expressed and actively transports chloride out of the neural cell, GABA remains excitatory. At that point, the GABA receptors switch to the normal inhibitory mode.

6.1.2. Age-Dependent Vulnerability of Anesthetics

Neurogenesis, neuronal morphogenesis, and synaptogenesis are the stages that comprise the progression of neural development. Progenitor cells, which multiply and differentiate into neurons or glial cells, are the first step in the process of neurogenesis. Subsequently, oligodendrocytes and astrocytes emerge, functioning as neurons' supporting cells. There is an excess of progenitor cells that mature into neural and glial cells during this proliferative (cell cycle) stage. To perform particular tasks, these cells can exit the cell cycle at various points. A subpopulation continues to be in the cell cycle and is not differentiated. Neurons can no longer replicate after going through terminal differentiation into a postmitotic state. Axons and dendrites emerge from the cell body to connect with other neurons in functional synapses. Up to 70% of neurons are destroyed early in development as a result of apoptosis, a programmed cell death, and other normal processes related to neurodevelopment. Programmed cell death after birth and early elimination during the embryonic stage control the development of CNS neurons. neurons and redundant neural progenitor cells that mismigrate or fail to form synapses.

Critical periods of plasticity during brain development are modulated by environmental cues and have been implicated in perceptual development in vision and speech. Likewise, the perioperative environment can influence brain development. Anesthetic drugs are powerful modulators of neuronal circuits and have an impact on the constant flux of CNS development and remodeling in both health and disease states. Because neurogenesis is ongoing throughout life, from the fetus to the elderly, these neural progenitor cells are vulnerable to the toxic effects of anesthetic drugs. Exposure to isoflurane produces neuronal cell death in brain regions where neural progenitor cells reside. Therefore, susceptibility to AIDN extends from the fetal period to late adulthood.

The period of rapid brain growth in most species is when they are most susceptible to AIDN, which typically coincides with the peak of synaptogenesis. In humans, this growth spurt occurs during the final trimester of pregnancy and continues until around 3 to 4 years old, making children especially sensitive to the negative effects of general anesthesia. Some debate surrounds this idea, but neuroinformatic research on the development of corticospinal tracts suggests that 7-day-old rat pups exhibit similar neurodevelopmental progress to 20- to 22-week-old human fetuses. This critical period is also when fetal alcohol syndrome poses the greatest risk, as exposure to alcohol during this time can interfere with brain development due to its effects as a GABA agonist and NMDA antagonist.

Species differences affect when the brain grows to its maximum during development. Since rodents are an altricial species, a large portion of their neurodevelopment happens after birth. This window of time spans approximately from postnatal day 6 to postnatal day 21. Simian species, such as humans, are generally regarded as precocial and have longer gestations due to the relatively advanced developmental stage at which offspring are born. Rhesus monkeys exposed as fetuses or as early as day 6 of life are vulnerable to anesthetic-induced neuroapoptosis. However, when the exposure takes place on day 35 postnatally, AIDN has not been proven. When given equivalent human concentrations of isoflurane (0.5%–0.5%) for four to six hours, with or without nitrous oxide, five-day-old rhesus monkeys showed extensive neuroapoptosis in the temporal, frontal, and hippocampus regions of the brain. On the other hand, rhesus monkeys exposed to high doses of ketamine over an extended time experience learning deficits in addition to an increase in neuroapoptosis.

Different neural fate patterns are produced depending on the exposure period during development. Pregnant rats exposed to anesthetics have more apoptotic cells in their developing brains. When newborn rodents are given anesthesia, their apoptosis increases and their axonal and dendritic arborization are stunted. On the other hand, exposure to anesthesia in young rat models increases synaptic density and dendritic formation but does not increase apoptosis. The similar altered dendritic morphologic appearance seen in neurologic and psychiatric disorders is concerning.

6.1.3. Characterization of AIDN

6.1.3.1. Pathologic Apoptosis

Rapid apoptosis is the characteristic feature of AIDN. Even though it is a crucial mechanism for regulating neural development, cellular stress can also trigger the apoptotic pathway (Figure 6.1).

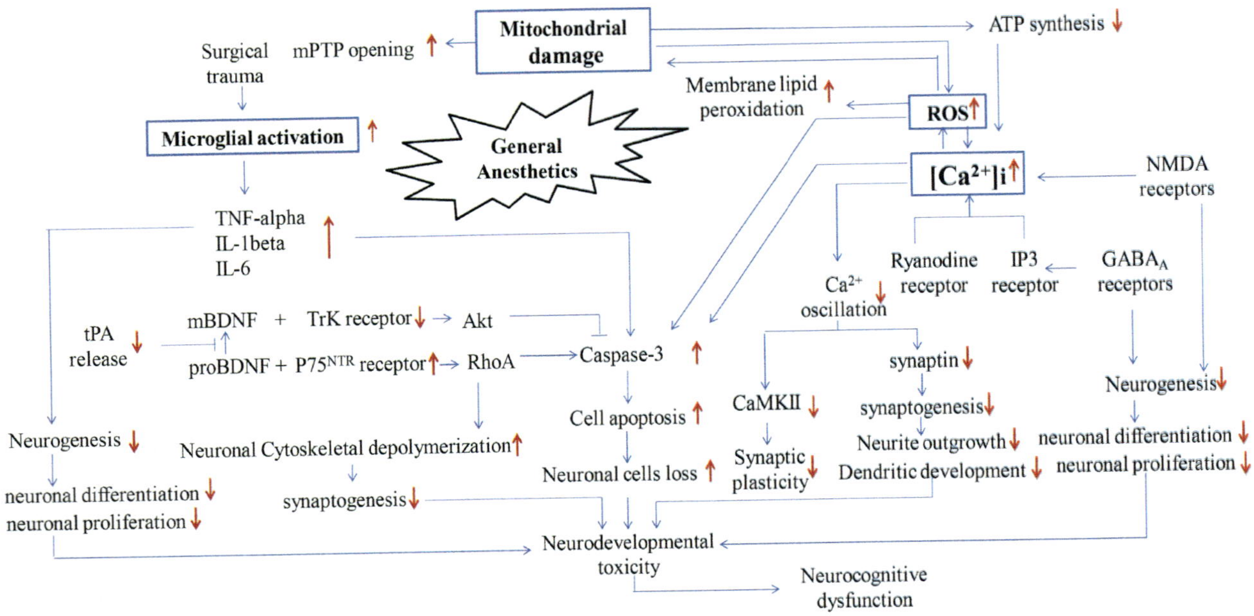

Figure 6.1. *Schematic diagram presenting possible pathways by which general anesthetics induce early neurotoxicity in developing brain and later neurocognitive dysfunction. Note: ATP: Adenosine triphosphate; ROS: Reactive oxygen species; NMDA receptor: N-methy-d-aspartate receptor; GABAA receptor: Gamma-aminobutyric acid type A receptor; IP3 receptor: Inositol triphosphate receptor; mPTP: Mitochondrial permeability transition pore; TNF-alpha: Tumor necrosis factor-alpha; IL-1beta: Interleukin-1beta; IL-6: Interleukin-6; tPA: Tissue plasminogen activator; mBDNF: Mature brain-derived neurotrophic factor; proBDNF: Brain-derived proneurotrophic factor; Akt: Phosphorylated serine/ threonine-specific protein kinase; CaMK II: Calcium/calmodulin-dependent Protein Kinase II; RhoA: Ras homolog gene family, member A; TrK receptor: Neurotrophic tyrosine kinase receptor; P75NTR receptor: Neurotrophin p75 receptor. ↑: increase; ↓: decrease; : block or inhibit.*

Source: *Lei X, Guo Q, Zhang J. Mechanistic Insights into Neurotoxicity Induced by Anesthetics in the Developing Brain. International Journal of Molecular Sciences. 2012; 13(6):6772-6799. https://doi.org/10.3390/ijms13066772.*

Glucocorticoids, heat, radiation, hunger, infection, low oxygen levels, pain, and anesthetics are a few examples of these stresses. The caspase enzymes, which are cysteine-dependent aspartate proteases that either start the apoptotic process (caspases 2, 8, 9, and 10) or modify it (caspases 3 and 7) are responsible for almost all cases of apoptosis. The extrinsic and intrinsic pathways are the two primary pathways. While the intrinsic pathway requires mitochondrial activation, the extrinsic pathway is mediated by death receptors on the cell membrane wall.

The Fas ligand to the Fas cell wall receptor, which subsequently becomes the Fas associated death domain, or FADD, is the extrinsic pathway. It combines with either procaspase 8 or 10 to form a signaling complex that induces death (DISC). Inducing cell death, this activates the effector caspase 3. Tumor necrosis factor-related apoptosis inducing ligand (TRAIL), which also activates FADD, DISC formation, and apoptosis, can also induce the extrinsic pathway. The mitochondria are part of the intrinsic pathway because they release proapoptotic proteins like apoptosis-inducing factor (AIF), endonuclease G, procaspases, Smac/Diablo, cytochrome c, and adenylate kinase-2 when under stress. Unlike other proteins, AIF can cause apoptosis without activating caspase. The increased permeability of the outer mitochondrial wall allows these proapoptotic proteins to be released from the gap between the inner and outer mitochondrial layers. The proapoptotic and prosurvival components of the Bcl-2 cytosolic proteins are assembled here. The Bax proteins (Bcl-2 proapoptotic) cause the outer wall permeability of the mitochondria, which releases cytochrome c and other proteins that activate caspase 9. Vaporous anesthetic exposure damages mitochondrial function, which activates the intrinsic apoptotic chain. This reaction is lessened by mitochondrial integrity restoration and reactive oxygen species (ROS) scavengers.

6.1.3.2. Impeded Neurogenesis

Animal neurogenesis is affected by anesthetics in a way that varies with age. In neonatal rats, isoflurane results in a decrease in neural stem cells and a reduction in neurogenesis; however, in adult rats, it causes a transient increase in neurogenesis. Similarly, in young rats, propofol reduces the proliferation of hippocampal cells, but not in adults. In young animals, exposure to isoflurane stunts astrocyte growth and delays their maturation. In animals, general anesthetic-induced inflammation may also result in a reduction in neurogenesis. Both in vivo and in vitro data suggest that general anesthetics, particularly in young and adult populations, may reduce the number of neural stem cells and their potential for self-renewal.

6.1.3.3. Altered Dendritic Development

Dendritic spines are small extensions of neurons that typically receive input from a single synapse and play a crucial role in synapse formation. Exposure to ketamine and isoflurane has been found to decrease synapse and spine density in very young infant rats. However, in slightly older rats (around postnatal days 15, 16, and 20), exposure to certain anesthetics such as propofol, midazolam, isoflurane, sevoflurane, desflurane, and ketamine actually increases dendritic spine formation. The implications of these findings are still unclear, but it is evident that the vulnerability of specific developmental stages plays a significant role in altering dendritic spine formation. Moreover, motor skill learning through activities like running on a rotarod has been shown to enhance dendritic development. On the other hand, exposure to ketamine and xylazine on postnatal day 14 resulted in reduced dendritic spine formation. In summary, the effects of anesthetics on dendritic morphogenesis vary depending on the age of exposure.

6.1.3.4. Aberrant Glial Development

The CNS's glial cells provide the scaffolding that directs the migration and synaptogenesis of developing neurons. Isoflurane exposure impairs astrocytes during neural development. Because of this anesthetic's interference with astrocytes' release of brainderived neurotrophic factor (BDNF), developing neurons are deprived of trophic support for axonal outgrowth. Additionally, in fetuses and newborn rhesus monkeys, isoflurane causes oligodendrocytes to undergo apoptosis.

6.1.3.5. Anesthetic Effects on Spinal Cord

When very young rat pups are exposed to general anesthetics (isoflurane, nitrous oxide), the spinal cord experiences an increase in apoptosis, with the ventral horns suffering the majority of the injuries. However, in exposed rats that were allowed to mature, no abnormalities related to motor function were found. When histologic examination of their spinal cords revealed increased apoptosis and microglial activation, postnatal day 3 rat pups that received an intrathecal ketamine injection had abnormal spinal function as adults. Analgesia was produced by intrathecal morphine, but the spinal cord did not undergo any histologic or functional changes. In the same population, exposure to bupivacaine, a local anesthetic, did not result in elevated apoptosis levels.

6.1.3.6. Neuroinflammation

The development of postoperative cognitive dysfunction may be influenced by the activation of neuroinflammatory cascades. It is evident that surgical trauma causes neuroinflammation. Thus, the use of anesthetics and analgesics during painful procedures such as surgery should reduce this reaction. Sevoflurane, however, elevates neuroinflammation markers in juvenile mice but not in adult mice. It's unclear if exposure to anesthesia and surgical trauma contributes to the development of neuroinflammation.

6.1.3.7. Alzheimer-Related Neuropathology

Preclinical reports show that the biological precursors of Alzheimer's disease are expressed. Mice undergoing experimental surgery had higher hippocampal β-amyloid accumulation. Furthermore, in rodent brains and cell culture, isoflurane exposure raises the levels of β-amyloid. A powerful combination of neuropathology associated with Alzheimer's disease and neuroinflammation may impair neurocognitive function.

6.1.3.8. Neurocognitive Function

In rodents, exposure to anesthetic drugs during fetal and neonatal stages is known to cause deficits in neurocognitive function. Standard behavioral tests for rodents include the prepulse inhibition of the startle reflex, the Morris water navigation test, the radial arm maze, startle, and odor recognition. Additionally, behavioral tests using an operant test battery or a human intruder paradigm were reported in rhesus monkeys exposed to ketamine or sevoflurane, respectively. While emotional reactivity is tested using the human intruder paradigm, motivation and recognition memory are assessed using the operant test battery. Following neonatal exposure to these drugs, both reports showed a decline in performance at an older age.

Anesthesia-related drug exposure also negatively affects neurobehavioral evaluations in older rats. In the radial arm maze test, rats anesthetized with isoflurane and nitrous oxide for six and twenty months, respectively, similarly developed persistent deficits. In another similar experimental paradigm, propofol did not, however, result in impaired radial arm maze test results. These reports unequivocally show that anesthesia-related exposure can result in neurobehavioral functional consequences later in life.

6.1.4. Relevant Anesthetic Durations and Concentrations

The duration of exposure may be more relevant than the concentration of exposure, although both are important. Almost all the animal studies involved an anesthetic exposure of at least 4 hours with some trials exposing primates to 24 hours of continuous anesthesia. Exposures of less than 1 hour regardless of the animal studied did not cause increased neuroapoptosis. Exposure to volatile anesthetics of 0.25% to 0.5% minimum alveolar concentration (MAC) for 6 hours increased caspase 3 marker levels, indicating an increase in cell death or apoptosis in rat pups. There is inconsistency about the relative neurotoxic potential of individual volatile anesthetics. Whether desflurane induces more neuroapoptosis than sevoflurane or halothane is not clear. Also, whether anesthetics given in combinations are more neurotoxic than solitary anesthetics is not known. Although nitrous oxide in combination with isoflurane is more neurotoxic than isoflurane alone, it may be because the total MAC exposure is higher when given in combination rather than a synergistic effect.

6.1.5. Anesthetic and Sedative Drugs

GABAA receptors are the target of GABAergic general anesthetics. GABA is an excitatory agent in the early stages of brain development, despite being inhibitory in the mature brain. A chloride influx caused by the immature Na/K/2Cl transporter protein NKCC1 results in neuron depolarization. Because of this, GABA stays excitatory until mature chloride transporter KCC2 is expressed, which actively moves chloride out of the neural cell, at which point GABA neurons transition to the normal inhibitory mode. In term human infants, this switch starts around the 15th postnatal week and lasts until the infant is about a year old.

Neurons contain the N-methyl-d-aspartate glutamate receptor (NMDAR), which is activated by the binding of glutamate, glycine, or d-serine. For synaptic plasticity, which is necessary for memory and learning, it is essential. Four subunits make up the structural makeup of the NMDAR protein: two GluN1 (previously known as NR1) and two GluN2 (previously known as NR2). Glycine is a coagonist that is bound by the GluN1 subunit, while glutamate is bound by the GluN2 subunit. Animal models of AIDN have been linked to ketamine, a noncompetitive NMDAR antagonist that upregulates the GluN1 subunit.

While repeated morphine administration over a 7-day period is linked to increased apoptosis in the sensory cortex and amygdala of neonatal rats, opioids generally do not increase neuroapoptosis. Nonetheless, postnatal day 7 rat pups did not experience an increase in neuroapoptosis when given a single dose of morphine. Moreover, dendritic morphologic appearance remained unchanged after receiving morphine daily for nine days in a row. These are not the brain regions that volatile and intravenous anesthetics affect; these anesthetics preferentially affect the hippocampal regions of developing brains, which are responsible for learning and memory.

6.1.6. Alleviation of AIDN

There are now several established molecular pathways explaining how anesthesia causes apoptosis. This discovery has prompted research to find out if there are neuroprotective techniques that can be used in clinical settings to lessen the harmful effects that general anesthetics have on young, developing patients. AIDN is lessened by a number of nonspecific medications with neuroprotective qualities, including lithium, melatonin, estrogen, erythropoietin, estradiol, and dexmedetomidine. Isoflurane-induced neuroapoptosis and behavioral impairment are lessened by dexmedetomidine. On the other hand, dexmedetomidine in high doses can cause neuroapoptosis. At clinical dosages, its neuroprotective effect most likely activates signaling pathways involved in cell survival. Ultimately, after a newborn is exposed to sevoflurane, neurobehavioral abnormalities are lessened in an improved and stimulating environment (Table 6.1).

Table 6.1. *AIDN and Dexmedetomidine-Clinical Trials*

First author	Study population	Number	Dex dosage and administration time	Scales used	Anesthesia induction	Anesthesia maintain	Conclusion
Dong Jun Kim	Orthopedic	115	100 mg/mL was administered at 0.4 μg kg − 1 h − 1(DEX)or Normal saline (0.1 mL kg − 1 h − 1)-Intra-operative	VAS, RSAS	Midazolam 30 min before anesthesia. Propofol, Sevoflorane, remifentanil, and rocuronium	Sevoflurane or propofol and remifentanil	Dexmedetomidine lowered the emergence agitation
Hong Hong	Orthopedic	712	Postoperative patient-controlled intravenous administration (IV) of either dexmedetomidine 200 μg or 0.9% saline and 200 μg sufentanil, diluted with 0.9% saline to 160 mL. The pump was programmed to deliver 2-ml boluses with a lockout interval of 8 min and a background infusion of 1 mL.h − 1.	RASS, Cam, Cam-ICU	Midazolam (1–3 mg), propofol or etomidate and sufentanil or remifentanil.	Propofol infusion, sevoflurane and/or nitrous oxide inhalation, and sufentanil or remifentanil	Low dose dexmedetomidine and supplemental intravenous analgesia did not reduce delirium. Although, it improved analgesia and sleep quality without aggravating adverse events.
Ting Huyan	Lung cancer	346	Dexmedetomidine (0.5 μg/kg) was administered in 20 min before the beginning of the operation followed by a continuous IV infusion at a rate of 0.1 μg/kg/h during the intraoperative period. The drug infusion was stopped 30 min before the end of the operation.	Intensive Care Delirium Screening Checklist (ICDSC)	Etomidate, Fentanyl, Rocuronium	Propofol, remifentanil and cisatracurium, sufentanil and atracurium cis-benzenesulfonate	Pre-operative and intra-operative administration of dexmedetomidine can lowered the incidence of delirium. Dexmedetomidine also lowered pain and improved sleep quality.
Xiaoyuan Sui	>4 h anesthesia laparotomy- non-cardiac	N/A	Dexmedetomidine hydrochloride is injected with a micro infusion pump within 15minutes before anesthesia induction with pre-injection loading dose (0.5μg/kg), followed by continuous infusion at a rate of 0.3μg/kg/h	MMSE VAS	Midazolam, etomidate, sufentanil, cisatracurium	Propofol and remifentanil (study was not finished)	This study will find out the efficacy and safety of dexmedetomidine in lowering POD
Stacie Deiner	Non-cardiac major surgeries	404	Dexmedetomidine infusion (0.5 μg/kg/h) during surgery and up to 2 h in the recovery room.	CAM, CAM ICU, MMSE	Avoided benzodiazepines and nitrous oxide, any other induction agents were permissible	Propofol, sevoflurane or both	Intra-operative infusion of dexmedetomidine does not decrease POD
Yuqin Lv	Hip re-placement	327	The treatment group was treated with 0.1 μg/kg/h DEX, while the placebo group was administered with an equal amount of normal saline solution intravenously within 72 h following THA surgery.	CAM	No pre-medications, along with a standard preoperative evaluation and the same general anesthesia protocol using IV midazolam (1–2 mg) and fentanyl (50–100 mg) for preoperative sedation	3–6 mg/kg IV fentanyl	Dexmedetomidine can reduce POD

First author	Study population	Number	Dex dosage and administration time	Scales used	Anesthesia induction	Anesthesia maintain	Conclusion
Bo-Jie Wang	Non-cardiac- >2 h	620	A loading dose dexmedetomidine (0.6 μg/kg) will be administered 10 min before anaesthesia induction, followed by a continuous infusion at a rate of 0.5 μg/kg/h until 1 h before the end of surgery.	CAM, CAM-ICU	Intravenous sufentanil and propofol	Intravenous sufentanil, propofol and inhalation of a 1:1 nitrous oxide–oxygen mixture. Rocuronium and/or cisatracurium are administered for muscle relaxation.	The study is investigating if dexmedetomidine use during general anesthesia can lower POD
Balachundhar Subramaniam *et al*	CABG/valve surgery in US	120	4 groups of patients: IV acetaminophen plus dexmedetomidine, IV acetaminophen plus propofol, Placebo plus dexmedetomidine and Placebo plus propofol. Dexmedetomidine group received an IV bolus dose of 0.5 to 1 μg/kg during chest closure, followed by a maintenance infusion of 0.1 to 1.4 μg/kg per hour. The IV propofol group received a maintenance dose of 20 to 100 μg/kg per minute. With placebo vs. acetaminophen administered within 1 h of ICU admission and thereafter every 6 h for 8 doses	CAM/CAM-ICU	Not found		Post-operative intravenous (IV) acetaminophen combined with IV propofol or dexmedetomidine reduced POD
Alparslan Turan	Cardiac	798	Either dexmedetomidine infusion or saline placebo started before the surgical incision at a rate of 0·1 μg/kg/ h then increased to 0·2 μg/kg/ h at the end of bypass, and postoperatively increased to 0·4 μg/kg/h, which was maintained until 24 h.	CAM-ICU	Midazolam, thiopental, etomidate, propofol, and sufentanil or fentanyl, or both, and	With volatile anaesthetics and a non-depolarising muscle relaxant	Dexmedetomidine infusion before surgical incision and continued for 24 h post-operatively did not decrease atrial fibrillation and POD
Mona Momeni	cardiac	420	Propofol infusion and dexmedetomidine (0.4 μg kg-1 h-1) or a propofol infusion and saline 0.9% (placebo group).	MMSE, CAM, CAM-ICU	Midazolam 0.03–0.06 $mgkg^{-1}$, sufentanil 0.30.5$μgkg^{-1}$, ketamine 0.3–0.5 $mg\,kg^{-1}$, and a bolus dose of propofol. A continuous infusion of sufentanil at a rate of 0.5–0.8 $μg\,kg^{-1}\,h^{-1}$ was administered for intraoperative analgesia.	Sevoflurane. Sevoflurane was continued during the CPB period.	The study does not recommend supplementing post-operative propofol with dexmedetomidine to reduce POD
George Djaiani	cardiac	185	Dexmedetomidine 0.4 μg/kg bolus followed by 0.2 to 0.7 $μg\,kg^{-1}\,h^{-1}$ infusion or propofol 25 to 50 $μg\,kg^{-1}\,h^{-1}$ infusion	CAM, CAM-ICU	10 to 12 μg/kg fentanyl, 0.5 to 2 mg/kg propofol, and 0.15 mg/kg pancuronium and	Maintained with 0.5 to 2.0% isoflurane.	Dexmedetomidine reduced incidence, delayed onset and shortened duration of POD

Source: Tsivitis A, Wang A, Murphy J, Khan A, Jin Z, Moore R, Tateosian V and Bergese S (2023) Anesthesia, the developing brain, and dexmedetomidine for neuroprotection. Front. Neurol. 14:1150135. doi: 10.3389/fneur.2023.1150135.

6.2. Clinical Evidence for Neurotoxicity

When considered collectively, three elements seem to cause AIDN in lab models: (1) vulnerability during a crucial developmental stage, (2) high anesthetic dosage, and (3) extended exposure time. It is difficult to extrapolate these lab results to a human neonate. A human brain takes years to develop, while a rat brain does so in a matter of weeks. A newborn rat pup under anesthesia for six hours might require weeks of anesthesia in a human newborn. This severe state is uncommon in clinical practice, except for sedation in patients receiving intensive care. It is therefore challenging to determine how an equivalent exposure affects the neurologic outcome in a neonate of human. The greatest incidence of neuroapoptosis and subsequent developmental delays in animals is caused by prolonged, repeated exposure to general anesthesia as well as early exposure. The neurotoxic effects of general anesthesia may be more likely in children who require frequent anesthetic examinations or radiation therapy for cancer.

The suggestion that pediatric anesthesia could be hazardous is restricted to epidemiological studies conducted after the fact. The effects of the underlying comorbid conditions and the surgery may complicate this evidence. Controlling for all known and unknown confounders is impossible due to the retrospective nature of these investigations, despite attempts to control for obvious confounders. Numerous epidemiological studies with roots in the Mayo Clinic have been conducted. Olmsted County, Minnesota, has a stable population, and researchers there have access to the medical and educational records of this population. In a retrospective cohort study involving more than 5,000 children born between 1976 and 1982, it was discovered that 593 patients who had anesthesia exposure before the age of four had greater learning disabilities in math, reading, and written language. Several anesthetic exposures and general anesthesia lasting longer than two hours were risk factors. In a related study, which used a matched cohort of 8530 kids from Olmsted County, it was discovered that the 64 kids under the age of two who experienced multiple anesthetic exposures were nearly twice as likely to have them.

Making use of the Medicaid billing codes for New York State, a database containing more than 200,000 children was created. Early research using this database showed that diagnoses for behavioral and developmental problems nearly tripled in children who had inguinal hernia repairs before turning one year old. Even after controlling for birth weight and gender, there was a nearly twofold increase in these problems in this group. However, a follow-up study that matched twins exposed to anesthesia with twin siblings not exposed to anesthesia discovered no correlation between receiving general anesthesia and developing neurologic and developmental issues later on. A brief retrospective cohort study of kids who underwent anesthesia before turning four years old was released. 53 children who were exposed were matched with an equal number of control children. Neurocognitive tests and cranial magnetic resonance imaging studies were performed on each child. They discovered that the children who had previously been exposed had considerably lower performance intelligence quotients (IQ) and listening comprehension scores. There was no significant loss of gray matter in previously identified vulnerable regions following exposure.

The general consensus is that children who have been exposed to anesthesia twice or more are at a higher risk. However, even a single general anesthesia exposure was linked to decreased performance on receptive and expressive language and cognitive tests conducted at age ten years, according to a 2012 prospectively followed cohort study from Australia involving 2608 children exposed to a wide variety of general anesthetics and surgical procedures before the age of three years. In a different prospective study, a comparable number of age- and gender-matched children who had not undergone anesthesia was compared to a smaller group of children who had been exposed to anesthesia before the age of one year. The anesthetized children did not differ in terms of familiarity, IQ, or Child Behavior Checklist scores, but they did exhibit deficits in measures of long-term recognition memory, according to the study.

Large database clinical investigations from Canada and Sweden reveal that exposure to surgery and anesthesia at an age older than 2 to 4 years increased the odds ratio of cognitive deficits, though not to the extent of previously published retrospective reports from smaller populations. Scrutiny of these large datasets reveals a lower percentage in academic achievement scores for toddlers undergoing ear, nose, and throat surgery. This finding suggests that early derangements in hearing and speech may have an impact on subsequent cognitive domains as assessed by school performance.

The relationship between early exposure to general anesthesia and subsequent academic difficulties has been questioned by other research. According to a Dutch study assessing the academic accomplishments of 1143 identical twin pairs, twin pairs whose members were all exposed to general anesthesia had lower educational accomplishments than twin pairs who were not. Nonetheless, discordant twin pairs' academic results (one exposed twin, one nonexposed twin) were comparable, suggesting that receiving general anesthesia was not a significant contributing factor. Similar to this, a sizable cohort study comprising 2689 Danish infants born between 1986 and 1990 who had inguinal hernioplasty as newborns was matched to control subjects chosen at random from an age-matched sample that accounted for 5% of the population. After accounting for known confounders, this study did not find any statistically significant differences between the children who were exposed and those who were not. There is evidence from two published large prospective cohort studies to suggest that anesthesia exposure has no effect on a child's subsequent neurocognitive domains. As far as prospective randomized controlled trials go, the GAS study is the only one that compares the benefits of regional anesthesia versus general anesthesia for early infancy inguinal hernia surgery. Compared to awake-regional anesthesia, this interim analysis did not find any evidence that a one-hour exposure to sevoflurane anesthesia during infancy increases the risk of a negative neurodevelopmental outcome by the time the child is two years old. The principal result, a five-year evaluation, is currently in progress.

The PANDA study looked at the effects of inguinal hernia surgery in babies under 36 months of age in a prospective manner. Every baby who was put under anesthesia was compared to a sibling who was not exposed to anesthesia using a comprehensive battery of neurocognitive tests. In the neurocognitive domains that were tested, there was no discernible difference when compared to a sibling cohort that had never had surgery or general anesthesia. The two negative studies only looked at the effects of brief surgical and general anesthesia exposures. These results are in line with the absence of AIDN in lab animals following brief exposures. In addition, all of the clinical reports' neurocognitive evaluations were carried out during childhood and adolescence rather than adulthood. Therefore, future research must address the connection between extended anesthetic drug exposure and neurocognitive performance in later life stages. On the other end of the age spectrum, elderly patients are at increased risk of developing postoperative cognitive dysfunction after surgery and anesthesia. (Stratmann, 2011).

6.3. Intraoperative Course and Neurocognitive Outcomes

However, anesthetic medication is not given in a vacuum during clinical settings. The growing central nervous system is a highly sensitive internal environment. The perioperative environment may have an impact on brain development because it modulates critical periods of plasticity during brain development. Anesthesia medications are potent neuronal circuit modulators that affect the ongoing development and remodeling of the central nervous system in both healthy and diseased conditions. Therefore, during these crucial stages of development, non-physiologic exposure to a variety of drugs and stressors (painful stimuli, maternal deprivation, hypoglycemia, hypoxia, and ischemia) may result in altered neuroplasticity and neuronal injury. Deterioration in long-term neurodevelopmental outcomes occurs in neonates undergoing surgery, which may result in congenital anomalies. Are there other confounding variables involved in this process? One should take into account the possible role of hitherto unidentified genetic syndromes linked to both developmental delay and infant surgery necessitating lesions.

Hemodynamic and metabolic changes in anesthetized or sedated patients undergoing painful procedures may impact the neurocognitive outcomes of patients exposed to general anesthesia. These factors may contribute to poor neurocognitive outcomes alone or in combination with the neurotoxic potential of general anesthetics. For infants undergoing general anesthesia, some of the factors linked to poor outcomes in neonates receiving intensive care may be relevant. These variables include temperature, serum glucose levels, carbon dioxide tensions, hyperoxia or hypoxia, and perioperative blood pressure. Seniors' cognitive function will also be impacted by the cognitive decline that comes with aging.

6.3.1. Arterial Blood Pressure

The various definitions of hypotension in the neonate and young infant make it difficult to determine the best course of action for managing arterial blood pressure in these fragile patients. A mean arterial blood pressure (MAP) below the 5th or 10th percentile for age, or for prematurely born infants, a MAP less than the infant's gestational age in weeks, are two commonly used definitions.

Additionally, during the first six weeks of life, the normal arterial blood pressure of very young infants increases rapidly, and then it remains relatively constant for the first year of life. For cerebral protection, it is best to keep arterial blood pressure within the range of cerebral autoregulation, though it is occasionally required to maintain sufficient cerebral perfusion below the range of cerebral autoregulation. The precise lower limits of cerebral autoregulation in neonates are unknown and probably vary. Moreover, there is probably a large range of interinfant variability. Given the infant's age in gestational weeks, the lower limits of cerebral autoregulation for some babies are in fact quite similar to the definition of hypotension. However, cerebral autoregulation at a MAP level significantly lower than their gestational age in weeks is present in certain premature infants. The lower limit of autoregulation in infants under 6 months of age occurred at 38 mm Hg, or a 20 percent decrease from baseline awake mean arterial pressure, according to a study done on children under 2 years old who were receiving sevoflurane anesthesia.

In contrast, the lower limit of autoregulation did not appear in infants older than six months until the arterial blood pressure dropped to forty percent of the normal arterial blood pressure. Although patients were not at risk for cerebral ischemia until the MAP was less than 35 mm Hg, a follow-up study on this group of children using near-infrared spectroscopy and Doppler flow technology revealed that the lower limits of autoregulation occurred at a MAP of 45 mm Hg. Therefore, after general anesthesia is induced, infants may be at risk for inadequate cerebral perfusion due to a decrease in arterial blood pressure because they have a lower cerebral autoregulatory reserve. Partial asphyxia may result from hypotension-induced inadequate perfusion. Sharp drops in arterial blood pressure are the primary cause of partial ischemia, which frequently results in damage to the watershed areas between the main cerebral blood vessels. The majority of general anesthetics result in hypotension, which can be lessened with surgical stimulation. Long-term hypotension in neonates can result from prolonged anesthesia inductions or surgical prep times.

6.3.2. Hypocapnia and the Brain

With its primary impact on the cerebral arteries, the partial arterial carbon dioxide pressure ($Paco_2$) is a significant modulator of cerebral blood flow (CBF). Hypocapnia causes cerebral vascular vasoconstriction, which lowers CBF. Hypocapnia-induced vasoconstriction can cause apoptotic cell death by changing cerebral energy metabolism, ischemia-induced tissue hypoxia and free radical generation, or by altering neuronal nuclear membranes and increasing nuclear Ca^{2+} influx. Hypocapnia, which results in cerebral alkalosis, reduces hemoglobin's capacity to release oxygen and lowers cerebral perfusion. The effects of hypocapnia may be more severe in premature infants. It is generally advised to maintain end-tidal CO_2 levels in infants and children under general anesthesia at or above 35 mm Hg.

6.3.3. Oxygen Management

When too much oxygen is given during general anesthesia, more reactive oxygen species (ROS) are produced, which can stress and kill cells. Normally, ROS and antioxidants in cells are in balance. Little infants have underdeveloped antioxidant defenses that makes it easy for them to override this balance. To prepare the fetus for the relatively hyperoxic environment after birth compared with the relatively hypoxic fetal environment, there is an increase in endogenous production of antioxidants during the final stages of fetal development as well as an increase in maternal-fetal transfer of antioxidants. Due to deficiencies in the two aforementioned factors, premature infants are more vulnerable to oxygen damage than term infants. Glutathione peroxidase, catalase, and superoxide dismutase are among the antioxidant enzymes that are involved. Reactive superoxide radicals are converted by these enzymes to hydrogen peroxide and subsequently to water. In young animals, hyperoxia causes neuroapoptosis, most likely as a result of oxidative stress and a drop in neurotrophin activity. Inflammatory cytokines that are triggered by oxygen can exacerbate cell stress. Neuroischemia can result from both hypoxia and anoxia. When glutamate is released from synaptic vesicles, neurons start to lose their electrochemical gradients and calcium enters the cytosol. This causes necrotic cell death to occur early. Nuclear enlargement, mitochondrial collapse, and inflammation are the signs of this. A fraction of stressed neurons undergo an apoptotic death at some point after the ischemia stress is removed, rather than dying instantly.

6.3.4. Temperature

One of the difficulties with pediatric anesthesia is maintaining temperature during the anesthesia. Babies lose heat more quickly through evaporative and radiant means due to their large skin surface area to body mass ratio and high basal metabolic rate. Moreover, during procedures, their radiant and conductive heat losses are increased by decreased subcutaneous fat and reduced vasoconstriction. Postoperative ventilation may be necessary for infants who are hypothermic at the end of anesthesia because they may not have the energy reserves to both rewarm themselves and ventilate on their own. For neonates who have already experienced hypoxic ischemic injury, mild hypothermia (core temperature of 32° to 34° C) is neuroprotective. When these same newborns were tested at the age of eighteen months, hyperthermia was linked to more neurocognitive impairments.

6.4. Current Evidence on Neonatal Neurotoxicity in Humans

Several animal studies have shown a relationship between anesthesia and neurotoxicity, but evaluating this effect in humans is challenging due to ethical constraints limiting randomized clinical trials in this area. Despite the inherent limitations of observational cohort studies, several human studies suggest an association between early exposure to anesthetics and poor cognitive performance later in life. Children receiving anesthesia before the age of three are more likely to have learning and behavior disorders compared to their peers without anesthesia. Early life exposure to anesthesia, especially if repeated or prolonged, adversely affects long-term neurodevelopmental outcomes in children. However, language and cognition deficits have been reported even after a single anesthetic exposure. Fetal exposure to anesthetics has also been linked to behavioral and psychiatric disturbances persisting into adulthood, including hyperactivity and attention deficit hyperactivity disorder (ADHD). Based on these studies, it is reasonable to speculate that the neuropathological changes observed in the developing brains of animals may similarly occur in the brains of infants and children following anesthesia. Nonetheless, some studies have shown no association between early anesthetic exposure or surgery and the development of cognitive or behavioral disturbances. Human neurobehavior is complex, and subtle impairments resulting from anesthesia may not be easily detected through current neuropsychological and neurobehavioral tests.

The currently available retrospective cohort studies in humans have limitations that prevent conclusive evidence. Children in these studies had surgery, making it difficult to separate the effects of comorbidities, surgical stress, and illness burden (e.g., school absenteeism) on learning, cognition, or behavior from anesthetic effects. Painful stimuli without analgesia and anesthesia have been shown to initiate a harmful stress response in young children and trigger neurotoxic effects in the developing brain, which anesthetics can blunt. Ongoing studies may clarify some of these issues. The GAS study (A Multi-site Randomized Controlled Trial Comparing Regional and General Anesthesia for Effects on Neurodevelopmental Outcome and Apnea in Infants) aims to separate the effects of general anesthesia from the surgical procedure. The MASK (Mayo Anesthesia Safety in Kids) study, a large cohort study, examines long-term cognitive development in children with no anesthetic exposure compared to those with single or multiple exposures before age three. The presence of several social and environmental confounding factors and long lag time may also influence the results. The Pediatric Anesthesia NeuroDevelopmental Assessment Study has undergone a feasibility study and is currently in the late planning stages. It compares a retrospective cohort of children who received anesthesia before age three with unanesthetized siblings in a prospective assessment of neurocognitive outcomes to reduce genetic and environmental contributions to cognitive performance.

The possibility of anesthesia-induced developmental neurotoxicity (AIDN) has significant implications for current anesthesia practices for pregnant women, infants, and children. If it is conclusively determined that anesthetic drugs injure developing brains, the major question will be what can be done about it.

Therefore, it is essential to develop and explore clinically relevant neuroprotective strategies in animals that are likely to mitigate the neurotoxic effects of anesthetics.

6.5. Methods of Protection Against AnaestheticInduced Neurotoxicitytheir Cellular and Molecular Mechanisms of Neuroprotection

Most commonly used anesthetics have demonstrated neurotoxic properties in preclinical studies. Several molecular mechanisms are involved in anesthetic-induced neurotoxicity and cognitive dysfunction. Interrupting this chain reaction may enable anesthetic drugs to reversibly depress neurons without triggering harmful cell death signals. Researchers have explored various neuroprotective strategies to prevent the histologic and developmental abnormalities caused by anesthetics. Peri-anesthesia treatment with reactive oxygen species (ROS) scavengers or mitochondrial protectants has been shown to prevent anesthesia-induced cognitive impairment. Additionally, several other mechanisms of action have been identified. Compounds such as erythropoietin (EPO), lithium, melatonin, 7-nitroindazole, L-carnitine, bumetanide, dexmedetomidine, and xenon have been found to reduce anesthetic-induced neurodegeneration in the developing brain.

Alpha2 Adrenoceptor Agonist

Alpha-2 adrenoceptor signaling plays a crucial trophic role during neurodevelopment and offers neuroprotection in various contexts of neuronal injury. The neuroprotective effects of dexmedetomidine appear to involve a reduction in cleaved caspase-3 levels and the reversal of isoflurane-induced decreases in anti-apoptotic Bcl-1, pERK1, and pERK2 protein expression in vivo. Additionally, the neuroprotective mechanisms of alpha-2 adrenoceptor signaling include the inhibition of calcium entry, scavenging of glutamate, and reduction in NMDA receptor activation.

Xenon

Although xenon is an antagonist at the NMDA-type glutamate receptor, its pretreatment has been shown to exert a neuroprotective effect. Xenon's neuroprotective properties may be attributed to its ability to inhibit intrinsic and common apoptotic pathways. In animal models, at low concentrations, xenon increased Bcl-2 expression, decreased cytochrome C release, and reduced P53 expression, thereby attenuating the neurotoxicity of isoflurane. However, an equipotent comparison of xenon with halogenated anesthetics revealed that xenon causes cell death in developing neurons at levels comparable to isoflurane and sevoflurane.

Brain Preconditioning with Anaesthetic

Prior exposure to low doses of anesthesia or shorter durations of anesthetic exposure can mitigate injury from high doses or prolonged anesthetic exposure in the developing brain. Preconditioning with isoflurane or propofol can protect against anesthetic-induced neurotoxicity. Sub-anesthetic doses of ketamine have been shown to reduce cell death and provide some degree of neuroprotection. Additionally, pretreatment with xenon can attenuate anesthesia-induced developmental neurotoxicity (AIDN).

Vitamins

Nicotinamide reduces the loss of neuronal cells in the developing rat brain caused by ketamine. Downregulation of Bax, inhibition of cytochrome c release from mitochondria into the cytosol, and a decrease in activated caspase-3 levels are all involved in this reduced neuroapoptosis. Nicotinamide exhibits strong inhibitory effects on proinflammatory cytokines as well. It may prevent neurodevelopmental disorders by blocking the rise in pro-inflammatory factors that isoflurane induces in levels of tumor necrosis factor alpha, interleukin-6 (IL-6), and IL-1β. One further defense against ketamine-induced neuroapoptosis is vitamin D3 (1-α-2, 5-dihydroxy-vitamin D3). Calcium within cells can be stabilized through the actions of trophic factor action or CaBP expression, both of which are induced by vitamin D3. Antioxidant vitamin C might be useful against AIDN as well.

Erythropoietin

In situations where there is brain damage, erythropoietin may have a direct neurotrophic and neuroprotective effect. It may also affect neurotransmitter release and be crucial for synaptic plasticity. Anaesthetics may cause neurotoxicity by preventing the production of EPO. Establishing the role of EPO is necessary.

Lithium

As an inhibitor of glycogen synthase kinase-3 β, lithium has demonstrated protective properties against drug-induced neuroapoptosis. Moreover, lithium therapy has the ability to dramatically raise serum levels of BDNF and inhibit neuroapoptosis in the central nervous system by blocking the BDNF-Akt-Bcl2 antiapoptotic signaling pathway.

Melatonin

Neuroprotective effect may be mediated by inhibition of mitochondriadependent apoptotic pathway.

AcetylLcarnitine

It is metabolized in the brain to acetyl coenzyme A, which subsequently enters the tricarboxylic acid cycle. It has been found to effectively block neuronal apoptosis caused by exposure to a combination of N_2O and isoflurane.

Activitydependent Neuroprotective Protein

Injection of NAP can inhibit anaestheticinduced caspase levels in dosedependent manner.

Bumetanide

Bumetanide is an inhibitor of the Cl^- importer NKCC ($Na^+K^+2Cl^-$ cotransporter) treatment, which suppresses depolarizing GABAergic responses.

Other Drugs

Cyclosporine A, Magnesium, and propofol have shown to attenuate the isofluraneinduced mPTP opening, caspase3 activation, and impairment of learning and memory by inhibition of mPTP opening. The ability to pharmacologically render the patients insensitive to neurotoxic effects of anesthetics will be a big breakthrough. A better understanding of the mechanisms of AIDN will certainly identify such candidate drugs and techniques.

A Closer Look

Neurotoxicity

Damage to the brain or peripheral nervous system resulting from exposure to hazardous substances, whether naturally occurring or man-made, is referred to as neurotoxicity. These poisons have the ability to change how the nervous system functions, which may damage or even kill nerves. Information transmission and processing in the brain and other parts of the nervous system depend on nerves. Neurotoxins most often cause damage to neurons because of their high metabolic rate. Microglia, oligodendrocytes, astroocytes, and capillary endothelium cells come next in risk order. A neurotoxin will damage specific areas or specific cellular components of the nervous system, depending on its chemical makeup. Since non-polar compounds are more soluble in lipids than polar compounds, which are less soluble in lipids, they have an easier time entering the nervous system. The affected neurotransmitter, the integrity of the cellular membrane, and the existence of detoxifying mechanisms are some of the variables that affect the body's reaction to neurotoxins.

Some examples of substances that can be neurotoxic to humans include:

- Chemotherapy drugs that are used to kill fast-growing cells
- Radiation
- Drug therapies or drugs of abuse
- Heavy metals such as mercury and lead
- Certain foods and food additives
- Insecticides/pesticides
- Cosmetics
- Industrial and cleaning solvents

Some examples of neurotoxic substances our environment has become polluted with and that it is difficult for people to avoid exposure to include:

- Mercury
- Cadmium
- Lead
- Insecticides
- Solvents
- Car exhaust
- Chlorine
- Formaldehyde

- Phenol

While some of the effects of neurotoxicity may show up right away, others may take months or even years to show symptoms. The properties of the neurotoxin, the dose an individual has been exposed to, their capacity to metabolize and excrete the toxin, the ability of the damaged mechanisms and structures to heal, and the susceptibility of a cellular target are just a few of the variables that affect how neurotoxicity manifests itself.

Some of the symptoms of neurotoxicity include:

- Paralysis or weakness in the limbs
- Altered sensation, tingling and numbness in the limbs
- Headache
- Vision loss
- Loss of memory and cognitive function
- Uncontrollable obsessive and/or compulsive behavior
- Behavioral problems
- Sexual dysfunction
- Depression
- Loss of circulation
- Imbalance
- Flu-like symptoms

Neurotoxicity can also lead to other conditions such as non-responsive asthma, chronic sinusitis, attention deficit hyperactivity disorder, and chronic fatigue syndrome. Additionally, some autoimmune diseases like rheumatoid arthritis and irritable bowel syndrome may have symptoms similar to these. Toxins that can cause neurotoxicity include glutamate, beta amyloid, and oxygen radicals, which are found naturally in the brain. Not only can neurotoxicity lead to movement disorders, cognitive decline, and autonomic nervous system dysfunction, but it has also been demonstrated to play a significant role in the advancement of neurological disorders like Alzheimer's disease. The nerve conduction test is the most effective way to determine whether the peripheral nervous system has been impacted. Pupillography, computerized balance, heart rate variability, triple-camera SPECT brain imaging, and neuropsychological testing are among the tests used to identify brain damage. Elimination or reduction of the toxic substance combined with therapy to support or alleviate symptoms is the treatment strategy for neurotoxicity. Eating, drinking, and air pollution avoidance may also be part of the treatment. Numerous therapies are employed to treat neurotoxicity, such as immune modulation, massage, and exercise. The degree of neural damage and the length and intensity of exposure to the toxic substance determine the outcome of neurotoxicity. In certain situations, exposure to neurotoxins can be lethal; in other cases, patients may live but may not fully recover. In other instances, patients recover fully from their treatments (American Society of Anesthesiologists)

Summary

- Anesthetic drugs are potent modulators of the central nervous system (CNS) and reversibly render patients insensate to painful procedures and surgery.
- Determining the root cause of the neurotoxic effect of CNS depressant drugs on the developing brain is complicated by the myriad of molecular targets and the still unknown mechanistic pathway to achieve general anesthesia.
- Neural development progresses through several steps that include neurogenesis, neuronal morphogenesis, and synaptogenesis. Neurogenesis starts with the creation of progenitor cells, which proliferate and differentiate into neurons or glial cells.
- Anesthetics affect neurogenesis in animals in an age-dependent manner. Isoflurane causes loss of neural stem cells and reduced neurogenesis in neonatal but not adult rats, where it causes a brief increase in neurogenesis.
- Dendritic spines are small protrusions of the neurons that typically receive input from a single synapse of an axon and are essential components of synaptogenesis. Exposure to ketamine and isoflurane decreases synapse and spine density in very young infant rats.
- Decrements in neurocognitive function clearly occur after fetal and neonatal exposure to anesthetic drugs in rodents. Standard behavioral measures in rodents include the Morris water navigation test, radial arm maze, startle, prepulse inhibition of the startle reflex, and odor recognition testing.
- The partial arterial carbon dioxide pressure ($Paco_2$) is an important modulator of the cerebral blood flow (CBF) with its main effect on cerebral arteries. Hypocapnia results in vasoconstriction of cerebral vessels leading to decreases in CBF.
- Potent inhaled anesthetics represent the mainstay of drugs used to maintain anesthesia in most clinical situations. They are easily titratable, reduce the autonomic response to noxious stimulation, and at clinically relevant doses can often provide sufficient muscle relaxation to facilitate surgical exposure.

References

1. Algie, C. M., Mahar, R. K., Tan, H. B., et al. (2015). Effectiveness and risks of cricoid pressure during rapid sequence induction for endotracheal intubation. *Cochrane Database of Systematic Reviews,* (11), CD011656.
2. Amrock, L. G., Starner, M. L., Murphy, K. L., & Baxter, M. G. (2015). Long-term effects of single or multiple neonatal sevoflurane exposures on rat hippocampal ultrastructure. *Anesthesiology, 122*, 87–95.
3. Andreae, M. H., & Andreae, D. A. (2013). Regional anesthesia to prevent chronic pain after surgery: A Cochrane systematic review and meta-analysis. *British Journal of Anaesthesia, 111*, 711–720.
4. Backeljauw, B., Holland, S. K., Altaye, M., & Loepke, A. W. (2015). Cognition and brain structure following early childhood surgery with anesthesia. *Pediatrics, 136*(1), e1–e12.
5. Bajic, D., Commons, K. G., & Soriano, S. G. (2013). Morphine-enhanced apoptosis in selective

brain regions of neonatal rats. *International Journal of Developmental Neuroscience, 31*, 258–266.

6. Barreveld, A., Witte, J., Chahal, H., et al. (2013). Preventive analgesia by local anesthetics: The reduction of postoperative pain by peripheral nerve blocks and intravenous drugs. *Anesthesia & Analgesia, 116*, 1141–1161.
7. Bartels, M., Althoff, R. R., & Boomsma, D. I. (2009). Anesthesia and cognitive performance in children: No evidence for a causal relationship. *Twin Research and Human Genetics, 12*, 246–253.
8. Bedford, P. D. (1955). Adverse cerebral effects of anesthesia on old people. *Lancet, 269*, 259–263.
9. Ben-Ari, Y. (2002). Excitatory actions of GABA during development: The nature of the nurture. *Nature Reviews Neuroscience, 3*, 728–739.
10. Berger, M., Nadler, J. W., Browndyke, J., et al. (2015). Postoperative cognitive dysfunction: Minding the gaps in our knowledge of a common postoperative complication in the elderly. *Anesthesiology Clinics, 33*(3), 517–550.
11. Bhananker, S. M., Posner, K. L., Cheney, F. W., et al. (2006). Injury and liability associated with monitored anesthesia care: A closed claims analysis. *Anesthesiology, 104*(2), 228–234.
12. Bittigau, P., Sifringer, M., Genz, K., et al. (2002). Antiepileptic drugs and apoptotic neurodegeneration in the developing brain. *Proceedings of the National Academy of Sciences U S A, 99*(23), 15089–15094.
13. Blomgren, K., Leist, M., & Groc, L. (2007). Pathological apoptosis in the developing brain. *Apoptosis, 12*, 993–1010.
14. Boscolo, A., Milanovic, D., Starr, J. A., et al. (2013). Early exposure to general anesthesia disturbs mitochondrial fission and fusion in the developing rat brain. *Anesthesiology, 118*, 1086–1097.
15. Boscolo, A., Ori, C., Bennett, J., et al. (2013). Mitochondrial protectant pramipexole prevents sex-specific long-term cognitive impairment from early anesthesia exposure in rats. *British Journal of Anesthesia, 110*(suppl 1), i47–i52.
16. Boscolo, A., Starr, J. A., Sanchez, V., et al. (2012). The abolishment of anesthesia-induced cognitive impairment by timely protection of mitochondria in the developing rat brain: The importance of free oxygen radicals and mitochondrial integrity. *Neurobiology of Disease, 45*, 1031–1041.
17. Brambrink, A. M., Back, S. A., Riddle, A., et al. (2012). Isoflurane-induced apoptosis of oligodendrocytes in the neonatal primate brain. *Annals of Neurology, 72*, 525–535.
18. Brambrink, A. M., Evers, A. S., Avidan, M. S., et al. (2012). Ketamine-induced neuroapoptosis in the fetal and neonatal rhesus macaque brain. *Anesthesiology, 116*, 372–384.
19. Briner, A., De Roo, M., Dayer, A., et al. (2010). Volatile anesthetics rapidly increase dendritic spine density in the rat medial prefrontal cortex during synaptogenesis. *Anesthesiology, 112*, 546–556.
20. Brown, C. H. T., Azman, A. S., Gottschalk, A., et al. (2014). Sedation depth during spinal anesthesia and survival in elderly patients undergoing hip fracture repair. *Anesthesia & Analgesia, 118*, 977–980.

21. Buss, R. R., Sun, W., & Oppenheim, R. W. (2006). Adaptive roles of programmed cell death during nervous system development. *Annual Review of Neuroscience, 29*, 1–35.

22. Cayabyab, R., McLean, C. W., & Seri, I. (2009). Definition of hypotension and assessment of hemodynamics in the preterm neonate. *Journal of Perinatology, 29*(suppl 2), S58–S62.

23. Cibelli, M., Fidalgo, A. R., Terrando, N., et al. (2010). Role of interleukin-1beta in postoperative cognitive dysfunction. *Annals of Neurology, 68*, 360–368.

24. Clancy, B., Kersh, B., Hyde, J., et al. (2007). Web-based method for translating neurodevelopment from laboratory species to humans. *Neuroinformatics, 5*, 79–94.

25. Cohen, N. A., & McMichael, J. P. (2004). What's new in ... Definitions of monitored anesthesia care. *American Society of Anesthesiologists Newsletter, 68*(6), 22–26.

26. Creeley, C. E., Dikranian, K. T., Dissen, G. A., et al. (2014). Isoflurane-induced apoptosis of neurons and oligodendrocytes in the fetal rhesus macaque brain. *Anesthesiology, 120*, 626–638.

27. Culley, D. J., Baxter, M. G., Yukhananov, R., & Crosby, G. (2004). Long-term impairment of acquisition of a spatial memory task following isoflurane-nitrous oxide anesthesia in rats. *Anesthesiology, 100*, 309–314.

28. Culley, D. J., Boyd, J. D., Palanisamy, A., et al. (2011). Isoflurane decreases self-renewal capacity of rat cultured neural stem cells. *Anesthesiology, 115*, 754–763.

29. Davidson, A. J., Disma, N., de Graaff, J. C., et al. (2015). GAS Consortium. Neurodevelopmental outcome at 2 years of age after general anesthesia and awake-regional anesthesia in infancy (GAS): An international multicenter, randomized controlled trial. *Lancet, 387*(10015), 239–250.

30. de la Rosa, J. L., & de Pablo, F. (2000). Cell death in early neural development: Beyond the neurotrophic theory. *Trends in Neurosciences, 23*, 454–458.

31. De Roo, M., Klauser, P., Briner, A., et al. (2009). Anesthetics rapidly promote synaptogenesis during a critical period of brain development. *PLoS One, 4*, e7043.

32. DiMaggio, C., Sun, L. S., Kakavouli, A., et al. (2009). A retrospective cohort study of the association of anesthesia and hernia repair surgery with behavioral and developmental disorders in young children. *Journal of Neurosurgical Anesthesiology, 21*, 286–291.

33. Dimaggio, C., Sun, L., & Li, G. (2011). Early childhood exposure to anesthesia and risk of developmental and behavioral disorders in a sibling birth cohort. *Anesthesia & Analgesia, 113*, 1143–1151.

34. Dzhala, V. I., Talos, D. M., Sdrulla, D. A., et al. (2005). NKCC1 transporter facilitates seizures in the developing brain. *Nature Medicine, 11*, 1205–1213.

35. Eckenhoff, J. E. (1953). Relationship of anesthesia to postoperative personality changes in children. *American Journal of Diseases of Children, 86*, 587–591.

36. Edwards, D. A., Shah, H. P., Cao, W., et al. (2010). Bumetanide alleviates epileptogenic and neurotoxic effects of sevoflurane in neonatal rat brain. *Anesthesiology, 112*, 567–575.

37. Flick, R. P., Katusic, S. K., Colligan, R. C., et al. (2011). Cognitive and behavioral outcomes after early exposure to anesthesia and surgery. *Pediatrics, 128*, e1053–e1061.

38. Franks, N. P. (2008). General anesthesia: From molecular targets to neuronal pathways of sleep and arousal. *Nature Reviews Neuroscience, 9*, 370–386.

39. Glatz, P., Sandin, R. H., Pedersen, N. L., et al. (2017). Association of anesthesia and surgery during childhood with long-term academic performance. *JAMA Pediatrics, 171*(1), e163470.

40. Glover, C. D., & Carling, N. P. (2014). Neuromonitoring for scoliosis surgery. *Anesthesia & Analgesia, 32*(1), 101–114.

41. Graham, M. R., Brownell, M., Chateau, D. G., et al. (2016). Neurodevelopmental assessment in kindergarten in children exposed to general anesthesia before the age of 4 years: A retrospective matched cohort study. *Anesthesiology, 125*(4), 667–677.

42. Guay, J. (2006). The effect of neuraxial blocks on surgical blood loss and blood transfusion requirements: A meta-analysis. *Journal of Clinical Anesthesia, 18*, 124–128.

43. Guay, J., Choi, P. T., Suresh, S., et al. (2014). Neuraxial anesthesia for the prevention of postoperative mortality and major morbidity: An overview of Cochrane Systematic Reviews. *Anesthesia & Analgesia, 119*, 716–725.

44. Hansen, T. G., Pedersen, J. K., Henneberg, S. W., et al. (2011). Academic performance in adolescence after inguinal hernia repair in infancy: A nationwide cohort study. *Anesthesiology, 114*(5), 1076–1085.

45. Head, B. P., Patel, H. H., Niesman, I. R., et al. (2009). Inhibition of p75 neurotrophin receptor attenuates isoflurane-mediated neuronal apoptosis in the neonatal central nervous system. *Anesthesiology, 110*, 813–825.

46. Hensch, T. K. (2005). Critical period plasticity in local cortical circuits. *Nature Reviews Neuroscience, 6*, 877–888.

47. Hofacer, R. D., Deng, M., Ward, C. G., et al. (2013). Cell-age specific vulnerability of neurons to anesthetic toxicity. *Annals of Neurology, 73*, 695–704.

48. Hovens, I. B., Schoemaker, R. G., van der Zee, E. A., et al. (2012). Thinking through postoperative cognitive dysfunction: How to bridge the gap between clinical and pre-clinical perspectives. *Brain, Behavior, and Immunity, 26*, 1169–1179.

49. Huang, L., & Yang, G. (2015). Repeated exposure to ketamine-xylazine during early development impairs motor learning-dependent dendritic spine plasticity in adulthood. *Anesthesiology, 122*, 821–831.

50. Ikonomidou, C., Bittigau, P., Ishimaru, M. J., et al. (2000). Ethanol-induced apoptotic neurodegeneration and fetal alcohol syndrome. *Science, 287*, 1056–1060.

51. Ikonomidou, C., Bosch, F., Miksa, M., et al. (1999). Blockade of NMDA receptors and apoptotic neurodegeneration in the developing brain. *Science, 283*, 70–74.

52. Ilfeld, B. M. (2011). Continuous peripheral nerve blocks: A review of the published evidence. *Anesthesia & Analgesia, 113*(4), 904–925.

53. Ing, C., DiMaggio, C., Whitehouse, A., et al. (2012). Long-term differences in language and cognitive function after childhood exposure to anesthesia. *Pediatrics, 130*, e476–e485.

54. Ishizawa, Y. (2011). Special article: General anesthetic gases and the global environment. *Anesthesia & Analgesia, 112*, 213–217.

55. Jagodic, M. M., Pathirathna, S., Joksovic, P. M., et al. (2008). Upregulation of the T-type calcium current in small rat sensory neurons after chronic constrictive injury of the sciatic nerve. *Journal of Neurophysiology, 99*, 3151–3156.

56. Jevtovic-Todorovic, V., Hartman, R. E., Izumi, Y., et al. (2003). Early exposure to common anesthetic agents causes widespread neurodegeneration in the developing rat brain and persistent learning deficits. *Journal of Neuroscience, 23*, 876–882.

57. Leslie, K., Myles, P. S., Kasza, J., et al. (2015). Nitrous oxide and serious long-term morbidity and mortality in the Evaluation of Nitrous Oxide in the Gas Mixture for Anesthesia (ENIGMA)-II Trial. *Anesthesiology, 123*(6), 1267–1280.

58. Lin, E. P., Soriano, S. G., & Loepke, A. W. (2014). Anesthetic neurotoxicity. *Anesthesia & Analgesia, 32*, 133–155.

59. Mashour, G. A., Shanks, A., Tremper, K. K., et al. (2012). Prevention of intraoperative awareness with explicit recall in an unselected surgical population: A randomized comparative effectiveness trial. *Anesthesiology, 117*(4), 717–725.

60. Massa, H., Lacoh, C. M., & Vutskits, L. (2012). Effects of morphine on the differentiation and survival of developing pyramidal neurons during the brain growth spurt. *Toxicological Sciences, 130*, 168–179.

61. McCann, M. E., & Soriano, S. G. (2012). Perioperative central nervous system injury in neonates. *British Journal of Anesthesia, 109*(suppl 1), i60–i67.

62. Meng, L., & Gelb, A. W. (2015). Regulation of cerebral autoregulation by carbon dioxide. *Anesthesiology, 122*, 196–205.

63. O'Leary, J. D., Janus, M., Duku, E., et al. (2016). A population-based study evaluating the association between surgery in early life and child development at primary school entry. *Anesthesiology, 125*, 272–279.

64. Ohnuma, S., & Harris, W. A. (2003). Neurogenesis and the cell cycle. *Neuron, 40*, 199–208.

65. Palanisamy, A., Baxter, M. G., Keel, P. K., et al. (2011). Rats exposed to isoflurane in utero during early gestation are behaviorally abnormal as adults. *Anesthesiology, 114*, 521–528.

66. Pancaro, C., Segal, B. S., Sikes, R. W., et al. (2016). Dexmedetomidine and ketamine show distinct patterns of cell degeneration and apoptosis in the developing rat neonatal brain. *Journal of Maternal-Fetal & Neonatal Medicine, 29*(23), 3827–3833.

67. Paule, M. G., Li, M., Allen, R. R., et al. (2011). Ketamine anesthesia during the first week of life can cause long-lasting cognitive deficits in rhesus monkeys. *Neurotoxicology and Teratology, 33*, 220–230.

68. Penzes, P., Cahill, M. E., Jones, K. A., et al. (2011). Dendritic spine pathology in neuropsychiatric disorders. *Nature Neuroscience, 14*, 285–293.

69. Quimby, K. L., Katz, J., & Bowman, R. E. (1975). Behavioral consequences in rats from chronic exposure to 10 ppm halothane during early development. *Anesthesia & Analgesia, 54*, 628–633.

70. Raper, J., Alvarado, M. C., Murphy, K. L., & Baxter, M. G. (2015). Multiple anesthetic exposure in infant monkeys alters emotional reactivity to an acute stressor. *Anesthesiology, 123*, 1084–1092.

71. Rappaport, B., Mellon, R. D., Simone, A., & Woodcock, J. (2011). Defining safe use of anesthesia in children. *New England Journal of Medicine, 364*, 1387–1390.

72. Rudolph, U., & Antkowiak, B. (2004). Molecular and neuronal substrates for general anesthetics. *Nature Reviews Neuroscience, 5*, 709–720.

73. Ryan, S. M., & Nielsen, C. J. (2010). Global warming potential of inhaled anesthetics: Application to clinical use. *Anesthesia & Analgesia, 111*, 92–98.

74. Ryu, Y. K., Khan, S., Smith, S. C., & Mintz, C. D. (2014). Isoflurane impairs the capacity of astrocytes to support neuronal development in a mouse dissociated coculture model. *Journal of Neurosurgery: Anesthesiology, 26*, 363–368.

75. Sanchez, V., Feinstein, S. D., Lunardi, N., et al. (2011). General anesthesia causes long-term impairment of mitochondrial morphogenesis and synaptic transmission in developing rat brain. *Anesthesiology, 115*, 992–1002.

76. Sanders, R. D., Sun, P., Patel, S., et al. (2010). Dexmedetomidine provides cortical neuroprotection: Impact on anesthetic-induced neuroapoptosis in the rat developing brain. *Acta Anesthesiologic Scandinavica, 54*, 710–716.

77. Sanders, R. D., Xu, J., Shu, Y., et al. (2008). General anesthetics induce apoptotic neurodegeneration in the neonatal rat spinal cord. *Anesthesia & Analgesia, 106*, 1708–1711.

78. Sanders, R. D., Xu, J., Shu, Y., et al. (2009). Dexmedetomidine attenuates isoflurane-induced neurocognitive impairment in neonatal rats. *Anesthesiology, 110*, 1077–1085.

79. Shen, X., Dong, Y., Xu, Z., et al. (2013). Selective anesthesia-induced neuroinflammation in developing mouse brain and cognitive impairment. *Anesthesiology, 118*, 502–515.

80. Shih, J., May, L. D., Gonzalez, H. E., et al. (2012). Delayed environmental enrichment reverses sevoflurane-induced memory impairment in rats. *Anesthesiology, 116*, 586–602.

81. Slikker Jr, W., Paule, M. G., Wright, L. K., et al. (2007). Systems biology approaches for toxicology. *Journal of Applied Toxicology, 27*, 201–217.

82. Slikker, W., Zou, X., Hotchkiss, C. E., et al. (2007). Ketamine-induced neuronal cell death in the perinatal rhesus monkey. *Toxicological Sciences, 98*, 145–158.

83. Soriano, S. G., Liu, Q., Li, J., et al. (2010). Ketamine activates cell cycle signaling and apoptosis in the neonatal rat brain. *Anesthesiology, 112*, 1155–1163.

84. Stratmann, G. (2011). Review article: Neurotoxicity of anesthetic drugs in the developing brain. *Anesthesia & Analgesia, 113*, 1170–1179.

85. Stratmann, G., Lee, J., Sall, J. W., et al. (2014). Effect of general anesthesia in infancy on long-term recognition memory in humans and rats. *Neuropsychopharmacology, 39*, 2275–2287.

86. Stratmann, G., Sall, J. W., May, L. D., et al. (2009). Isoflurane differentially affects neurogenesis and long-term neurocognitive function in 60-day-old and 7-day-old rats. *Anesthesiology, 110*, 834–848.

87. Sun, L. S., Li, G., Miller, T. L., et al. (2016). Association between a single general anesthesia exposure before age 36 months and neurocognitive outcomes in later childhood. *JAMA, 315*, 2312–2320.

88. Tang, J. X., Mardini, F., Janik, L. S., et al. (2013). Modulation of murine Alzheimer pathogenesis and behavior by surgery. *Annals of Surgery, 257*, 439–448.

89. Tau, G. Z., & Peterson, B. S. (2010). Normal development of brain circuits. *Neuropsychopharmacology, 35*, 147–168.

90. Terrando, N., Eriksson, L. I., & Eckenhoff, R. G. (2015). Perioperative neurotoxicity in the elderly: Summary of the 4th International Workshop. *Anesthesia & Analgesia, 120*, 649–652.

91. Terrando, N., Monaco, C., Ma, D., et al. (2010). Tumor necrosis factor-alpha triggers a cytokine cascade yielding postoperative cognitive decline. *Proceedings of the National Academy of Sciences U S A, 107*, 20518–20522.

92. Torvik, A. (1984). The pathogenesis of watershed infarcts in the brain. *Stroke, 15*, 221–223.

93. Urban, B. W., & Bleckwenn, M. (2002). Concepts and correlations relevant to general anesthesia. *British Journal of Anesthesia, 89*(1), 3–16.

94. Vacas, S., Degos, V., Feng, X., & Maze, M. (2013). The neuroinflammatory response of postoperative cognitive decline. *British Medical Bulletin, 106*, 161–178.

95. Vavilala, M. S., Lee, L. A., Lee, M., et al. (2003). Cerebral autoregulation in children during sevoflurane anesthesia. *British Journal of Anaesthesia, 90*, 636–641.

96. Vutskits, L. (2012). General anesthesia: A gateway to modulate synapse formation and neural plasticity? *Anesthesia & Analgesia, 115*, 1174–1182.

97. Vutskits, L., Gascon, E., Potter, G., et al. (2007). Low concentrations of ketamine initiate dendritic atrophy of differentiated GABAergic neurons in culture. *Toxicology, 234*, 216–226.

98. Vutskits, L., Gascon, E., Tassonyi, E., & Kiss, J. Z. (2005). Clinically relevant concentrations of propofol but not midazolam alter in vitro dendritic development of isolated gamma-aminobutyric acid positive interneurons. *Anesthesiology, 102*, 970–976.

99. Vutskits, L., Gascon, E., Tassonyi, E., & Kiss, J. Z. (2006). Effect of ketamine on dendritic arbor development and survival of immature GABAergic neurons in vitro. *Toxicological Sciences, 91*, 540–549.

100. Walker, S. M., Westin, B. D., Deumens, R., et al. (2010). Effects of intrathecal ketamine in the neonatal rat: Evaluation of apoptosis and long-term functional outcome. *Anesthesiology, 113*, 147–159.

101. Wang, C., Sadovova, N., Hotchkiss, C., et al. (2006). Blockade of N-methyl-D-aspartate receptors by ketamine produces loss of postnatal day 3 monkey frontal cortical neurons in culture. *Toxicological Sciences, 91*, 192–201.

102. Wang, S., Peretich, K., Zhao, Y., et al. (2009). Anesthesia-induced neurodegeneration in fetal rat brains. *Pediatric Research, 66*, 435–440.

103. Werker, J. F., & Hensch, T. K. (2015). Critical periods in speech perception: New directions. *Annual Review of Psychology, 66*, 173–196.

104. Westin, B. D., Walker, S. M., Deumens, R., et al. (2010). Validation of a preclinical spinal safety model: Effects of intrathecal morphine in the neonatal rat. *Anesthesiology, 113*, 183–199.

105. Wilder, R. T., Flick, R. P., Sprung, J., et al. (2009). Early exposure to anesthesia and learning disabilities in a population-based birth cohort. *Anesthesiology, 110*, 796–804.

106. Xie, Z., & Vutskits, L. (2016). Lasting impact of general anesthesia on the brain: Mechanisms and relevance. *Nature Reviews Neuroscience, 17*(11), 705–717.

107. Xie, Z., Culley, D. J., Dong, Y., et al. (2008). The common inhalation anesthetic isoflurane induces caspase activation and increases amyloid beta-protein level in vivo. *Annals of Neurology, 64*, 618–627.

108. Xie, Z., Dong, Y., Maeda, U., et al. (2006). Isoflurane-induced apoptosis: A potential pathogenic link between delirium and dementia. *Journal of Gerontology A: Biological Sciences and Medical Sciences, 61*, 1300–1306.

109. Xu, Z., Dong, Y., Wang, H., et al. (2014). Age-dependent postoperative cognitive impairment and Alzheimer-related neuropathology in mice. *Scientific Reports, 4*, 3766.

110. Yahalom, B., Athiraman, U., Soriano, S. G., et al. (2011). Spinal anesthesia in infant rats: Development of a model and assessment of neurologic outcomes. *Anesthesiology, 114*, 1325–1335.

111. Zhang, L. L., Pathak, H. R., Coulter, D. A., et al. (2006). Shift of intracellular chloride concentration in ganglion and amacrine cells of developing mouse retina. *Journal of Neurophysiology, 95*, 2404–2416.

Chapter 7

ANESTHESIA DELIVERY SYSTEMS

Contents

Introduction

The anesthesia workstation, also known as the anesthesia machine, and the anesthetic breathing system, also known as the anesthetic circuit, make up an anesthesia delivery system. Together, they allow for the removal of carbon dioxide from the patient's body and the administration of known concentrations of oxygen and inhaled anesthetics. Either chemical neutralization or washout—a gas flow from the anesthesia machine of more than 5 L/min—can be used to eliminate carbon dioxide. To safely and effectively administer anesthetic agents during surgical procedures and other medical interventions, anesthesia delivery systems are essential parts of contemporary medical practice. To provide the best possible anesthesia depth, patient comfort, and safety, these systems are made to precisely control the delivery of anesthetic gases and vapors.

Delivering a precise blend of anesthetic agents and oxygen to the patient's respiratory system is the main purpose of anesthesia delivery systems. This concoction is designed to provide the right amount of anesthesia and to keep it there while maintaining proper ventilation and oxygenation. Vaporizers, flowmeters, breathing circuits, and monitoring devices are common parts of anesthesia delivery systems. These components cooperate to control the patient's delivery, concentration, and gas flow rates. These systems are available in a variety of configurations, from straightforward setups for easy procedures to complex machines for intricate surgeries. They are made to accommodate the various requirements of various patient demographics, clinical environments, and surgical specializations. Features like automated drug delivery, integrated monitoring, and ergonomic design are examples of how anesthesia delivery system advancements continue to improve clinical outcomes and patient safety. Furthermore, continued innovation and research aims to enhance anesthesia care delivery while lowering environmental impact and increasing efficiency (American Society of Anesthesiologists, 1987; American Society of Anesthesiologists Committee on Equipment and Facilities, 2008).

Orientation and Directional Terms

Term	Definition	Illustration
Anesthesia delivery system	An anesthetic machine must control fresh gas flow, provide a means of delivering the fresh carrier gas to the patient (breathing circuit), and control the concentration of anesthetic vapor delivered.	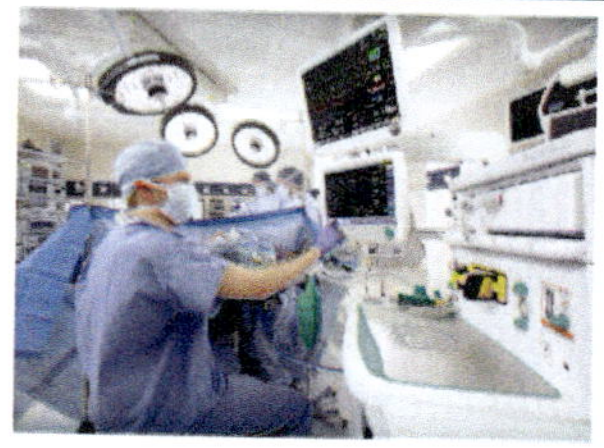
Diameter-index safety system	The diameter-index safety system was developed as a standard to provide non-interchangeable connections where removable, exposed, threaded connections are employed. It is used in conjunction with individual gas lines of medical gas administering equipment at pressures of 200 psig or less.	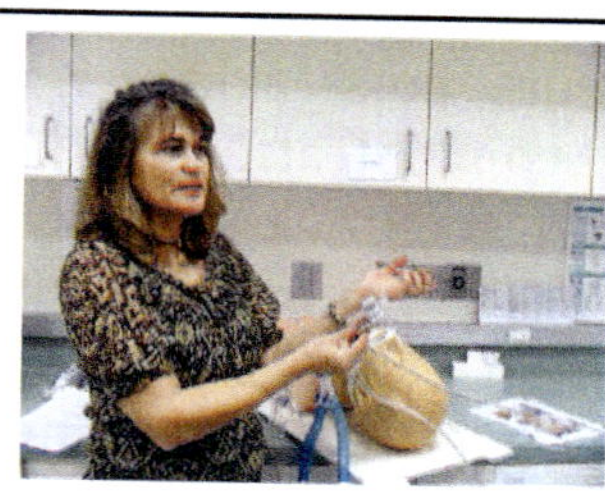
Anesthesia breathing system	Anesthesia breathing systems serve as a conduit to deliver anesthetic and other gases to a patient. Various designs of breathing systems have been created to serve this function. One method of classifying anesthesia breathing systems is based on how gas flows: open, semi-open, semi-closed, and closed systems.	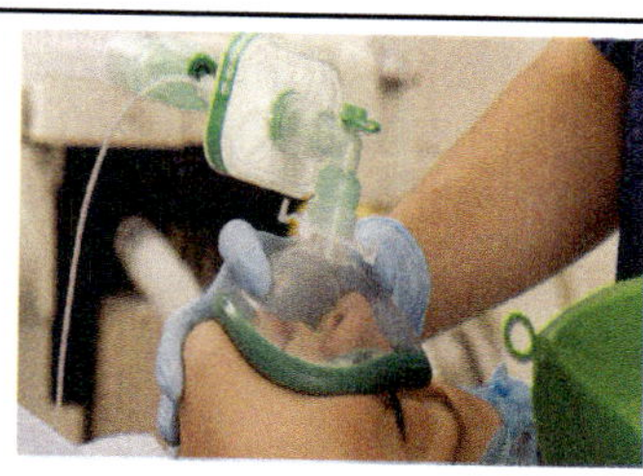
Bain circuit	Bain circuit is a type of breathing circuit commonly used in anesthesia for delivering and monitoring the patient's inhaled and exhaled gases during surgery or other medical procedures.	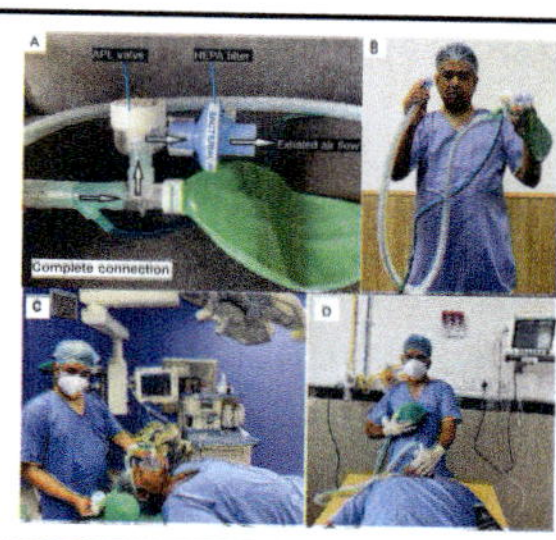
Adjustable pressure-limiting (APL)	As anesthetic and fresh gases are delivered to the system, pressure will build if the gas inflow is greater than inspired volumes. Thus, the system also contains an adjustable pressure-limiting valve (APL valve) which allows gases to exit the breathing system.	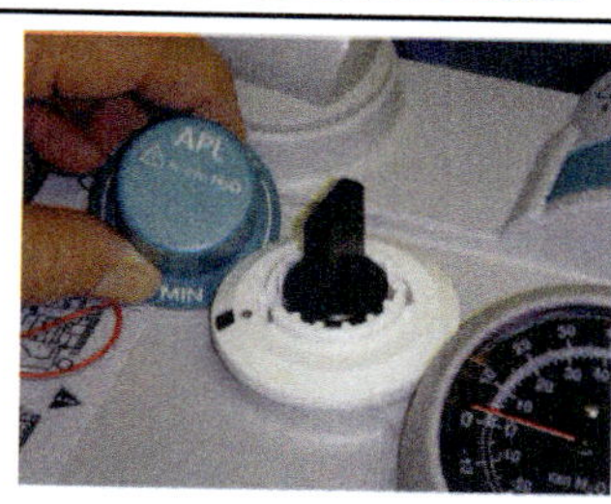

7.1. Anesthesia Workstation

From a basic pneumatic device to a sophisticated integrated computer-controlled multicomponent workstation, the anesthesia machine has undergone evolution. The anesthesia workstation's parts work together harmoniously to provide the patient with known concentrations of inhaled anesthetics. The ventilator, scavenging system, anesthesia breathing circuit, vaporizers, an electrocardiogram, arterial blood pressure, temperature, pulse oximeter, and inhaled and exhaled concentrations of oxygen, carbon dioxide, anesthetic gases, and vapors are among the numerous components of the anesthesia workstation that were previously referred to as the anesthesia machine (the pressure-regulating and gas-mixing components). Included are alarm systems to indicate apnea or to disconnect the patient's anesthetic breathing system. The workstation's alarms, which include a capnograph and pulse oximeter, must be operational and audible to the anesthesia provider. The majority of anesthetic machines are pneumatically and electrically powered.

The medical gases and volatile anesthetic vapors at known concentrations are ultimately delivered to the common gas outlet by the anesthesia workstation. These gases enter the breathing system responsible for administering anesthesia to the patient, either through mechanical or spontaneous ventilation. Exhaled gases are either recycled back to the patient via a CO_2 absorbent or they leave the system through the scavenging system (Figure 7.1).

Common Features of Anesthesia Machines:

- An inlet of hospital pipeline for compressed gases (oxygen, nitrous oxide, and air)
- An inlet of compressed gas cylinders
- Pressure regulators to reduce pipeline and cylinder pressure to safe and consistent levels
- Fail-safe device
- Flowmeters to control the amount of gases delivered to the breathing limb
- Vaporizers for adding volatile anesthetic gas to the carrier gas
- Common gas line through which compressed gases mixed with a volatile agent enter the breathing limb
- Breathing limb, including an oxygen analyzer, inspiratory one-way valve, circle system, gas sampling line, spirometer to measure the respiratory rate and volume, expiratory one-way valve, adjustable pressure-limiting valve, carbon dioxide absorbent, reservoir bag, mechanical ventilator, and scavenging system

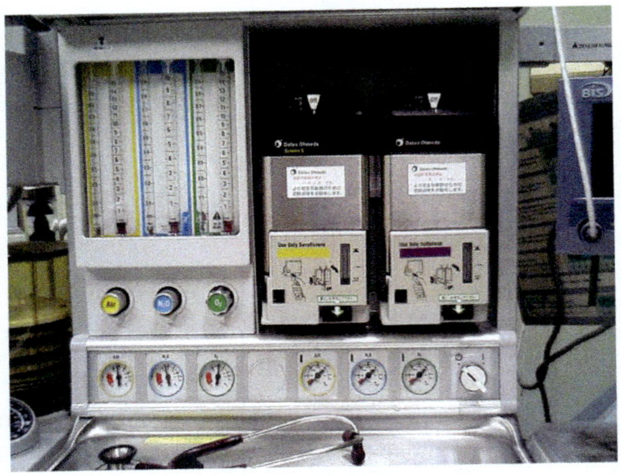

Figure 7.1. *An anesthesia delivery system.*

Source: By Ignis - Own work, CC BY-SA 3.0, https://commons.wikimedia.org/w/index.php?curid=379540.

7.1.1. Fail-Safe Valve

A fail-safe valve built into anesthesia machines is intended to stop the machine from delivering hypoxic gas mixtures in the event that the oxygen supply fails. When the pressure in the oxygen delivery line falls to less than 30 psi, this valve closes or proportionately reduces the flow of all gases. This safety feature guards against oxygen delivery from a central source or cylinder attached to the anesthesia machine running out of oxygen without the user realizing it. However, when gas pressure is maintained in the anesthesia machine's circuit and oxygen flow is zero, this valve does not stop the delivery of 100% nitrous oxide. An oxygen analyzer is required in this case in order to identify the delivery of a hypoxic gas mixture. An alert anesthesia provider is far more beneficial than a fail-safe valve or an oxygen analyzer.

7.1.2. Compressed Gases

The anesthesia machine typically receives its supply of gases (oxygen, nitrous oxide, and air) from a central supply source situated within the hospital. Through pipelines to wall outlets with color coding (green for oxygen, blue for nitrous oxide, and yellow for air), hospital-supplied gases are brought into the operating room from a central Source. Pipeline gas misconnections are avoided by using quick connects or the non-interchangeable diameter index safety system (DISS) fittings to connect color-coded pressure hoses to wall outlets. The anesthesia machine's ventilator can also be powered pneumatically by air or oxygen from a central supply source (Figure 7.2).

To reduce the chance of a misconnection, gas enters the anesthesia machine through pipeline inlet connections that are gas specific (threaded noninterchangeable connections). The machine's flowmeters need the gas to be supplied at a suitable pressure (roughly 50 psi) from the central supply source in order to operate (Figure 7.3).

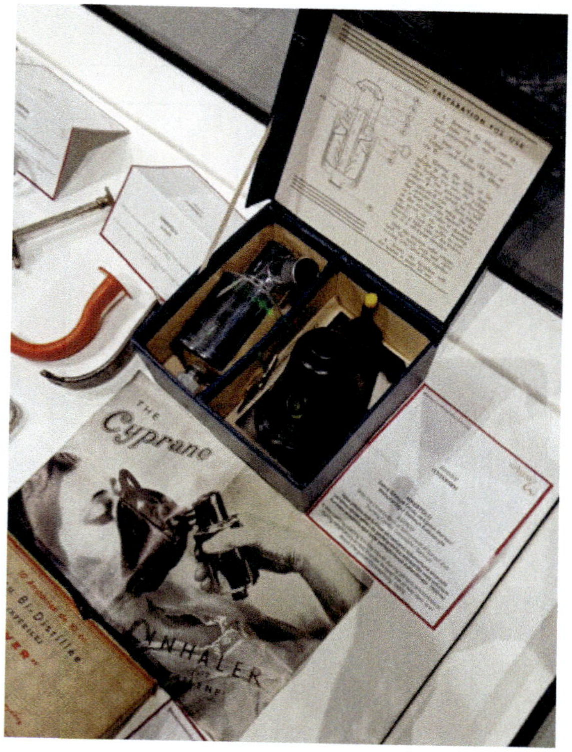

Figure 7.2. *Another system.*

Source: htt By - Own work, CC0, https://commons.wikimedia.org/w/index.php?curid=143970787.

Nitrous oxide and oxygen cylinders are also fitted to anesthesia machines in case the central gas supply fails. A hanger yoke assembly—a device that consists of two metal pins that match holes in the gas cylinder's valve casing—attaches color-coded cylinders to the anesthesia machine (pin indexed safety system [PISS]). Because of its design, the anesthesia machine cannot have an oxygen cylinder attached to any yoke other than the one intended for oxygen. Alternatively, the oxygen yoke could have a cylinder attached to it that held nitrous oxide, which would release the gas when the oxygen flowmeter was turned on. The anesthesia machine has color-coded pressure gauges that show the gas pressure in the corresponding gas cylinder (green for oxygen, blue for nitrous oxide).

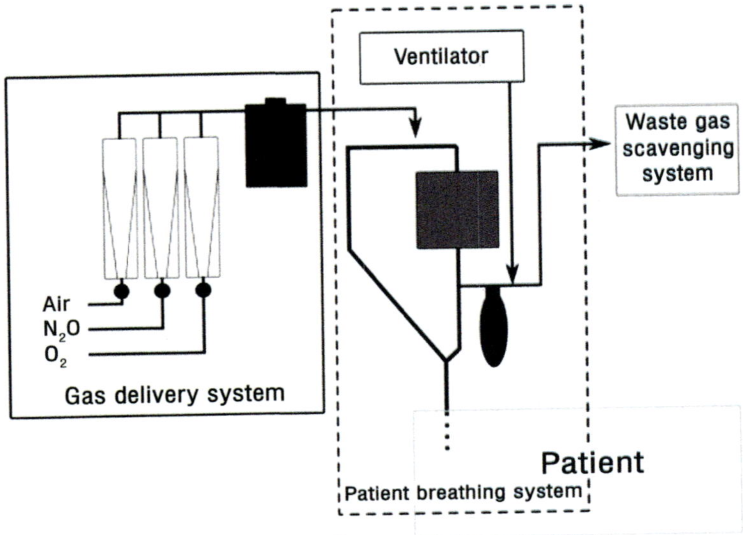

Figure 7.3. *Schematic diagram of the internal circuitry of an anesthesia machine. Oxygen and nitrous oxide enter the anesthesia machine through a central supply line (most common); alternatively (infrequently), they are provided from gas cylinders attached to pin-indexed yokes on the machine. Check valves prevent transfilling of gas cylinders or flow of gas from cylinders into the central supply line. Pressure regulators decrease pressure in the tubing from the gas cylinders to about 50 psi. The fail-safe valve prevents flow of nitrous oxide if the pressure in the oxygen supply circuit decreases to less than 30 psi. Needle valves control gas flow to rotameters (flowmeters). Agent-specific vaporizers provide a reliable means to deliver preselected concentrations of a volatile anesthetic. An interlock system allows only one vaporizer to be in the "on" (delivery) setting at a time. After mixing in the manifold of the anesthesia machine, the total fresh gas flow enters the common outlet for delivery to the patient through the anesthetic breathing system (circuit).*

Source: By TwoOneTwo - Own work, CC BY-SA 3.0, https://commons.wikimedia.org/w/index.php?curid=3559500.

7.1.2.1. Calculation of Cylinder Contents

The volume of oxygen in an oxygen cylinder is directly correlated with its pressure. For instance, at 2000 psi, a full E size oxygen cylinder holds roughly 625 L of oxygen; at 1000 psi, the volume decreases to half. As a result, it is possible to calculate the amount of time that an oxygen flow rate can be sustained before the cylinder runs out of fuel. Unlike oxygen, which has a pressure gauge that shows how much gas is left in the cylinder, nitrous oxide has a gas cylinder that keeps its pressure at 750 psi as long as there is liquid nitrous oxide present. To keep the pressure inside the cylinder constant, more liquid is vaporized as the nitrous oxide leaves the cylinder as a vapor.

It can be inferred that approximately 75% of the gas cylinder's contents have been used up when the pressure starts to drop after all of the liquid nitrous oxide has evaporated. When the pressure gauge starts to drop from its previously steady value of 750 psi, about 400 L of nitrous oxide remain because a full nitrous oxide cylinder (E size) contains roughly 1590 L. Heat is taken from the metal cylinder and the surrounding air by the vaporization of a liquefied gas (nitrous oxide) and the expansion of a compressed gas (oxygen). Because of this, atmospheric water vapor frequently condenses as frost in valves and on gas cylinders, especially when these tanks are producing a lot of gas. Due to the absence of water vapor in compressed gases, internal icing does not happen.

7.1.3. Flowmeters

The anesthesia machine's flowmeters precisely regulate and measure the gas flow to the common gas inlet. Gas flow is measured using the proportionality principle, which states that the flow through a resistance equals the pressure. Gas flow usually enters the bottom of a glass flow tube that is tapered (the cross-sectional area increases upward from the site of gas entry) and positioned vertically. A bobbin- or ball-shaped float is raised when gas enters the flowmeter tube. When the float's reduction in pressure equalizes gravity, the float comes to rest. The bobbin's upper end or the ball's equator displays the gas flow rate in milliliters or liters per minute. The physical characteristics of the gas (density and viscosity) and the resistance of the tube dictate the proportionality between pressure and flow. At the factory, the flowmeters are first calibrated for the gas that is indicated. Flowmeters cannot be used with other gases since few gases have the same density and viscosity. An oxygen flowmeter's accompanying scale is green, while a nitrous oxide flowmeter's scale is blue.

After leaving the flowmeters, gas flows into a manifold, or mixing chamber, which is situated above the flowmeters. The last gas to be added to the manifold should be oxygen since the oxygen flowmeter should be the last in the series of flowmeters. This configuration minimizes the chance that leaks in the device near the oxygen inlet will lower the supplied oxygen content, while leaks farther away from that location cause volume loss without affecting the mixture's quality. However, regardless of the flowmeter tube arrangement, a leaky oxygen flowmeter tube can result in a hypoxic mixture. Indeed, the delicate design of this anesthesia machine component makes flowmeter tube leaks a potential hazard. Errors in the delivered flow may arise from subtle cracks that are missed.

The anesthesia machine's manifold mixes the gases, which then flow to an outlet port where they are either directed into a vaporizer or an anesthetic breathing system. An oxygen flush valve that avoids the flowmeters and manifold is designed to deliver a significant amount of oxygen (35 to 75 L/min) to the outlet port in an emergency. Direct communication between the low-pressure and high-pressure oxygen circuits is made possible by the oxygen flush valve. When the oxygen flush valve is opened during a mechanical inspiration from the anesthesia machine ventilator, high airway pressure can be transferred to the patient's lungs, potentially leading to barotrauma (American Society of Anesthesiologists, 1987; American Society of Anesthesiologists Committee on Equipment and Facilities, 2008)

7.2. Vaporizers

Liquids at room temperature and atmospheric pressure are volatile anesthetics. The process of turning a liquid into a vapor, or vaporization, happens in a closed container called a vaporizer. Delivering the vapor concentration that emerges from vaporizing a volatile liquid anesthetic to the patient requires the same level of precision and consistency as administering other gases, such as oxygen or nitrous oxide.

7.2.1. Physics of Vaporization

A liquid's constituent molecules are always moving randomly. The molecules at the liquid-oxygen interface in a vaporizer holding a volatile liquid anesthetic are subjected to an asymmetrical arrangement of intermolecular forces. This asymmetric arrangement causes the surface molecules to be drawn into the liquid phase by a net attractive force. In order for surface molecules to move into the gas phase, where their comparatively low density makes vapor, this force must be overcome. Heat provides the energy required for molecules to escape the liquid. The amount of calories needed at a given temperature to turn one gram of liquid into vapor is known as the heat of vaporization of a liquid. As the liquid's temperature drops, more heat of vaporization is required for molecules to escape the liquid phase.

In a vaporizer that is closed, vaporization stops when the number of molecules leaving the liquid phase equals the number of molecules returning, indicating that equilibrium has been reached between the liquid and vapor phases. Pressure is produced as a result of collisions between the molecules in the vapor phase and the container walls. Vapor pressure is the name given to this pressure, which varies depending on the volatile anesthetic. In addition, the temperature of the liquid affects the vapor pressure, meaning that a drop in temperature corresponds to a decrease in vapor pressure and a reduction in the number of molecules in the vapor phase. The liquid anesthetic cools, which indicates that heat (heat of vaporization) has been lost, depleting the energy needed for vaporization. Because it reduces the vapor pressure and the possible vapor concentration, this cooling is undesirable.

7.2.2. Vaporizer Classification and Design

Agent-specific, variable-bypass, flow-over, temperature-compensated (having an automated temperature-compensating device that helps maintain a constant vaporizer output over a wide range of temperatures), and out-of-circuit vaporizers are the different categories into which vaporizers fall. With a vapor pressure of about 1 atm (664 mm Hg) at 20° C, desflurane cannot be safely vaporized with these modern vaporizers. Because of this, a desflurane vaporizer is pressurized to 1500 mm Hg using a backpressure regulator and electrically heated to 23 to 25 degrees Celsius. This creates an environment where the volatility of the anesthetic is relatively lower but still predictable.

The term "variable bypass" refers to separating the entire fresh gas flow through the vaporizer into two halves. Twenty percent or less of the fresh gas flow is directed into the vaporizing chamber of the vaporizer, where the liquid anesthetic vapor causes the chamber to become saturated (flow-over). The vaporizer's bypass chamber is where the second part of the fresh gas flow goes. At the anesthesia machine's patient outlet side, both parts of the fresh gas flow mix. The concentration control dial controls how much fresh gas flow is diverted through the vaporizing chamber and, consequently, how much volatile anesthetic is given to the patient. The volume percent scale for the particular anesthetic drug is displayed on the concentration control dial. When the temperature of the vaporizer varies, an expansion element or a temperature-sensitive bimetallic strip affect how much gas is proportioned between the bypass and vaporizing chambers (temperature compensated). For instance, the temperature sensing elements in the vaporizer chamber permit increased gas inflow to counteract the effect of the liquid anesthetic's decreasing temperature.

To further reduce heat loss, vaporizers are frequently made of metals with high thermal conductivity, such as copper and bronze. Consequently, the output of the vaporizer is almost linear between 20°C and 35°C. The vaporizers' designation as agent specific and out of circuit highlights the fact that they are separate from the anesthetic breathing system and specifically calibrated to handle a single volatile anesthetic.

Vaporizers that are tipped over may leak liquid anesthetic into the bypass chamber from the vaporizing chamber, increasing the amount of vapor that escapes the device. However, because vaporizers are fixed to the anesthesia machine and don't need to be moved often, the chance of tipping is reduced. The most common cause of vaporizer leaks is a loose filler cap.

The anesthesia machine usually has two or three vaporizers dedicated to a particular anesthetic. Only one vaporizer at a time can be turned on thanks to a safety interlock mechanism. Depressing a release button on the concentration dial and rotating it counterclockwise are the steps involved in turning on a vaporizer. By doing this, the dial cannot unintentionally turn from the off to the on position. The filler port's placement on the lower part of the vaporizer reduces the possibility that liquid anesthetic will be overfilled into the vaporizing chamber (>125 mL). The amount of liquid anesthetic in the vaporizing chamber can be seen visually through a window next to the filler port. A liquid anesthetic other than the one for which the vaporizer was calibrated cannot be put into the vaporizing chamber unless an anesthetic-specific keyed filler device is used. Due to the fact that desflurane has a vapor pressure of almost one atmosphere, it is especially crucial to avoid overdosing on anesthetics in modern vaporizers. Similar to anesthesia machines, vapori manufacturers advise periodic maintenance, typically done every 12 months.

7.3. Anesthetic Breathing Systems

The purpose of anesthetic breathing systems is to remove carbon dioxide from the patient's air while also providing oxygen and anesthetic gases. The anesthetic breathing apparatus is conceptually a tubular extension of the patient's upper airway. Since peak flows of up to 60 L/min are reached during spontaneous inspiration, anesthetic breathing systems can significantly increase the resistance to inhalation. Connections and unidirectional valves have an impact on this resistance. To reduce this breathing resistance, the breathing system's components—especially the tracheal tube connector—should have the largest lumen possible. Curved connectors should be used in place of right-angle connectors in order to reduce resistance. The increased resistance to inhalation caused by anesthetic breathing systems can be countered by replacing spontaneous breathing with regulated ventilation of the patient's lungs (American Society of Anesthesiologists, 1987; American Society of Anesthesiologists Committee on Equipment and Facilities, 2008) (Table 7.1).

Table 7.1. *Systems and Effects*

	Functional connectivity	Effective connectivity	Topological properties	Evoked responses—sensory processing	Spatio-temporal dynamics
Propofol	Disruption of within- and between-network functional connectivity in large-scale brain networks (particularly fronto-parietal connectivity; Boveroux et al., 2010)	Reduced amplitude and complexity of long-distance cortical communication (Gómez et al., 2013; Sarasso et al., 2015)	Increased local efficiency (parietal regions; Kim et al., 2016; Lee et al., 2017)	Generalized alteration in short-latency evoked electrocorticographic responses to auditory novelty within higher-order cortical areas, outside the auditory cortex (Nourski et al., 2018)	Alteration of dynamics and directionality of effective connectivity (Lee et al., 2009; Untergehrer et al., 2014; Sanders et al., 2018)
	Suppression of the complexity of regions sparsely connected with large-scale brain networks (Pappas et al., 2019)	Disruption of effective connectivity in large-scale brain networks (Lee et al., 2009; Boly et al., 2012; Lee et al., 2018; Untergehrer et al., 2014; Guldenmund et al., 2016; Sanders et al., 2018)	Fewer small-world properties (Barttfeld et al., 2015)	Suppression of long-latency responses to novelty (Nourski et al., 2018)	Reduced complexity and randomness of the electroencephalographic signal (Wang et al., 2017; Darracq et al., 2018b)
	Disruption of thalamo-cortical connectivity within higher-order networks (Boveroux et al., 2010)	Alteration of effective connectivity in lower-order sensory networks (Gómez et al., 2013)	Limitation of connectivity configuration repertoire (Barttfeld et al., 2015; Cavanna et al., 2018)	Reconfiguration of cortical functional connectivity networks involved in nociception, despite activation of spinal cord and cortex by noxious stimulation (Lichtner et al., 2018a,b)	Synchronization of local activity (Huang et al., 2018)
	Preservation of connectivity in lower-order sensory networks (Boveroux et al., 2010)		Traffic of information constrained to inflexible patterns (Mashour, 2018; Uhrig et al., 2018)		Prolongation of long-distance communication timescales (Gómez et al., 2013; Huang et al., 2018)
			Remoteness from criticality, with preserved scale-free organization (Liu et al., 2014; Tagliazucchi et al., 2016; Alonso et al., 2019) Disturbance of posterior parietal hub activity (Lee et al., 2013)		
Halogenated vapors	Breakdown of functional connectivity in higher-order resting-state consciousness networks (Palanca et al., 2015) Disruption of thalamo-cortical connectivity within higher-order networks (Palanca et al., 2015)	Disruption of fronto-parietal anterior to posterior effective connectivity (Lee et al., 2013)	Limitation of connectivity configuration repertoire (Cavanna et al., 2018; Uhrig et al., 2018)	No information	Augmentation of temporal persistence in neuronal oscillation amplitude (Thiery et al., 2018) Disruption of intermediate strength spatio-temporal patterns of functional connectivity within and between consciousness networks (Kafashan et al., 2016)
			Remoteness from criticality (Lee et al., 2018)		
	Preservation of connectivity in lower-order sensory networks (Ranft et al., 2016)				Preservation of higher strength spatio-temporal patterns within networks (Kafashan et al., 2016)

	Functional connectivity	Effective connectivity	Topological properties	Evoked responses—sensory processing	Spatio-temporal dynamics
Ketamine	Global increase in functional connectivity, with network reorganization (Driesen et al., 2013b) Disruption of functional connectivity in all higher-order consciousness networks but not in the executive control network (Bonhomme et al., 2016) Preservation of functional connectivity in sensory networks (Bonhomme et al., 2016) Long-term effect on the interactions between the default mode network and networks involved in depression? and restoration of the abnormal connectivity of depressed patients (Li et al., 2018; Vutskits, 2018) Transient effect on working memory network (Driesen et al., 2013a)	Disruption of fronto-parietal anterior to posterior effective connectivity (Lee et al., 2013; Vlisides et al., 2017) Reduced alpha power in the precuneus and temporo-parietal junction (possibly related to disconnected consciousness; Vlisides et al., 2018; Darracq et al., 2018a)	No information	TMS-evoked communication complexity close to the waking state (Sarasso et al., 2015)	No information
Dexmedetomidine	Reduced within-network and thalamic connectivity in higher-order consciousness networks (Guldenmund et al., 2017) Preservation of lower-order sensory networks functional connectivity (Guldenmund et al., 2017) Better preservation of functional connectivity between thalamus, medial anterior cingulate cortex, and mesopontine area as compared to sleep and propofol unresponsiveness (Guldenmund et al., 2017)	No information	Reduced local and global large-scale network efficiency (Hashmi et al., 2017) Reduced large-scale network connectivity strength (Hashmi et al., 2017) No impairment in node degree (Hashmi et al., 2017)	No information	No information
Benzodiazepines	Disruption of higher-order consciousness networks (Greicius et al., 2008; Liang et al., 2018) Preservation of lower-order sensory networks (Frolich et al., 2017)	Disruption of effective connectivity in large-scale brain networks (Greicius et al., 2008; Ferrarelli et al., 2010; Liang et al., 2018)	No information	Reduced auditory cortex activation by sounds (Frolich et al., 2017) Reduced duration and propagation of evoked TMS cortical response (Ferrarelli et al., 2010)	No information
Xenon	No information	No information	Remoteness from criticality (Colombo et al., 2019)	TMS-evoked high amplitude slow waves with low complexity (Sarasso et al., 2015)	Slowing down and smoothing of the temporal profile of the EEG signal (Colombo et al., 2019)

Source: Bonhomme V, Staquet C, Montupil J, Defresne A, Kirsch M, Martial C, Vanhaudenhuyse A, Chatelle C, Larroque SK, Raimondo F, Demertzi A, Bodart O, Laureys S and Gosseries O (2019) General Anesthesia: A Probe to Explore Consciousness. Front. Syst. Neurosci. 13:36. doi: 10.3389/fnsys.2019.00036.

The presence or absence of (1) a gas reservoir bag in the circuit, (2) rebreathing of exhaled gases, (3) a method to chemically neutralize exhaled carbon dioxide, and (4) unidirectional valves determines the classification of anesthetic breathing systems as open, semi-open, semi-closed, and closed. The Mapleson F (Jackson-Rees) system, the Bain circuit, and the circle system are the three most widely utilized anesthetic breathing systems.

7.3.1. Mapleson Breathing Systems

In 1954, Mapleson analyzed and described five different arrangements of fresh gas inflow tubing, reservoir tubing, face mask, reservoir bag, and an expiratory valve to administer anesthetic gases. These five different semi-open anesthetic breathing systems are designated Mapleson A to E. The Mapleson F system, which is a Jackson-Rees modification of the Mapleson D system, was added later. The Bain circuit is a modification of the Mapleson D system.

7.3.1.1. Flow Characteristics

The lack of chemical carbon dioxide neutralization and valves to direct gases to or from the patient are characteristics of the Mapleson systems. Rebreathing happens when inspiratory flow surpasses fresh gas flow because there is no discernible difference between inspired and expired gases. The amount of rebreathing determines the makeup of the inspired mixture. The fresh gas flow rate has a major impact on how much rebreathing each system does. Determining the ideal fresh gas flow may be challenging. It is necessary to modify the fresh gas flow when transitioning from controlled and spontaneous ventilation. The most effective way to find the ideal fresh gas flow is to monitor end-tidal CO_2. The best way to understand how well these circuits work is to look at the gas composition during controlled and spontaneous ventilation's final exhalation.

7.3.2. Mapleson F (Jackson-Rees) System

The distal end of the gas reservoir bag has an adjustable pressure-limiting overflow valve, and this is part of the T-piece configuration that makes up the Mapleson F (Jackson-Rees) system. When utilizing this anesthetic breathing system, the degree of rebreathing is determined by the ventilation technique (controlled versus spontaneous) and the pressure-limiting overflow valve adjustment (venting). It is advised to provide fresh gas flow equivalent to two or three times the patient's minute ventilation in order to avoid the patient rebreathing exhaled gases.

7.3.2.1. Flow Characteristics

Exhaled gases travel down the expiratory limb during spontaneous ventilation and combine with inhaled gases. The exhaled gases are forced down the expiratory limb by the fresh gas during the expiratory pause. The inhaled gas mixture during the subsequent inspiration originates from the reservoir bag, the expiratory limb, and the fresh gas flow.

7.3.2.2. Clinical Uses

When tracheally intubated patients are being transported, the Mapleson F system is frequently utilized for controlled ventilation. Circuit dead space and resistance are low since the pressure-limiting overflow valve is the only moving component.

This is ideal for pediatric anesthesia. The Mapleson F system may be used for both spontaneous and controlled ventilation. It is inexpensive, can be used with a face mask or endotracheal tube, is lightweight, and can be repositioned easily. Pollution of the atmosphere with anesthetic gases when using this system can be decreased by adapting it to scavenging systems.

7.3.2.3. Disadvantages

The Mapleson F system has three drawbacks: (1) high fresh gas intake required to stop rebreathing; (2) high air pressure and barotrauma possible if the overflow valve obstructs; and (3) no humidification. One way to counteract dehydration is to let the fresh gas flow through an inline heated humidifier.

7.3.3. Bain System

The Bain circuit is a coaxial variation of the Mapleson D system, wherein the corrugated expiratory tubing is positioned inside the fresh gas supply tube. Although the fresh gas is supplied at the patient end of the circuit, the fresh gas tube enters the circuit close to the reservoir bag. The overflow valve next to the reservoir bag is where the exhaled gases are released. It is possible to utilize the Bain circuit for both regulated and uncontrolled ventilation. A fresh gas flow of 200 to 300 mL/kg/min is necessary to prevent rebreathing during spontaneous ventilation, whereas a flow of only 70 mL/kg/min is necessary during controlled ventilation.

7.3.3.1. Advantages

The Bain circuit has the following benefits: (1) partial rebreathing conserves moisture; (2) the surrounding exhaled gases in the corrugated expiratory tube warm the fresh gas inflow; and (3) the overflow valve makes it easier to scavenge waste anesthetic gases. It is portable, reusable, and easily sterilized. It comes in handy during head and neck surgeries and other situations where patient access is restricted.

7.3.3.2. Disadvantages

The inner fresh gas tube may unintentionally disconnect or kink, which is one of the risks associated with the Bain circuit. To enable examination of the inner tube, the outer expiratory tube ought to be transparent.

7.3.4. Circle System

In the US, the circle system is the most widely used anesthetic breathing technique. Its primary parts are arranged in a circle, which gives it its name. The circle system uses carbon dioxide absorbents and chemical neutralization to stop carbon dioxide from being breathed again.

7.3.4.1. Classification

The type of circle system—open, semiclosed, or closed—depends on how much new gas is introduced. To stop gases from rebreathing, a semiopen system uses a very high fresh gas flow. The most widely used method involves rebreathing of gases using a semiclosed system. In a closed system, the patient's gas consumption and the inflow gas match precisely. When the fresh gas inflow rate is set at less than the patient's minute ventilation, rebreathing of exhaled gases in the semiclosed and closed circle systems leads to (1) some conservation of body heat and moisture in the airways and (2) decreased pollution of the surrounding atmosphere with anesthetic gases.

7.3.4.2. Disadvantages

The circle system's drawbacks include: (1) more difficulty breathing due to unidirectional valves and carbon dioxide absorbent; (2) bulkiness and decreased portability; and (3) a higher risk of malfunction due to the intricate design of the device.

7.3.4.3. Impact of Rebreathing

In a semi-closed circle system, breathing back exhaled gases affects the concentrations of these gases in the anesthetic that is inhaled. Rebreathing of exhaled gases depleted of anesthetic, for instance, greatly dilutes the concentration of anesthetic in the fresh gas inflow when uptake of the anesthetic gas is high, as during induction of anesthesia. In clinical practice, this dilution effect of absorption is counteracted by raising the anesthetic concentration delivered. The effect of dilution on the inspired concentration caused by rebreathing exhaled gases decreases as anesthetic uptake declines.

7.3.4.4. Components

A fresh gas inlet, inspiratory and expiratory unidirectional check valves, inspiratory and expiratory corrugated tubing, a Y-piece connector, an adjustable pressure-limiting (APL) valve—also called an overflow or pop-off valve—a reservoir bag, a canister holding carbon dioxide absorbent, a bag/vent selector switch, and a mechanical anesthesia ventilator are the components that make up the circle system.

Fresh Gas Inlet and Unidirectional Valves

Through a connection from the anesthesia machine's common gas outlet, fresh gas is introduced into the circle system. The corrugated tubing has two unidirectional valves, one for inhalation and one for exhalation, located in separate limbs. These valves have two functions: (1) they allow positive-pressure breathing to occur, and (2) they stop exhaled gases from breathing again until they have gone through the carbon dioxide absorbent canister and had their oxygen content restored. If the unidirectional valves become stuck in the open position, it can lead to rebreathing and hypercapnia; if it happens in the closed position, the circuit can become completely blocked. The expiratory valve may become stuck in the closed position, which can lead to barotrauma and breath stacking. The only dead space in the circle system, assuming the unidirectional valves are operating as intended, is between the patient and the Y-piece.

Corrugated Tubing

The patient's gases are delivered to and from the inspiratory and expiratory corrugated tubes. Their large bore offers little resistance, and their corrugations are flexible, kink-resistant, and encourage turbulent flow as opposed to laminar flow. A smaller delivered tidal volume results from positive pressure ventilation because part of the delivered gas compresses inside the circuit and some distends the corrugated tubing.

Y-Piece Connector

At the patient end of the circuit, a Y-piece connector has three features: an inner diameter of 15 mm that fits onto an endotracheal tube connector, an outer diameter of 22 mm that fits inside a face mask, and a curved elbow.

Adjustable Pressure-Limiting Valve

APL (overflow or pop-off) valves allow excess gas from the breathing system to be vented into the waste gas scavenging system when the bag/vent selector switch is set to "bag." They can also be adjusted to enable the anesthesia provider to provide controlled or assisted ventilation of the patient's lungs by manually compressing the gas reservoir bag. When spontaneous ventilation occurs, the APL valve should be fully open to ensure that circuit pressure is minimal during inspiration and expiration.

Reservoir Bag

When the bag/vent selector switch is set to "bag," the gas reservoir bag maintains an available reserve volume of gas to satisfy the patient's spontaneous inspiratory flow rate (up to 60 L/min), which greatly exceeds conventional fresh gas flows (commonly 3 to 5 L/min) from the anesthesia machine. The bag also serves as a safety device because its distensibility limits pressure in the breathing circuit to less than 60 cm H_2O, even when the APL valve is closed (Figure 7.4).

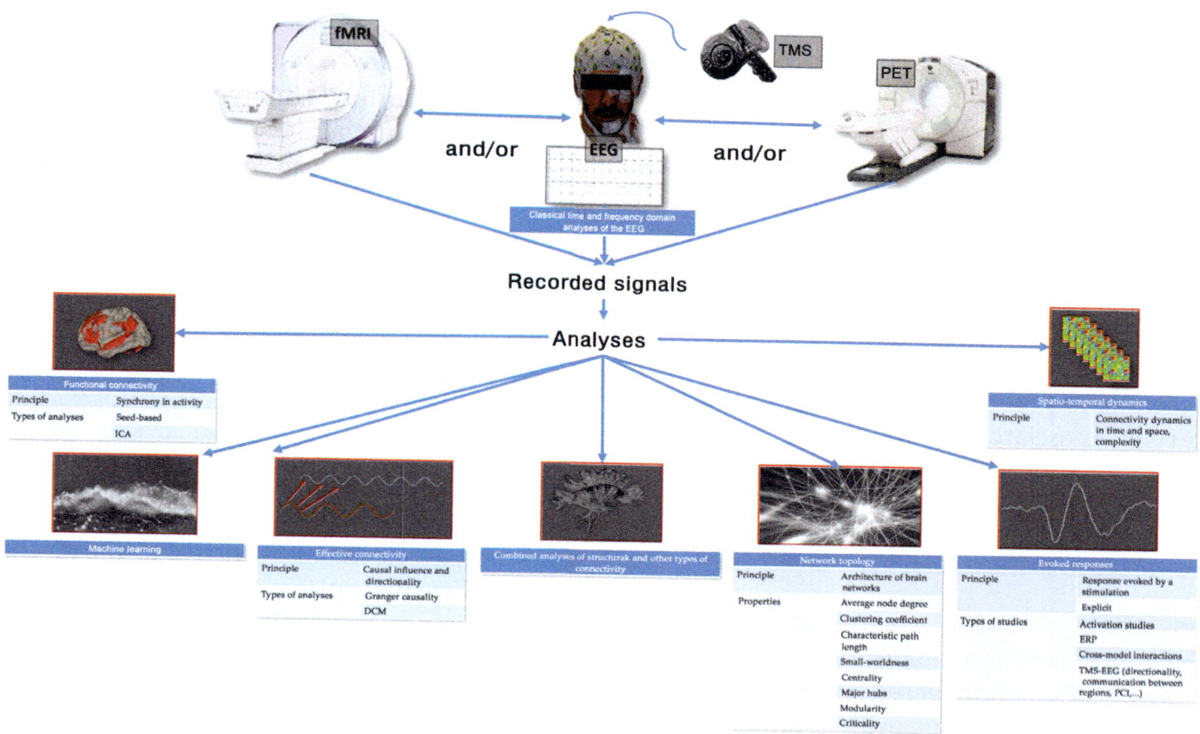

Figure 7.4. *Studying the effects of anesthesia.*

Source: Bonhomme V, Staquet C, Montupil J, Defresne A, Kirsch M, Martial C, Vanhaudenhuyse A, Chatelle C, Larroque SK, Raimondo F, Demertzi A, Bodart O, Laureys S and Gosseries O (2019) General Anesthesia: A Probe to Explore Consciousness. Front. Syst. Neurosci. 13:36. doi: 10.3389/fnsys.2019.00036.

7.3.5. Closed Anesthetic Breathing System

When carbon dioxide is absorbed, all exhaled gases are completely rebreathed in a closed anesthetic breathing system, and the ventilator's APL or relief valve is closed. When the patient's metabolic oxygen requirements—which range from 150 to 250 mL/min during anesthesia—are met by the fresh gas inflow into the circle system (150 to 500 mL/min) and anesthetic gases lost due to tissue uptake, the system is said to be closed. In order to maintain a closed system when using sidestream gas analyzers, the analyzed gas that exits the analyzer needs to be added back to the breathing system.

7.3.5.1. Advantages

Advantages of a closed circle anesthetic breathing system over a semiclosed circle anesthetic breathing system include (1) maximal humidification and warming of inhaled gases, (2) less pollution of the surrounding atmosphere with anesthetic gases, and (3) economy in the use of anesthetics.

7.3.5.2. Disadvantages

A disadvantage of a closed circle anesthetic breathing system is an inability to rapidly change the delivered concentration of anesthetic gases and oxygen because of the low fresh gas inflow.

7.3.5.3. Dangers of Closed Anesthetic Breathing System

The delivery of (1) unpredictable and potentially inadequate oxygen concentrations and (2) unknown and potentially excessive concentrations of potent anesthetic gases are the main risks associated with a closed anesthetic breathing system.

Unpredictable Concentrations of Oxygen

When using a closed anesthetic breathing system, the likelihood of unpredictable and possibly insufficient delivered concentrations of oxygen increases if nitrous oxide is added to the fresh gas inflow. For instance, a decrease in the concentration of oxygen in the alveoli may arise from a gradual decrease in the tissue's uptake of nitrous oxide combined with an unchanged uptake of oxygen. Therefore, when nitrous oxide is administered through a closed anesthetic breathing system, the use of an oxygen analyzer mounted on the inspiratory or expiratory limb of the circle system is required.

Unknown Concentrations of Potent Anesthetic Gases

When a closed anesthetic breathing system is used, the majority of the inhaled gases are made up of exhaled gases, which are carbon dioxide-free. This indicates that the concentration found in the exhaled gases affects the makeup of the gases that are inhaled. The amount of anesthetic in exhaled gases indicates how much of the drug is absorbed by the tissue. At first, there is minimal anesthetic concentration in the exhaled gases and maximum tissue uptake. The amount of anesthetic that the patient inhales is diluted when they rebreathe these exhaled gases. Therefore, in order to counteract maximal tissue uptake, high anesthetic inflow concentrations are required. On the other hand, when tissue uptake has decreased, minimal amounts of anesthetic need to be added to the inflow gases. Estimating the inhaled concentration given to the patient through a closed anesthetic breathing system is challenging due to the unknown influence of tissue uptake on the anesthetic concentration in exhaled gases. This drawback can be somewhat mitigated by starting a closed anesthetic breathing system approximately 15 minutes after a higher fresh gas inflow (3 L/min). This method allows nitrogen to be expelled from the lungs and coincides with the anesthetic's peak tissue absorption (American Society of Anesthesiologists, 1987; American Society of Anesthesiologists Committee on Equipment and Facilities, 2008).

7.4. Anesthesia Machine Ventilators

The patient's ventilation is provided by the mechanical anesthesia ventilator when the bag/vent selector switch is set to "vent," which removes the gas reservoir bag and APL valve from the circle anesthetic system. Anesthesia ventilators can run on electricity, compressed gas, or both. The majority of traditional anesthesia machine ventilators operate pneumatically using pressurized oxygen or air that is directed toward the area inside the ventilator casing between the rigid casing and the compressible bellows during the inspiratory phase. The bellows is forced to release its contents into the patient's lungs through the inspiratory limb of the breathing circuit when pressurized air or oxygen enters this area. The ventilator relief valve closes as a result of the pressurized air or oxygen, preventing inspiratory anesthetic gas from escaping into the scavenging system. When it comes to ventilator driving gas, oxygen is better than air because it increases the fraction of inspired oxygen in the event of a bellows leak. Peak inspiratory pressures will increase in a ventilator powered by 50 psi oxygen or air if there is a leak in the bellows. The bellows refills as the patient exhales, and the driving gas is either vented into the room or directed to the scavenging system. Some more recent anesthesia machines have piston-type ventilators that are powered mechanically. The piston gives the patient the appropriate tidal volume or airway pressure by acting similarly to a syringe's plunger.

7.4.1. Bellows

Because the bellows won't rise (fill) in the event of an anesthesia breathing system leak or an unintentional disconnect, ventilators with standing or ascending bellows—which rise during exhalation—are the preferred option. Because the bellows will continue to rise and fall during a disconnection, ventilators with bellows that descend during exhalation—also known as hanging or descending bellows—may be dangerous. Every time a ventilator is used, an audible disconnect alarm needs to be set off (Figure 7.5).

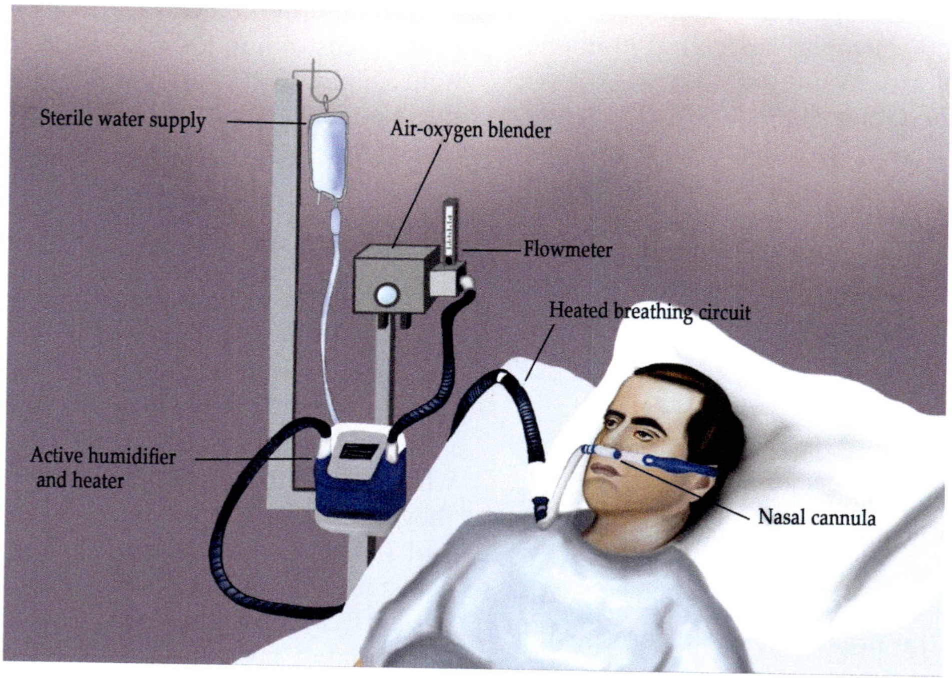

Figure 7.5. *An illustration of one of the techniques by which HFOT can be administered, showing a nasal cannula device, which consists of an air–oxygen blender, allowing for FiO2 ranging from 0.21 to 1.0 and a flowmeter that generates up to 60 L/min flow. The gas is then humidified and heated in the active humidifier and heater and is delivered via the heated breathing circuit to the patient (i.e., through a soft wide-bore nasal cannula).*

Source: *Al-Husinat L, Jouryyeh B, Rawashdeh A, Alenaizat A, Abushehab M, Amir MW, Al Modanat Z, Battaglini D, Cinnella G. High-Flow Oxygen Therapy in the Perioperative Setting and Procedural Sedation: A Review of Current Evidence. Journal of Clinical Medicine. 2023; 12(20):6685. https://doi.org/10.3390/jcm12206685.*

7.4.2. Humidity and Heat Exchange in the Breathing Circuit

The primary heat and moisture exchanger (HME) for bringing inspired gas to body temperature and 100% relative humidity during its passage to the alveoli is the upper respiratory tract, particularly the nose. Medical gases (whether piped or in cylinders) are depleted of water to avoid condensation and corrosion. The task of heating and humidifying inspired gases falls to the tracheobronchial mucosa when tracheal intubation or the use of a laryngeal mask airway bypasses the upper airway. In patients on intubation, humidification of inspired gases by the lower respiratory tract may result in mucosal dehydration, compromised surfactant and ciliary function, secretion inspissation, atelectasis, and an increase in the alveolar-to-arterial gradient. Patients who are intubated may lose heat and water when they breathe in dry, room-temperature gases. Since general anesthesia renders infants and children poikilothermic, reducing heat loss and the resulting drops in body temperature is the primary reason to provide heated humidification to intubated patients. Heat loss is more significant than water loss.

7.4.3. Humidification

To reduce the amount of water and heat lost during vaporization, humidification involves adding moisture, or water vapor, to the gases that the anesthetic breathing system delivers. The gases in the breathing circuit are heated and made more humid by the water that forms and the heat produced by the chemical neutralization of carbon dioxide. (1) HME humidifiers, (2) heated water vaporizers and humidifiers, and (3) nebulizers are the types of humidifiers used in the intensive care unit and for anesthesia.

7.4.3.1. Heat and Moisture Exchanger Humidifiers

HME humidifiers are apparatuses that retain a portion of the heat and water exhaled and return it to the inspired gases when positioned between the Y-piece of the circle system and the endotracheal tube. They have a porous membrane that is either hygroscopic or hydrophobic, which allows the patient to breathe in while the humidified gases are trapped and returned. Heat and moisture exchanging filters (HMEFs) can be created by adding bacterial and viral filters to HME humidifiers.

Advantages

HME humidifiers have several advantages over other kinds of humidifiers, including being: (1) lightweight; (2) simple and easy to use; (3) not requiring an external power source; (4) disposable; and (5) inexpensive.

Disadvantages

HME humidifiers have the following drawbacks: (1) they are less effective at regulating patient temperature than heated water vaporizers and humidifiers; (2) they add resistance and make breathing harder, so they should be used carefully when a patient is spontaneously ventilating; (3) they can clog with patient secretions or blood; and (4) they can increase dead space, which can significantly increase rebreathing in young patients. There are specific low-volume HMEs for pediatric patients.

7.4.3.2. Heated Water Vaporizers and Humidifiers

To provide a relative humidity that is higher than that provided by HME humidifiers, heated water vaporizers and humidifiers are utilized. Patients in intensive care units and pediatric anesthesia are the ones who use heated water vaporizers more frequently. Humidifiers and heated water vaporizers can cause thermal injury, nosocomial infections, increased breathing effort, and an increased chance of malfunction because of their intricate designs.

7.4.3.3. Nebulizers

Nebulizers create a mist made up of tiny water droplets floating in a gaseous medium. The carrier gas's temperature has no bearing on how many water droplets can be delivered. Nebulizers can provide medicine to peripheral airways in addition to water.

7.5. Pollution of the Atmosphere with Anesthetic Gases

Operating room staff may be at risk for health problems if they are exposed to low concentrations of inhaled anesthetics on a regular basis. There are currently no mandatory exposure limits for nitrous oxide and volatile anesthetics according to the Occupational Safety and Health Administration (OSHA). OSHA advises that exposure concentrations of volatile anesthetics in the operating room not surpass 2 ppm and that nitrous oxide concentrations not surpass 25 ppm. The American Society of Anesthesiologists has issued guidelines about waste anesthetic gases.

Scavenging of waste anesthetic gases, routine preventive maintenance of anesthesia equipment, observance of anesthetic techniques, and sufficient ventilation of operating rooms are all necessary for controlling the pollution of the atmosphere with anesthetic gases.

7.5.1. Scavenging Systems

The process of gathering and then removing released gases from the operating room is known as scavenging. If the bag/vent selector switch is set to "bag," the excess gas originates from the APL valve; otherwise, it comes from the ventilator relief valve. Through these valves, all of the patient's extra gas leaves the breathing apparatus. Furthermore, certain anesthetic breathing systems route the drive gas within the bellows canister to the scavenging system when the bag/vent selector switch is set to "vent." The amount of gas administered to a patient during anesthesia typically far exceeds what the patient requires. To guarantee sufficient scavenging, the anesthesia provider needs to make sure the scavenging system is in working order and is adjusted appropriately. When using sidestream gas analyzers, the analyzed gas that comes out of the device needs to be either fed back into the breathing system or directed toward the scavenging system.

There are two types of scavenging systems: active and passive. The hospital's vacuum system is linked to an active system, and a vacuum pulls gases out of the apparatus. The hospital's ventilation duct is linked to a passive system, which allows waste gases to exit the machine naturally. Many anesthesia machines have a waste gas receiver mounted on the side that allows for scavenging. A few of the system's benefits are as follows: (1) a needle valve that lets the doctor manually control how much vacuum is passed through the scavenging system; (2) a needle valve that can be adjusted so that the 3-L reservoir bag will be slightly inflated and seem to "breathe" with the patient; and (3) in contrast to other active scavenging systems, a waste gas receiver that runs without a powerful vacuum.

7.5.1.1. Hazards

Scavenging systems can cause negative pressures in the breathing system or excessive positive pressure in the breathing circuit if they are blocked from doing their job. Scavenging systems can also cause negative pressures in the breathing circuit if they are subjected to an excessive amount of vacuum. Two relief valves are included in scavenging systems to reduce these risks. The positive-pressure scavenge relief valve opens when the pressure reaches 10 cm H_2O to let the gas escape into the room in the event that gas builds up in the scavenging system and is unable to exit the anesthesia machine as intended. The negative pressure scavenge relief valve opens when negative pressure is applied to the scavenging system, allowing room air to be drawn in rather than gas from the patient. Furthermore, the excess waste anesthetic gas leaves the scavenging system through the positive-pressure relief valve and contaminates the operating room if the amount of fresh gas flow exceeds the scavenging system's capacity.

7.5.2. Periodic Preventive Maintenance of Anesthesia Equipment

Nitrous oxide leaks at high pressure can be caused by malfunctioning yokes connecting the anesthesia machine to the nitrous oxide tank or by loose connections between the anesthesia machine and the central nitrous oxide gas supply. Low-pressure anesthetic gas leaks can result from leaks between the anesthesia machine and the patient as well as from leaks inside the machine. The anesthesia machine should have regular preventive maintenance performed by trained service representatives.

7.5.3. Anesthetic Technique

Anesthetic techniques that can cause pollution in the operating room include: (1) wearing face masks that are too small; (2) flushing the anesthetic delivery circuit; (3) filling anesthetic vaporizers; (4) using endotracheal tubes that are not cuffed; (5) failing to turn off the nitrous oxide flow or vaporizers at the end of the anesthetic; and (6) using semi-open breathing circuits, which are difficult to scavenge.

7.5.4. Adequate Room Ventilation

The air in the operating room should be exchanged at least 15 times per hour by the operating room ventilation system. This rate should be checked periodically by the hospital's clinical engineering department.

7.6. Elimination of Carbon Dioxide

All exhaled gases are vented to the atmosphere in open and semiopen breathing systems, which eliminate carbon dioxide. Through chemical neutralization, carbon dioxide is eliminated by semi-closed and closed breathing systems. The exhaled gases are directed through a carbon dioxide absorber, which is made up of a canister filled with carbon dioxide absorbent granules, to achieve chemical neutralization. Typically, during exhalation, gas moves from top to bottom through the absorber. Dust and water are able to collect at the base of the absorber, below the canister.

7.6.1. Carbon Dioxide Absorbents

Calcium hydroxide (Ca[OH]2) is the neutralizing base for carbon dioxide generated during respiration and is used by all carbon dioxide absorbents. For effective and secure carbon dioxide absorption, water is a fundamental component shared by all carbon dioxide absorbents. The various absorbents' varying safety profiles and absorptive qualities are caused by catalysts, which are also present in carbon dioxide absorbents.

7.6.1.1. Traditional Carbon Dioxide Absorbents: Soda Lime

The main ingredients of soda lime granules are calcium hydroxide, water, and trace amounts of the strong bases potassium hydroxide (KOH) and sodium hydroxide (NaOH), which act as catalysts for the absorption of carbon dioxide.

Granules of soda lime break easily and release an alkaline dust that, if breathed in, can cause bronchospasm. To give the granules hardness and reduce the formation of alkaline dust, silica is added. When carbon dioxide reacts with the water in the soda lime granules, carbonic acid is created, which is the first step in neutralizing carbon dioxide with soda lime. The hydroxides in the soda lime granules are then reacted by the carbonic acid to produce carbonates, water, and heat (with bicarbonates acting as intermediates).

The alkaline bases in the soda lime granules are leached by the water created by neutralizing carbon dioxide, the water in the granules, and the water condensed from the patient's exhaled gases, resulting in a slurry that contains NaOH and KOH at the canister's bottom. These univalent bases have the potential to corrode skin. The breakdown of inhaled anesthetics to clinically significant concentrations of carbon monoxide and of sevoflurane to compound A can occur due to the strong base NaOH and KOH catalysts found in soda lime.

7.6.1.2. New-Generation Carbon Dioxide Absorbents: Amsorb Plus and Litholyme

In contrast to soda lime, Amsorb Plus and Litholyme are new-generation carbon dioxide absorbents made of calcium hydroxide and water, without the presence of strong bases like NaOH or KOH. Rather than converting sevoflurane to compound A or inhaled anesthetics to carbon monoxide, they contain chemically inert catalysts. Neutralization of carbon dioxide with Amsorb Plus or Litholyme begins with reaction of carbon dioxide with water present in the granules and the subsequent formation of carbonic acid. The calcium hydroxide in the granules then reacts with the carbonic acid to produce calcium carbonate, water, and heat.

7.6.1.3. Heat of Neutralization

Humidifying the gases and releasing some of the heat produced in these exothermic reactions are two beneficial uses for the water that is created when carbon dioxide is neutralized with soda lime, Amsorb Plus, and Litholyme. The canister's warmth indicates the heat produced during the neutralization of carbon dioxide. If the anesthesia provider notices that the canister is not warming up, there's a chance that the carbon dioxide is not being chemically neutralized.

7.6.2. Efficiency of Carbon Dioxide Neutralization

The size of the carbon dioxide granules and the existence or lack of channeling in the carbon dioxide canister have an impact on the efficiency of carbon dioxide neutralization.

7.6.2.1. Absorbent Granule Size

The ideal size of absorbent granules strikes a balance between airflow resistance and absorptive efficiency in the carbon dioxide absorbent canister. Because more surface area comes into contact with carbon dioxide when absorbent granule size decreases, absorbent efficiency increases. However, the less space there is for gas to pass through and the higher the flow resistance, the smaller the absorbent granules. Mesh size, which is the number of openings per linear inch in a sieve that allow granular particles to pass through, is the term used to describe absorbent granule size. In the context of anesthesia, carbon dioxide absorbents are typically granularized to a size between 4 and 10 mesh, which maximizes absorbent efficiency while minimizing resistance. A 4-mesh screen has four quarter-inch apertures for every inch of linear space. There are ten tenth-inch apertures per linear inch on a 10-mesh screen.

7.6.2.2. Channeling

Channeling is the process by which exhaled gases are preferentially allowed to pass through the carbon dioxide absorber canister through low-resistance pathways, thereby avoiding the majority of the carbon dioxide absorbent granules. Before using, gently shake the canister to ensure that the absorbent granules are packed firmly, thereby minimizing channeling that may arise from loose packing. The purpose of carbon dioxide absorbent canisters is to allow exhaled gas to pass through the absorbent granules uniformly.

7.6.2.3. Absorptive Capacity

The most carbon dioxide that 100 g of carbon dioxide absorbent can absorb determines the absorptive capacity of the material. Their effectiveness may be significantly reduced if exhaled gases pass through the absorbent granules. The structural design of the carbon dioxide absorbent canister affects the absorbent's absorptive capacity.

7.6.2.4. Indicators

When the carbon dioxide absorbent granules are depleted, a pH-sensitive indicator dye in the carbon dioxide absorbents changes color. When the granules' absorptive components run out, carbonic acid builds up and changes the pH and, consequently, the color of the indicator dye. When the soda lime's indicator dye runs out, the granules turn purple instead of white. Though absorptive capacity does not regain with time, depleted soda lime granules may eventually return to their original white color. Reusing the dye causes the purple color shift to occur again very quickly. On the other hand, Amsorb Plus and Litholyme both have an indicator dye in them that, when depleted, turns the color of the granules from white to purple and stays that way.

7.6.3. Degradation of Inhaled Anesthetics

Soda lime breaks down sevoflurane into nephrotoxic compounds (compound A) when it is wet and contains a typical water complement or when it is dry. Desflurane, enflurane, or isoflurane may be converted to carbon monoxide by desiccated soda lime. On the other hand, dehydrated or moist Litholyme and Amsorb Plus do not break down inhaled anesthetics.

7.6.3.1. Generation of Compound A

A dose- and time-dependent nephrotoxin known as compound A can be produced when soda lime breaks down sevoflurane. Three factors increase the amount of compound A produced with soda lime: (1) low fresh gas flows; (2) higher sevoflurane concentrations; and (3) higher absorbent temperatures. Thus far, there hasn't been any evidence of clinically noteworthy kidney damage linked to sevoflurane usage. By contrast, sevoflurane is not broken down to compound A by Amsorb Plus or Litholyme.

7.6.3.2. Generation of Carbon Monoxide

The colorless, odorless gas known as carbon monoxide (CO) is toxic because it causes carboxyhemoglobin to form in the blood when oxygen from hemoglobin is removed. Desiccated soda lime has the ability to degrade inhaled anesthetics, producing carbon monoxide concentrations that can rise to 30% or more and substantial amounts of carboxyhemoglobin. The inhaled anesthetic used (desflurane = enflurane > isoflurane >> halothane = sevoflurane), low fresh gas flows, higher concentrations of inhaled anesthetics, higher absorbent temperatures, and, most importantly, the degree of dryness of the absorbent (desiccation) all lead to an increase in the production of carbon monoxide and carboxyhemoglobin. \Soda lime dehydrates more quickly, converting inhaled anesthetics to carbon monoxide. Desiccation necessitates high dry gas flow for an extended length of time (often 48 hours) in between cases. If the breathing bag is not turned on, the desire gets worse. The fresh gas in this case follows the retrograde path of least resistance, which passes through the bottom, top, and 22 mm breathing bag mount of the absorbent canister, as the inspiratory valve creates resistance to forward flow. As a result, patients who were anesthetized on Monday after an unintentional continuous flow of oxygen (flowmeter left on) through the soda lime carbon dioxide absorbent over the weekend tend to have higher blood concentrations of carboxyhemoglobin. On the other hand, inhaled anesthetics do not break down into carbon monoxide when using Amsorb Plus or Litholyme.

7.6.3.3. Fire and Extreme Heat in the Breathing System

When sevoflurane is used in the circle system, desiccation of the carbon dioxide absorbent Baralyme—which is no longer clinically available—can result in fire. Sevoflurane and Baralyme's poorly understood chemical reaction has the potential to produce enough heat and combustible degradation products to cause fires to spontaneously start in the breathing circuit and carbon dioxide absorber canister. Desiccated soda lime has been linked to cases of extreme heat without fire that have been documented in Europe. Anesthesia professionals should try their best to avoid using desiccated carbon dioxide absorbents to avoid this issue. (Olympio, 2005)

7.6.3.4. Recommendations Regarding Safe use of Carbon Dioxide Absorbents

The Anesthesia Patient Safety Foundation has published suggested steps regarding the selection of carbon dioxide absorbents and steps to take should desiccation of the carbon dioxide absorbent be a potential risk (Figure 7.6).

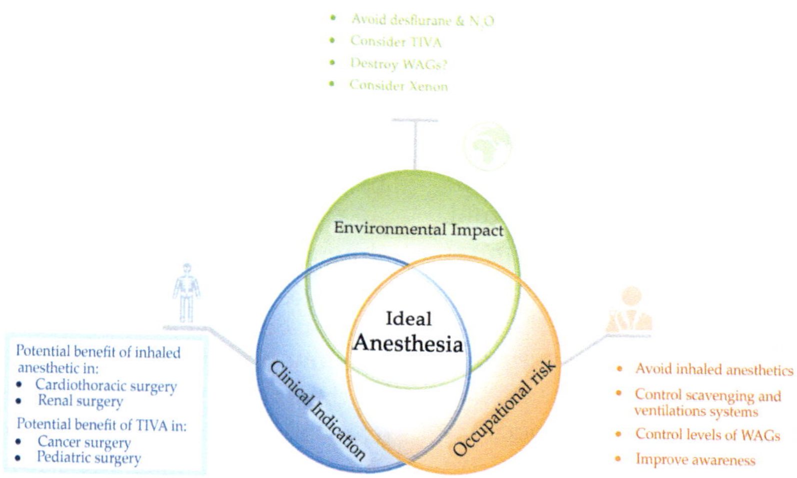

Figure 7.6. *Schematic view of the three different perspectives in choosing an anesthesia technique. Abbreviations: N2O: Nitrous oxide; TIVA: Total intravenous anesthesia; WAG: Waste anesthetic gas.*

Source: *Gaya da Costa M, Kalmar AF, Struys MMRF. Inhaled Anesthetics: Environmental Role, Occupational Risk, and Clinical Use. Journal of Clinical Medicine. 2021; 10(6):1306. https://doi.org/10.3390/jcm10061306.*

7.7. Checking Anesthesia Machine and Circle System Function

A higher risk of severe morbidity and mortality related to anesthesia care has also been linked to improperly inspecting anesthesia equipment before use, which can cause harm to patients. The Food and Drug Administration created the preanesthesia checkout (PAC) in 1993, and it has since gained widespread recognition as a crucial stage in the process of getting ready to provide anesthesia care. Since then, anesthesia delivery systems have developed to the point where not all of the anesthesia delivery systems available today can be used with the same checkout process.

7.7.1. ASA 2008 Recommendations for Preanesthesia Checkout Procedures

To provide guidelines that could be applied to all anesthesia delivery systems, the American Society of Anesthesiologists created new Recommendations for Pre-Anesthesia Checkout Procedures in 2008. This allowed individual departments to create PACs that were tailored to the anesthesia delivery systems that were being used at their facilities and could be completed quickly and consistently. Particularly, items that are not assessed by the automated checkout must be identified and additional manual checkout procedures added as necessary for more recent anesthesia delivery systems that have automated checkout features. Every day before the first case, a thorough anesthesia machine and circle system function checkout procedure should be carried out. Before every use that day, a quick checkout should be completed. The most crucial preoperative procedures are as follows: (1) confirm that a self-inflating manual ventilation device (Ambu bag) and an auxiliary oxygen cylinder are available and operational; (2) check for leaks in the machine's low-pressure system; (3) calibrate the oxygen monitor; and (4) check for positive-pressure leaks in the breathing system.

7.7.1.1. Verification That Auxiliary Oxygen Cylinder and Manual Ventilation Device are Available and Functioning

One of the main factors contributing to anesthesia-related morbidity and mortality is inadequate ventilation. As equipment malfunctions can happen at any time, making it impossible to ventilate the patient, a self-inflating manual ventilation device (such as an Ambu bag) should be available at all anesthetizing locations and should be regularly inspected to ensure it is operating properly. A backup oxygen supply, such as an oxygen cylinder with a regulator and a way to open the cylinder valve, should also be readily available and inspected. This source of oxygen should be kept apart from the anesthesia machine and pipeline supply.

7.7.1.2. Leak Check of the Machine's Low-Pressure System

The integrity of the anesthesia machine is verified by performing a leak check on the low-pressure system, which runs from the flowmeters to the common gas outlet. It assesses the part of the anesthesia apparatus that is located downstream of all safety equipment, except the oxygen monitor. Due to the components' increased susceptibility to leaks and breakage, the low-pressure circuit is the most fragile part of the anesthesia machine. Leaks in this circuit can cause hypoxia, patient awareness, or both. Therefore, the machine's low-pressure system needs to be inspected.

Certain anesthesia machine designs have different leak tests for the low-pressure system; the anesthesia provider should consult the operator's manual for details. The low-pressure system of more recent anesthesia machines is automatically checked, but unless each vaporizer is turned on separately during the low-pressure system self-test, internal vaporizer leaks might not be discovered.

7.7.1.3. Calibration of the Oxygen Monitor

The oxygen monitor is the sole machine safety instrument that can identify issues after the flowmeters. The proportioning system, the oxygen supply failure alarm, and the fail-safe valve are the other machine safety features that are located upstream of the flowmeters.

7.7.1.4. Positive-Pressure Leak Check of the Breathing System

Before any procedure, the breathing system must have a positive-pressure leak checked. The unidirectional valves' integrity is not tested by this test since a breathing system will pass the leak check even if the unidirectional valves are malfunctioning or stuck closed (American Society of Anesthesiologists, 1987; American Society of Anesthesiologists Committee on Equipment and Facilities, 2008)

A Closer Look

Anesthetic Vaporizer

Anesthetic vaporizers are indispensable components of anesthesia machines, pivotal in delivering volatile liquid anesthetics to patients undergoing surgical or medical procedures. Functioning as gas blenders and flow regulators, these devices convert liquid anesthetic agents into a vaporized form, ensuring precise and controlled administration tailored to individual patient needs. These vaporizers are engineered with meticulous design features, including temperature-compensated flow control valves and bypass systems, to maintain consistent and accurate delivery of anesthetic gases.

Conduct Science's vaporizer system has a 120 cc liquid capacity with a large sight glass to allow liquid level monitoring at-a-glance. The apparatus has an automated flow rate (0.2 to 10,000 cc/min) and temperature compensation (10° to 35° C) capabilities and is equipped with 50kPa pressure tolerance tanks. To prevent unintentional engagement, the system comes with an integrated safety lock. These vaporizers are designed to be used with isoflurane (0 to 5% output) and sevoflurane (0 to 8% output) and are available as pour-fill, easy attachment-fill, and cage mount-fill styles.

The vaporizer system is composed of a concentration control dial, the bypass chamber, the vaporizing chamber, the filler port, and the filler cap.

Vaporizers are designed to be used with specific anesthetic agents and are equipped with filling systems to enforce the same. The filler tubes are agent-specific. The fittings on the vaporizer and the collar of the bottles are specific to the agent too. This precaution is built into the design to prevent the mixing of the anesthetic agents.

Most modern vaporizers can be seen fitted to the back bar of the anesthetic machines using special mounting systems. These set-ups allow a quick and easy exchange of vaporizers between anesthetic machines. Although multiple vaporizers can be fitted to the anesthetic machine, as a cautionary measure most back bar systems restrict usage to only one vaporizer at a time.

The variable bypass vaporizers are the most commonly used vaporizers. Their working principle involves splitting the fresh gas flow and saturating a small portion completely with the volatile anesthetic before recombining into the main gas flow. This process is achieved by setting the anesthetic concentration using the control dial and the pressurized chamber of the plenum vaporizers. These devices are also equipped with thermo-compensation capabilities for a steady vaporizer output.

Precision vaporizers are renowned for their ability to deliver an exact concentration of anesthetic, adjustable in minute increments, and are frequently employed with volatile agents like isoflurane, sevoflurane, and desflurane. Variable bypass vaporizers offer flexibility by adjusting gas flow rates, indirectly impacting the concentration of vaporized anesthetic reaching the patient, while non-variable bypass vaporizers provide a fixed concentration of anesthetic gas determined by the flow rate of carrier gas. Despite differences in design, all types of vaporizers undergo stringent testing and calibration to ensure their precision and safety. Regular maintenance and calibration routines are imperative to uphold accuracy and minimize the risk of under- or overdosing patients.

Anesthetic vaporizers integrate numerous safety features to mitigate risks associated with anesthesia delivery. Automatic shutoff mechanisms and interlocks prevent the administration of excessive concentrations of anesthetic gases, enhancing patient safety during procedures. Additionally, vaporizers are equipped with alarms and monitoring systems to alert anesthesia providers of potential malfunctions or deviations from intended settings. These safety measures, combined with meticulous training and adherence to best practices, contribute to the overall safety and efficacy of anesthesia administration.

In the dynamic landscape of healthcare technology, ongoing advancements in anesthetic vaporizer design continue to enhance precision, safety, and user experience. Integration with anesthesia machine software allows for real-time monitoring and data recording, facilitating quality assurance and enhancing patient care. Moreover, the development of vaporizers compatible with a broader range of anesthetic agents provides clinicians with more options for tailoring anesthesia delivery to individual patient needs.

Anesthetic vaporizers represent a cornerstone of modern anesthesia practice, facilitating the precise and controlled delivery of volatile liquid anesthetics. Through meticulous design, rigorous testing, and ongoing advancements, these devices contribute to the safety, efficacy, and quality of anesthesia care, ensuring optimal patient outcomes in surgical and medical settings.

Summary

- An anesthesia delivery system consists of the anesthesia workstation (anesthesia machine) and anesthetic breathing system (circuit), which permit the delivery of known concentrations of inhaled anesthetics and oxygen to the patient, as well as the removal of the patient's carbon dioxide.
- Anesthesia delivery systems are integral components of modern medical practice, facilitating the safe and effective administration of anesthesia agents during surgical procedures and other medical interventions.
- The anesthesia machine has evolved from a simple pneumatic device to a complex integrated computer-controlled multicomponent workstation. The components within the anesthesia workstation function in harmony to deliver known concentrations of inhaled anesthetics to the patient.
- Anesthesia machines are equipped with a fail-safe valve designed to prevent the delivery of hypoxic gas mixtures from the machine in the event of a failure of the oxygen supply. This valve shuts off or proportionally decreases the flow of all gases when the pressure in the oxygen delivery line decreases to less than 30 psi.
- Gases used in the administration of anesthesia (oxygen, nitrous oxide, air) are most often delivered to the anesthesia machine from a central supply source located in the hospital.
- Volatile anesthetics are liquids at room temperature and atmospheric pressure. Vaporization, which is the conversion of a liquid to a vapor, takes place in a closed container, referred to as a vaporizer.
- Vaporizers are classified as agent-specific, variable bypass, flow-over, temperature-compensated (equipped with an automatic temperature-compensating device that helps maintain a constant vaporizer output over a wide range of temperatures), and out-of-circuit.
- The function of anesthetic breathing systems is to deliver oxygen and anesthetic gases to the patient and to eliminate carbon dioxide. Conceptually, the anesthetic breathing system is a tubular extension of the patient's upper airway.
- The Mapleson systems are characterized by the absence of valves to direct gases to or from the patient and the absence of chemical carbon dioxide neutralization.
- The Bain circuit is a coaxial version of the Mapleson D system in which the fresh gas supply tube runs coaxially inside the corrugated expiratory tubing. The fresh gas tube enters the circuit near the reservoir bag, but the fresh gas is actually delivered at the patient end of the circuit.
- Fresh gas enters the circle system through a connection from the common gas outlet of the anesthesia machine.
- Exhaled gases, devoid of carbon dioxide, form a major part of the inhaled gases when a closed anesthetic breathing system is used. This means that the composition of the inhaled gases is influenced by the concentration present in the exhaled gases.

- Ventilators with bellows that rise during exhalation (standing or ascending bellows) are preferred because the bellows will not rise (fill) if there is a leak in the anesthesia breathing system or the system becomes accidentally disconnected.
- Humidification is a form of vaporization in which water vapor (moisture) is added to the gases delivered by the anesthetic breathing system to minimize water and heat loss.
- High-pressure leakage of nitrous oxide can occur as a result of faulty yokes attaching the nitrous oxide tank to the anesthesia machine or faulty connections from the central nitrous oxide gas supply to the anesthesia machine.
- Soda lime granules consist of calcium hydroxide, water, and small amounts of the strong bases sodium hydroxide (NaOH) and potassium hydroxide (KOH) that serve as catalysts for carbon dioxide absorption.

References

1. American Society of Anesthesiologists. (1987). *Check-Out: A Guide for Preoperative Inspection of An Anesthetic Machine* (pp. 1–14). Park Ridge, IL: American Society of Anesthesiologists.
2. Andrews, J. J. (1988). *Understanding Anesthesia Machines*. Cleveland, OH: International Anesthesia Research Society Review Course Lectures.
3. Andrews, J. J. (1998). *The Circle System: A Collection of 30 Color Illustrations*. Washington, DC: Library of Congress.
4. Andrews, J. J., Johnston, R. V., & Kramer, G. C. (1993). Consequences of misfilling contemporary vaporizers with desflurane. *Canadian Journal of Anesthesia, 40*, 71–74.
5. Arbous, M. S., Meursing, A. E., van Kleef, J. W., & de Lange, J. J. (2005). Impact of anesthesia management characteristics on severe morbidity and mortality. *Anesthesiology, 102*, 257–268.
6. Bain, J. A., & Spoerel, W. E. (1972). A streamlined anesthetic system. *Canadian Anesthetists' Society Journal, 19*, 426–435.
7. Baxter, P. J., Garton, K., & Kharasch, E. D. (1998). Mechanistic aspects of carbon monoxide formation from volatile anesthetics. *Anesthesiology, 89*, 929–941.
8. Brockwell, R. C., & Andrews, J. J. (2006). Delivery systems for inhaled anesthetics. In P. G. Barash, B. F. Cullen, & R. K. Stoelting (Eds.), *Clinical Anesthesia* (pp. 557–594). Philadelphia: Lippincott Williams & Wilkins.
9. Brockwell, R. C., & Andrews, J. J. (2010). Inhaled anesthetic delivery systems. In R. D. Miller (Ed.), *Miller's Anesthesia* (7th ed., pp. 667–718). Philadelphia: Churchill Livingstone.
10. Cooper, J. B., Newbower, R. S., & Kitz, R. J. (1984). An analysis of major errors and equipment failures in anesthesia management: Considerations for prevention and detection. *Anesthesiology, 60*, 34–42.
11. Food and Drug Administration. (1993). *Anesthesia Apparatus Checkout Recommendations*. Rockville, MD: Food and Drug Administration.
12. Kharasch, E. D., Frink, E. J., Artru, A., et al. (2001). Long-duration low-flow sevoflurane and isoflurane effects on postoperative renal and hepatic function. *Anesthesia & Analgesia, 93*, 1511–1520.

13. Lester, M., Roth, P., & Eger, E. I. (2004). Fires from the interaction of anesthetics with desiccated absorbent. *Anesthesia & Analgesia, 99*, 769–774.

14. McGregor, D. G., Baden, J. M., Bannister, C., et al. (1999). *Waste Anesthetic Gases: Information For the Management in Anesthetizing Areas and The Post Anesthesia Care Unit (PACU)*. Park Ridge, IL: American Society of Anesthesiologists.

15. Olympio, M. A. (2005). Carbon dioxide absorbent desiccation safety conference convened by APSF. *Anesthesia Patient Safety Foundation Newsletter, Summer, 20*(2), 25–29. Retrieved from: www.apsf.org (accessed on 29 July 2024).

16. Sykes, M. K. (1968). Rebreathing circuits: A review. *British Journal of Anaesthesia, 40*, 666–674.

17. Willis, B. A., Pender, J. W., & Mapleson, W. W. (1975). Rebreathing in a T-piece: Volunteer and theoretical studies of Jackson-Rees modification of Ayre's T-piece during spontaneous respiration. *British Journal of Anaesthesia, 47*, 1239–1246.

Chapter

SPINAL, EPIDURAL, AND CAUDAL ANESTHESIA

8

Contents

Introduction

In today's anesthetic practice, spinal, epidural, and caudal anesthesia techniques are essential for providing efficient anesthesia and pain relief for a variety of surgical procedures and obstetric care. In order to block sensation and motor function in the targeted body parts, these regional anesthesia techniques entail injecting local anesthetics into the spinal canal, caudal canal, or epidural space.

A local anesthetic is injected into the subarachnoid space during spinal anesthesia, also referred to as subarachnoid block, which produces a quick and deep anesthesia extending down to the umbilicus. Surgery on the lower extremities, pelvis, and lower abdomen frequently uses it. The process of administering local anesthetics via intermittent bolus injection or continuous infusion involves inserting a catheter into the epidural space. This method, which is commonly used for labor analgesia, postoperative pain management, and anesthesia for surgeries involving the thorax, abdomen, and lower extremities, offers greater flexibility in the depth and duration of anesthesia.

Using the sacral hiatus, a local anesthetic is injected into the caudal epidural space to provide anesthesia for surgeries and procedures on the lower extremities, genitalia, and perineum in both adult and pediatric patients. These regional anesthesia techniques are important parts of contemporary anesthesia practice because they provide benefits over general anesthesia alone, such as better pain control, decreased opioid consumption, and improved recovery outcomes.

Orientation and Directional Terms

Term	Definition	Illustration
Caudal block	Caudal epidural block is a commonly used technique for surgical anesthesia in children and chronic pain management in adults.	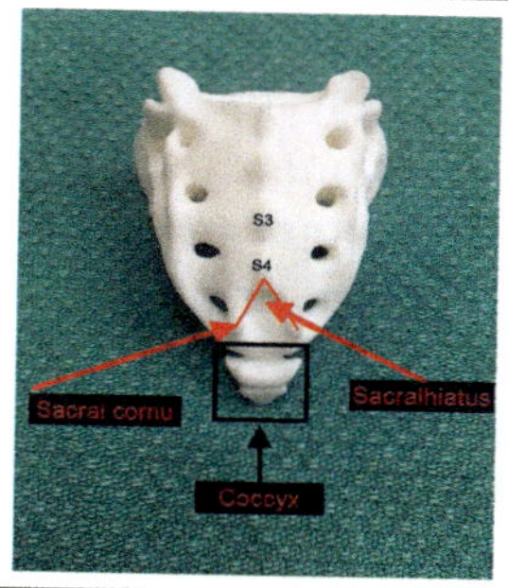
Chronic pain	Chronic pain is long standing pain that persists beyond the usual recovery period or occurs along with a chronic health condition, such as arthritis. Chronic pain may be "on" and "off" or continuous.	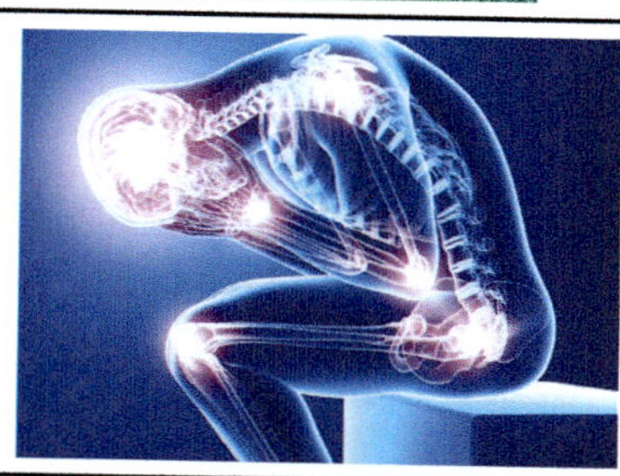
Spinal cord	A column of nerve tissue that runs from the base of the skull down the center of the back. It is covered by three thin layers of protective tissue called membranes. The spinal cord and membranes are surrounded by the vertebrae (back bones).	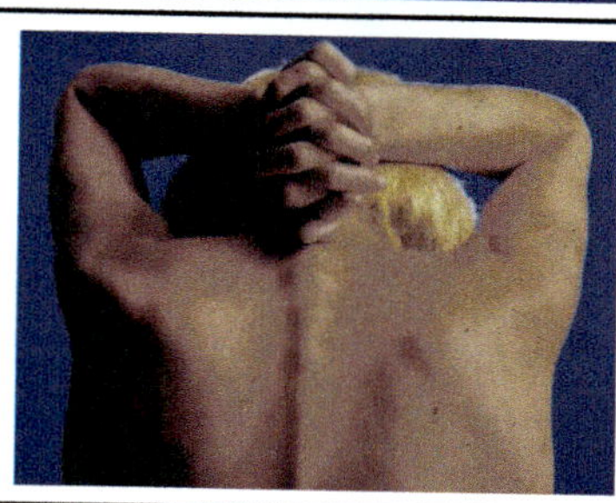
Anterior spinal artery	Anterior spinal artery is a major artery providing nutrient-rich blood supply to the entire spinal cord section except for the dorsal columns. This artery runs along the entire length of the spinal cord anastomosing with other arteries.	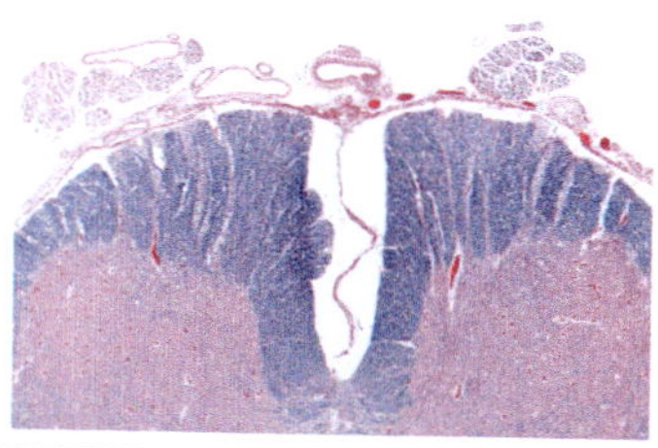
Systemic vascular resistance (SVR)	Systemic vascular resistance (SVR) is the resistance in the circulatory system that is used to create blood pressure, the flow of blood and is also a component of cardiac function. When blood vessels constrict (vasoconstriction) this leads to an increase in SVR.	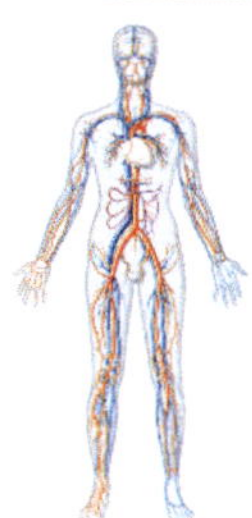

8.1. Principles

Central neuraxial blocks are the collective term for spinal, epidural, and caudal blocks. The methods differ significantly in terms of pharmacology, physiology, and technique, but they all lead to one or more combinations of motor, sensory, and sympathetic blockade. A tiny quantity of medication is needed for spinal anesthesia to provide quick, strong, consistent, but limited sensory analgesia. On the other hand, epidural anesthesia acts more slowly, usually lasts longer with the use of a catheter, and needs a lot of local anesthetic. Moreover, it might have complications and systemic side effects that are not present with spinal anesthesia. While adding flexibility to clinical care, combined spinal and epidural techniques blur some of these distinctions (Figure 8.1).

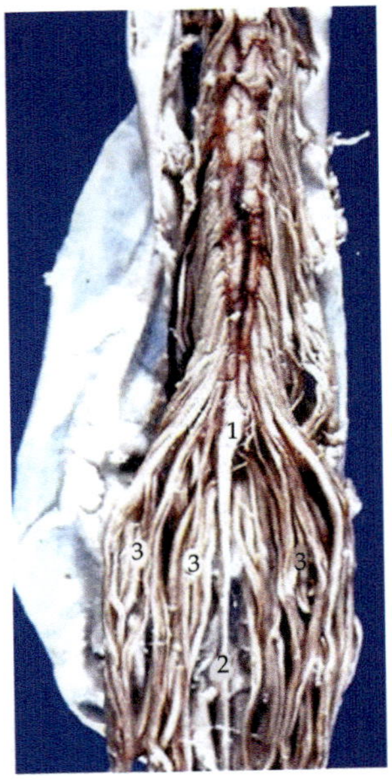

Figure 8.1. *Terminal spinal cord and cauda equina.*

Source: By John A Beal, PhD, Dep't. of Cellular Biology & Anatomy, Louisiana State University Health Sciences Center Shreveport - http://www.healcentral.org/healapp/showMetadata?metadataId=40566, CC BY 2.5, https://commons.wikimedia.org/w/index.php?curid=1020191.

8.2. Practice

In obstetrics, surgery, acute postoperative pain management, and chronic pain relief, neuraxial blockade is frequently used. For surgery on the lower abdomen, pelvic organs (such as the bladder), or both, single-injection spinal or epidural anesthesia is frequently utilized (e.g., thoracic, abdominal, lower limb).

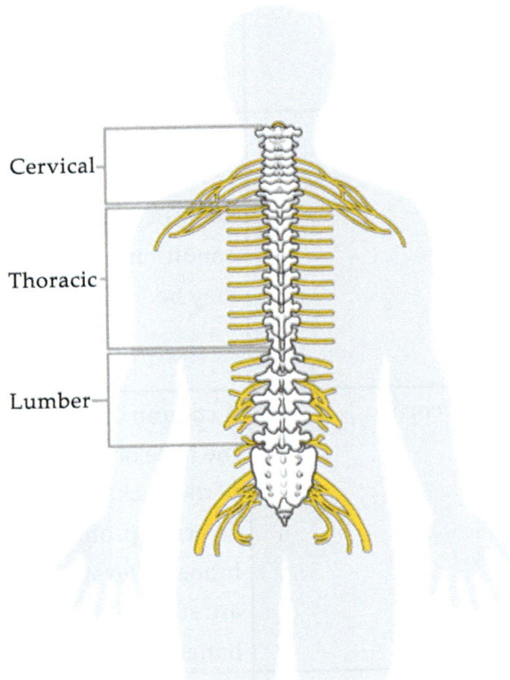

Figure 8.2. *The spine.*

Source: By Cancer Research UK - Original email from CRUK, CC BY-SA 4.0, https://commons.wikimedia.org/w/index.php?curid=34332941.

Continuous catheter-based epidural infusions are used to relieve postoperative pain for several days following major surgery (e.g., obstetric labor analgesia). While pulmonary and potentially cardiac morbidity can be decreased with neuraxial analgesia, the benefits to mortality seem to be negligible. In more recent times, the focus of epidural analgesia has shifted to aiding in the quick recovery following surgery. Caudal blocks are primarily used in children for surgical anesthesia and analgesia, and in adults with chronic pain for therapeutic analgesia. Long-term indwelling spinal catheters can be implanted to treat both malignant and nonmalignant chronic pain. (Covino et al., 1999) (Figure 8.2).

8.3. Anatomy

The spinal cord ends distally in the conus medullaris as the filum terminale (fibrous extension) and the cauda equina (neural extension), continuing proximally with the medulla oblongata. From the lower border of L1 in adults to L3 in infants, this distal termination varies. Three membranes encircle the spinal cord inside the bony vertebral column: the pia mater, arachnoid mater, and dura mater, which run from inner to outer. The subarachnoid, or intrathecal, space between the pia and arachnoid maters is home to cerebrospinal fluid, or CSF. The brain and spinal cord are closely surrounded by the highly vascular pia mater membrane. The dura is a strong fibroelastic membrane, and the arachnoid mater is a delicate, nonvascular membrane that serves as the main barrier to drugs entering and exiting the CSF-4.

The epidural space, which stretches from the foramen magnum to the sacral hiatus, envelops the dura. The ligamentum flavum borders the posterior longitudinal ligament, the pedicles and intervertebral foramina border it laterally, and the posterior longitudinal ligament borders it anteriorly. Blood vessels, fat, areolar tissue, lymphatics, and nerve roots are among its contents (Figure 8.3).

The sacral hiatus is also reached by the ligamentum flavum, also referred to as the "yellow ligament," which runs from the foramen magnum. Despite being depicted in classical art as a single ligament, it is actually made up of the left and right ligamenta flava, which come together to form a ventral opening and an acute midline angle.

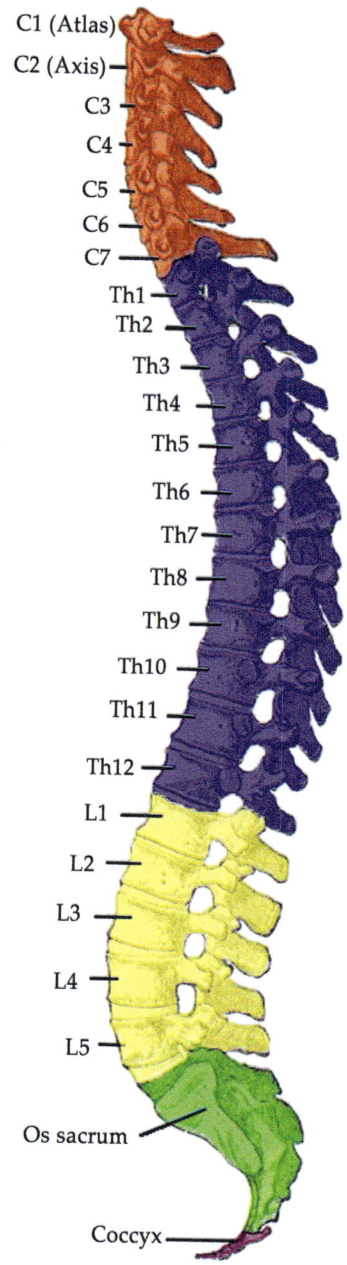

Figure 8.3. *The vertebral column from a lateral view exhibits four curvatures.*

Source: By Henry Vandyke Carter - Vertebral column image.- From: Henry Gray (1918) Anatomy of the Human Body (See "Book" section below)- Altered by User:Uwe Gille, Public Domain, https://commons.wikimedia.org/w/index.php?curid=1282158.

The thickness, skin-to-dura distance, and ligamentum flavum distance all change depending on where in the vertebral canal one is located. The vertebral canal is circular in shape and has the smallest area at the thoracic levels, and it is triangular in shape at the lumbar levels. The lamina of the vertebral bodies or the interspinous ligaments (which join the spinous processes) are located directly posterior to the ligamentum flavum. The supraspinous ligament, which connects to the vertebral spines and runs from the external occipital protuberance to the coccyx, is the last structure (Figure 8.4).

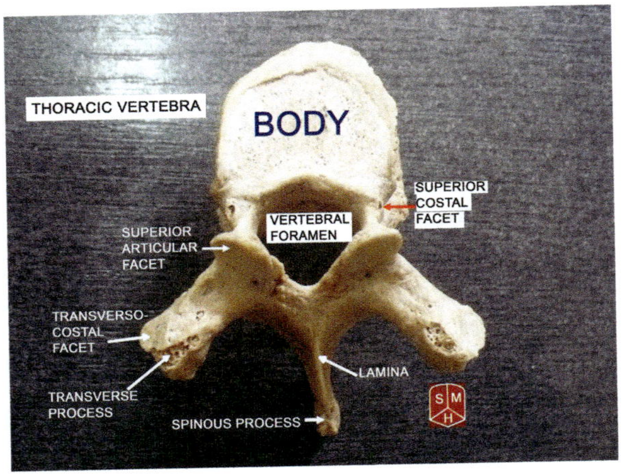

Figure 8.4. *Typical thoracic vertebra.*

Source: By Anatomist90 - Own work, CC BY-SA 3.0, https://commons.wikimedia.org/w/index.php?curid=17155527.

There is a sacrum in addition to 7 cervical, 12 thoracic, and 5 lumbar vertebrae. The anterior element of the vertebra is the vertebral body, while the posterior elements are the vertebral arch, spinous process, pedicles, and laminae. The zygapophyseal (facet) joints and the fibrocartilaginous joints, which have central disks containing the nucleus pulposus, connect the vertebrae anteriorly and posteriorly, respectively. Unlike the lumbar spinous processes, which are angulated almost horizontally, the thoracic spinous processes are angulated more steeply caudad. For the purpose of inserting and advancing needles, the clinical distinctions between the lumbar and caudal spinous processes are significant. The terminal segment of the dural sac, which normally ends at S2 in adults and lower in children, is located in the sacral canal. A venous plexus is also present in the sacral canal.

8.3.1. Spinal Nerves

To form spinal nerves, dorsal (afferent) and ventral (efferent) nerve roots combine distal to the dorsal root ganglion. The spinal nerves are divided into 31 pairs: 8 cervical, 12 thoracic, 5 lumbar, 5 sacral, and 1 coccygeal. After passing through the intervertebral foramen, the dura, arachnoid, and pia encase the nerves, eventually giving rise to the epineurium, perineurium, and endoneurium, in that order. Originating in the intermediolateral gray columns between T1 and L2, preganglionic sympathetic fibers travel via the ventral nerve root to the paravertebral sympathetic ganglia and farther-reaching plexuses (Figure 8.5).

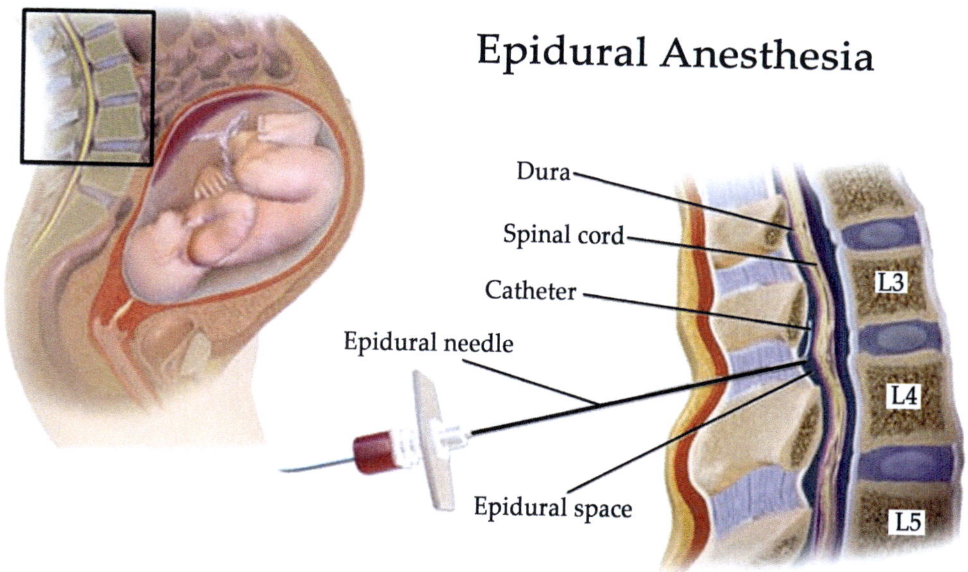

Figure 8.5. *Lumbar and thoracic epidural technique. The increased angle of needle insertion during thoracic epidural cannulation may provide a slightly longer distance of "needle travel" before entering the epidural space. In contrast to lumbar epidural cannulation, the distance traveled is modified by a more perpendicular angle of needle insertion.*

Source: Althobaiti M, Ali S, Hariri NG, Hameed K, Alagl Y, Alzahrani N, Alzahrani S, Al-Naib I. Recent Advances in Smart Epidural Spinal Needles. Sensors. 2023; 23(13):6065. https://doi.org/10.3390/s23136065.

8.3.2. Blood Supply

One anterior spinal artery supplies the anterior two thirds of the spinal cord, while two posterior spinal arteries supply the posterior one third. The artery of Adamkiewicz, which emerges from the aorta and enters an intervertebral foramen between T7 and L4 on the left, is one of the biggest anastomotic feeder arteries to the anterior system. Anterior spinal artery syndrome, which is characterized by anterior horn motor neuron damage and disruption of pain and temperature perception below the affected level, is caused by ischemia within the anterior system. Any one or a combination of hemorrhage, vasculopathy, mechanical obstruction, and profound hypotension can cause ischemia. Before draining into the internal vertebral venous plexus in the medial and lateral components of the epidural space, longitudinal anterior and posterior spinal veins connect with segmental anterior and posterior radicular veins. These flow into the azygos venous system.

8.3.3. Anatomic Variations

Variations in CSF volume and the size and structure of the spinal nerve roots can affect the quality, height, and regression time of the spinal blocks. Likewise, the epidural space is less homogeneous and more segmented than previously thought, which could contribute to the unpredictable spread of drugs. Lastly, the contents of the epidural space can also differ and affect how much local anesthetic is needed (Figure 8.6 and 8.7).

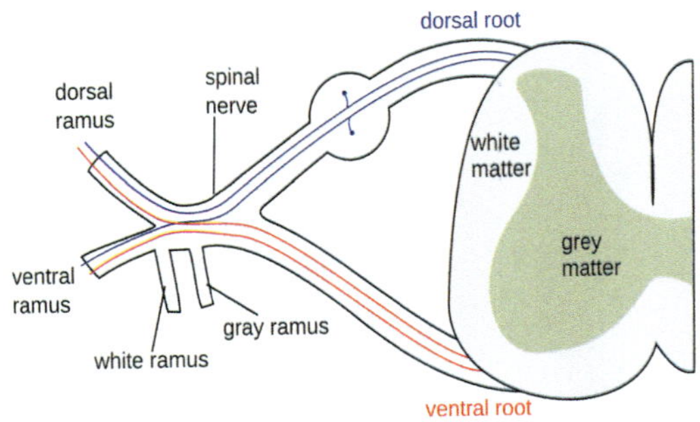

Figure 8.6. *The spinal cord and nerve roots.*

Source: By Mysid (original by Tristanb) - Vectorized in CorelDraw by Mysid on an existing image at en-wiki by Tristanb., CC BY-SA 3.0, https://commons.wikimedia.org/w/index.php?curid=1420508.

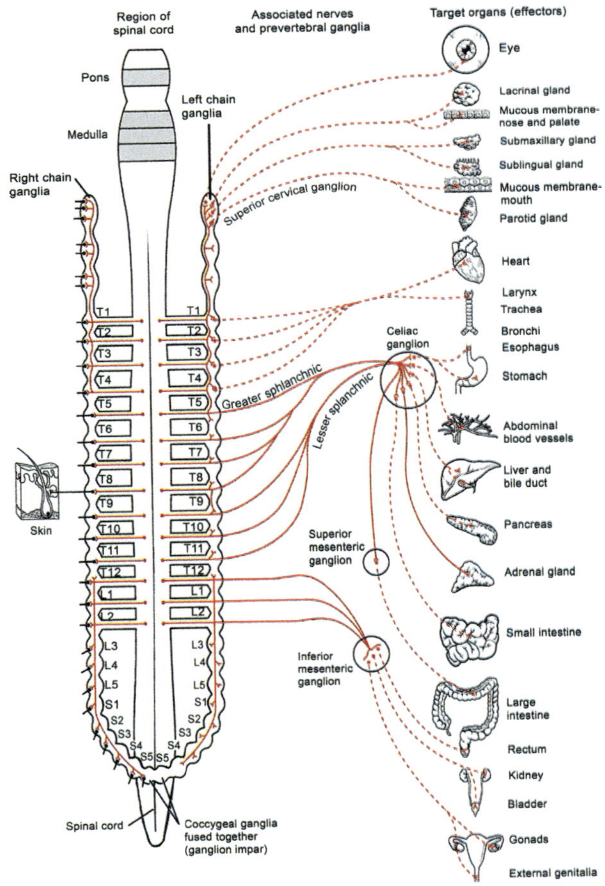

Figure 8.7. *Cell bodies in the thoracolumbar portion of the spinal cord (T1-L2) give rise to the peripheral sympathetic nervous system. Preganglionic efferent fibers travel in the ventral root and then via the white ramus communicans to paravertebral sympathetic ganglia or more distant sites such as the celiac ganglion. Afferent fibers travel via the white ramus communicans to join somatic nerves, which pass through the dorsal root to the spinal cord.*

Source: By OpenStax College - Anatomy & Physiology, Connexions Web site. http://cnx.org/content/col11496/1.6/, Jun 19, 2013., CC BY 3.0, https://commons.wikimedia.org/w/index.php?curid=30148017.

8.4. Mechanism of Action

Local anesthetics interfere with nerve signals going through the dorsal root ganglia, spinal nerve roots, and spinal cord. Unlike extradural nerves, which are frequently covered in dura mater, also known as the "dural sleeve," subarachnoid nerves are easily anesthetized, even with a small dose of local anesthetic. The size, surface area, and level of myelination of the nerve fibers exposed to the local anesthetic determine how quickly the blockade occurs. The most sensitive to local anesthetic blockade are the small preganglionic sympathetic fibers (B fibers, 1 to 3 μm, minimally myelinated). It is easier to block the cold temperature-sensing C fibers (0.3 to 1 μm, unmyelinated) than the myelinated A-delta pinprick sensation fibers (1 to 4 μm). The last sensory fibers to be affected are the myelinated A-beta fibers (5 to 12 μm) that conduct touch sensation. The most resilient to local anesthetic blockade are the larger, myelinated A-alpha motor fibers, which range in size from 12 to 20 μm (Figure 8.8).

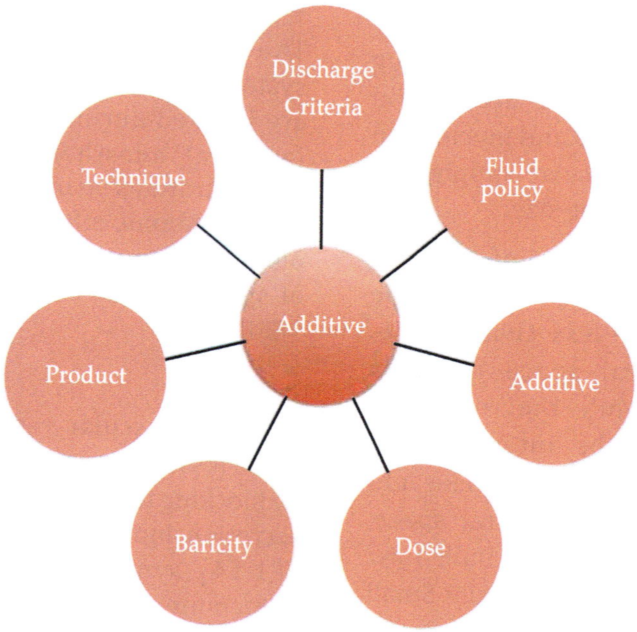

Figure 8.8. *Spinal anesthesia variables.*

Source: Barbara Breebaart, M. (2020). Local Anaesthetics for Spinal Anaesthesia in Day-Case Surgery. IntechOpen. doi: 10.5772/intechopen.89018.

The opposite sequence is followed by the regression of blockade, or "recovery.." Differential sensory block refers to the maximum block height that varies based on each sensory modality. As a result, cold sensation, which is also a good indicator of sympathetic blockade, is primarily cephalad and typically occurs one to two spinal segments above the level of pinprick anesthesia, which is itself one to two spinal segments above touch anesthesia. (Covino et al., 1999)

8.4.1. Drug Uptake and Distribution

Direct injection of a local anesthetic into the CSF causes it to diffuse toward other spinal cord segments from high concentration areas. The CSF circulation time is connected to rostral spread, which is frequently noticeable in 10 to 20 minutes. In order to reach the deeper dorsal root ganglia, the local anesthetic also diffuses through the pia mater and passes through the spaces of Virchow-Robin, which are extensions of the subarachnoid space that accompany the blood vessels that invade the spinal cord from the pia mater. A fraction of the subarachnoid medication diffuses outward and enters the epidural space, while a portion is absorbed by the pia and dura mater blood vessels.

Drug penetration and uptake are directly proportionate to the drug mass, CSF drug concentration, contact surface area, lipid content (high in the spinal cord and myelinated nerves), and local tissue vascular supply, but inversely related to nerve root size.

The uptake and distribution of epidural drugs are more intricate. A portion of the injected local anesthetic—less than 20%—moves from the epidural space into the CSF to block neurons, while the remaining portion is lost through the intervertebral foramina, vascular absorption, or uptake into the epidural fat. Within the epidural space, other local anesthetics diffuse by bulk flow both longitudinally and circumferentially. Small caliber (greater spread in the thoracic space), decreased epidural space compliance, decreased epidural fat content, and decreased local anesthetic leakage through the intervertebral foramina (e.g.) are factors that may enhance the distribution of local anesthetic within the epidural space. As in spinal stenosis and the elderly), and elevated epidural pressure (e.g., in the course of pregnancy). The vertebral level affects the direction in which drugs spread as well. In the lumbar and low thoracic regions, spread is primarily cephalad; however, following a high thoracic injection, it becomes caudad.

8.4.2. Drug Elimination

In the CSF, drug metabolism does not occur. A decrease in CSF drug concentration brought on by non-neural tissue uptake and, most crucially, vascular absorption causes regression of neural blockade. A shorter duration of action results from the drug being exposed to a larger area for vascular absorption when it spreads more widely. Lipid-soluble local anesthetics (e.g., bupivacaine) can slow vascular absorption by binding to epidural fat and creating a depot.

8.5. Physiologic Effects

The somatic (sensory and motor) nervous systems and the sympathetic nervous system are blocked during neraxial anesthesia. Except for local anesthetic blood levels reaching concentrations strong enough to independently cause systemic effects, the physiological effects of epidural anesthesia are comparable to those of spinal anesthesia.

8.5.1. Cardiovascular

Systemic vascular resistance (SVR) and, to a much lesser extent, cardiac output are decreased by blocking the adrenal medullary catecholamine secretion and the peripheral (T1-L2) and cardiac (T1-T4) sympathetic fibers. Several factors determine how much the spinal or epidural technique lowers arterial blood pressure.

8.5.1.1. Systemic Vascular Resistance

The baseline sympathetic tone (i.e., a larger hemodynamic shift is associated with higher sympathetic tone in the elderly) and the degree of sympathectomy (i.e., such as the block's height). When spinal anesthesia is used, the sympathectomy usually extends two to six dermatomes above the sensory block level; when epidural anesthesia is used, the extent is the same. Even in cases of near-total sympathectomy, SVR in healthy normovolemic patients should only drop by 15% to 18%

following neuraxial blockade if normal cardiac output is preserved.

8.5.1.2. Cardiac Output

Heart rate plus stroke volume equals cardiac output, which is typically either maintained or slightly reduced when spinal anesthesia kicks in. Preload (venous return) and afterload (SVR) are decreased by venous and arterial vasodilation, respectively. The venous system contains 75% of the total blood volume, so the venodilation effect is predominant and the stroke volume is decreased. The decrease in venous return and right atrial filling causes a compensatory baroreceptor-mediated sympathetic response (vasoconstriction and elevated heart rate) above the level of blockade, but this also decreases signal output from intrinsic atrial and great vein chronotropic stretch receptors, increasing parasympathetic activity. Unless neuraxial anesthesia is extended to the T1 level, the two opposing responses result in a minimal change in heart rate. In this case, blockade of the cardioaccelerator fibers may cause severe bradycardia and even asystole, along with a marked reduction in venous return. After spinal anesthesia, the Bezold-Jarisch reflex can also result in profound bradycardia and circulatory collapse, particularly when there is hypovolemia and a small endsystolic left ventricular volume.

8.5.1.3. Coronary Blood Flow

A reduction in coronary blood flow corresponds with a decrease in mean arterial pressure. In patients with ischemic heart disease, however, a high thoracic block may be advantageous. After all, it can improve both regional and global myocardial function and reverse ischemic changes because it lowers myocardial oxygen demand and left ventricular afterload.

8.5.2. Central Nervous System

Regional cerebral blood flow (CBF) may be reduced in older patients and those with preexisting hypertension due to hypotension brought on by spinal anesthesia. On the other hand, none of the patients' postoperative cognitive function changed in studies showing a drop in cerebral perfusion. Nonetheless, it would seem wise to avoid hypotension.

8.5.3. Respiratory

Clinical significance is typically not attached to changes in pulmonary variables during neuraxial block. A decrease in diaphragmatic or phrenic function precedes a decrease in vital capacity, which is linked to a reduction in expiratory reserve volume caused by paralysis of the abdominal muscles required for forced exhalation. These alterations may impact patients with severe respiratory conditions and are more pronounced in obese patients. Hypoperfusion of the respiratory centers in the brainstem can sporadically cause respiratory arrest, but once cardiac output and arterial blood pressure are restored, this almost always goes away.

8.5.4. Gastrointestinal

When splanchnic sympathetic innervation to the gastrointestinal tract is disrupted by neuraxial blockade from T6 to L1, unopposed parasympathetic (vagal) activity causes a contracted gut and hyperperistalsis. Up to 20% of patients may experience vomiting and nausea. When treating nausea brought on by deep (T5) subarachnoid anesthesia, atropine works well. The effect of thoracic epidural anesthesia (TEA) on intestinal perfusion is directly influenced by arterial blood pressure. Systemic hypotension corrected with vasopressor therapy (e.g., reduced colonic perfusion is corrected by norepinephrine. However, after emergency laparotomy, esophageal surgery, and other gastrointestinal interventions, TEA may even lower the rate of anastomotic leak. It may also improve anastomotic mucosal blood flow in patients having esophagectomy.

8.5.5. Renal

Although neuraxial blockade is associated with a predictable decrease in renal blood flow, this decrease has minimal physiological significance. It is dubious to believe that neuraxial blocks usually result in urine retention.

8.6. Indications

8.6.1. Neuraxial Anesthesia

Spinal anesthesia administered by single injection is helpful for known-duration procedures involving the lower extremities, lower abdomen, perineum, or pelvic girdle. Additionally, it might be recommended if patients want to stay conscious or if there are coexisting medical conditions that raise the risks of general anesthesia use, like a serious respiratory illness or a potentially problematic airway. By using a catheter to administer local anesthetic, epidural anesthesia enables longer-lasting surgical anesthesia. Although less common, indwelling catheter-based spinal anesthesia may be helpful in situations where it is difficult to insert an epidural catheter or in cases of severe cardiac disease where more hemodynamically stable incremental dosing is needed to ensure the safety of a single-shot spinal anesthetic.

8.6.2. Neuraxial Analgesia

When combined with other additives, such as opioids, intrathecal or epidural local anesthetics can offer superior, long-lasting intra- and postoperative analgesia during and after hip or knee replacement, labor and delivery, laparotomy, thoracotomy, and increasingly, cardiac surgery. They could also be applied to the treatment of persistent pain. (Covino et al., 1999)

8.7. Contraindications

8.7.1. Absolute

The three most significant issues are localized sepsis, drug allergy to any of the prescribed medications, and patient refusal. Neuraxial techniques may be absolutely contraindicated in cases where a patient is unable to remain motionless during a needle puncture, as this could expose the neural structures to traumatic injury. Moreover, increased intracranial pressure may theoretically predispose to brainstem herniation.

8.7.2. Relative

Relative contraindications can be approached by the system and must be weighed against the potential benefits of neuraxial blockade.

8.7.2.1. Neurologic

Myelopathy or Peripheral Neuropathy

The risk-benefit ratio of performing neuraxial techniques should be taken into consideration, particularly in patients with preexisting central or peripheral neurologic diseases such as multiple sclerosis (MS) or diabetic polyneuropathy, even though it has never been conclusively shown to increase susceptibility to injury following neuraxial anesthesia or analgesia (the double-crush phenomenon). Neuraxial blockade is not contraindicated in cases of chronic low back pain without a neurologic deficit.

Spinal Stenosis

Spinal stenosis has been linked to nerve damage after neuraxial procedures; however, it is unclear how much the natural course of the spinal disease and surgical factors contributed.

Spine Surgery

Patients are not more vulnerable to neurologic complications after prior spine surgery. However, needle access to the CSF or epidural space and epidural catheter insertion may be difficult or impossible in the presence of scar tissue, adhesions, hardware, or bone grafts. Furthermore, the subsequent distribution of the local anesthetic can be erratic and incomplete, especially in the CSF or epidural space.

Multiple Sclerosis

MS patients may show a prolonged motor and sensory blockade and be more sensitive to neuraxial local anesthetics. There is insufficient evidence to support any association between neuraxial anesthesia and worsening MS symptoms.

Spina Bifida

The risk of traumatic needle injury to the spinal cord may increase with the severity of the neural tube defect. Local anesthetic distribution can vary significantly in the CSF and, if present, the epidural space. Under any of these conditions, a thorough assessment of neurologic status needs to be done and documented, along with the conversation about the advantages and disadvantages.

8.7.2.2. Cardiac

Aortic Stenosis or Fixed Cardiac Output

In patients who are dependent on preload, there is a theoretical risk of a swift and notable decrease in SVR following spinal anesthesia, which could potentially lead to a hazardous reduction in coronary perfusion. Neuraxial anesthesia in the setting of aortic stenosis requires careful consideration for each patient, taking into account the severity of the condition, the function of the left ventricle, and the urgency of the case. Improved hemodynamic control might be possible with a catheter-based neuraxial anesthetic combined with several tiny local anesthetic doses.

Hypovolemia

An exaggerated hypotensive response because of vasodilatory effects may occur.

8.7.2.3. Hematologic

Thromboprophylaxis and Anticoagulants

There have been devastating instances of spinal hematomas linked to low-molecular-weight heparin (LMWH)-induced paralysis. The guidelines from professional societies and the American Society of Regional Anesthesia and Pain Medicine (ASRA) regarding neuraxial techniques (including catheter removal) in patients undergoing thrombolytic or antithrombotic therapy can be referred to.

Inherited Coagulopathy

In patients with known hemophilia, von Willebrand disease, or idiopathic thrombocytopenic purpura, hemorrhagic complications following neuraxial techniques are rare when factor levels exceed 0.5. IU/mL for factor VIII, von Willebrand factor, and ristocetin cofactor activity, or when the platelet count exceeds 50×10^9/L prior to block performance. In both the obstetric and general populations, the minimum safe factor levels and platelet count for neuraxial blockade are still unknown.

8.7.2.4. Infection

In the context of a systemic infection, there are theoretical worries about iatrogenic neuraxis seeding, especially if a catheter is left in place. This may be enough justification, combined with significant vasodilation, to forego neuraxial techniques in patients experiencing severe bacteremia or septic shock. While lumbar punctures are an essential part of the investigation of fever of unknown origin, some healthcare professionals avoid using neuraxial techniques on febrile patients. After antibiotic therapy has shown a response, patients with systemic infection evidence can safely be put under neuraxial anesthesia. (Covino et al., 1999)

8.8. Spinal Anesthesia

8.8.1. Factors Affecting Block Height

The spinal segment innervation of intra-abdominal structures, including the peritoneum (T4), bladder (T10), and uterus (T10), may be significantly more cephalad than the corresponding skin incision used to perform surgery on these structures. There can be significant interpatient variability in the distribution of local anesthetic spread within the intrathecal space due to drug, patient, and procedural factors, all of which are not under the anesthesia provider's control. The most crucial factors are ultimately dosage, baricity, and patient positioning.

8.8.1.1. Drug Factors

Baricity

The density of a local anesthetic solution divided by the density of CSF is known as baricity. The standard definition of it is 37°C because density is inversely related to temperature. For example, bupivacaine 0 percent may be isobaric at 24 °C but slightly hypobaric at 37 °C. CSF has a density of 1.00559 g/L. Isobaric refers to local anesthetic solutions with the same density as CSF; hyperbaric refers to solutions with a higher density than CSF; hypobaric refers to solutions with a lower density. Local anesthetic solutions are frequently made hyperbaric or hypobaric by adding dextrose and sterile water, respectively. Hyperbaric solutions exhibit a more consistent distribution pattern, with a preference for the dependent areas of the spinal canal. Whereas isobaric solutions typically aren't affected by gravity, hypobaric solutions tend to spread to nondependent regions. This means that the dependent side will be affected more favorably when hyperbaric local anesthetic is administered to patients in the lateral decubitus position. When patients are placed in the horizontal supine position right after intrusion, the natural curvatures of the vertebral column affect how the local anesthetic spreads.

Dose, Volume, and Concentration

Although volume × concentration = dose, dose is the most accurate factor in determining the local anesthetic spread (and consequently, block height) of isobaric and hypobaric solutions. The main factor affecting hyperbaric local anesthetic injections is baricity. If all other variables are under control, the choice of additive medications (apart from opioids) or local anesthetics has no effect on the spread. Because of pharmacologic enhancement at the extremes of the spread where the local anesthetic block alone would have been subclinical, opioids may increase mean spread.

8.8.1.2. Patient Factors

The number of spinal levels that are anesthetized (blocked) by a spinal anesthetic depends on a variety of patient factors. Extremes in height (tall or short), weight (thin or obese), age (young children or old), and gender are some of these variables. The height of a patient has no bearing on how quickly spinal anesthesia spreads among "normal-sized" adults. But the dosage should be influenced by the length of the vertebral column, which is connected to the spread of the local anesthetic. The lumbosacral CSF pressure is relatively constant, but patient-to-patient variations in CSF volume affect peak block height and regression. The CSF volume itself does not correlate well with basic anthropomorphic measurements other than body weight, even though block height varies indirectly with CSF volume. Theoretically, a decrease in CSF volume could lead to an increase in the spread of local anesthetic and block height in obese patients due to their larger abdominal mass and potentially higher epidural fat (Tables 8.1 and 8.2).

Table 8.1. *Complications in Children*

Kokki 2000	Post-puncture headache
Puncuh 2004	Blockade failure, arterial hypotension, desaturation, airway obstruction, post-puncture headache.
Kokki 2005	Block failure, bradycardia, hypotension, desaturation, post-puncture headache
Imbelloni 2006	Blockade failure, bradycardia, hypotension, bronchospasm, and post-puncture headache
Williams 2006	Blockade failure, bradycardia, desaturation
Kachko 2007	Bradycardia, block failure, high block, apnea.
Ecoffey 2010	High spinal block

Source: Hernández-Cortez, E., M. Martínez-Barragán, Y., & L. Iñiguez-Lopéz, K. (2022). Spinal Anesthesia in Pediatrics. IntechOpen. doi: 10.5772/intechopen.100590.

Table 8.2. *Advantages of Spinal Anesthesia*

1.	Cardiorespiratory stability in preterm
2.	Short stay in the neonatal care unit
3.	Quick recovery of gastrointestinal function
4.	Less response to surgical-anesthetic stress
5.	Hemodynamic stability
6.	Accelerates awakening
7.	Postoperative analgesia
8.	Good immune response
9.	Quick onset of action

CSF, Cerebrospinal fluid.

Source: Hernández-Cortez, E., M. Martínez-Barragán, Y., & L. Iñiguez-Lopéz, K. (2022). Spinal Anesthesia in Pediatrics. IntechOpen. doi: 10.5772/intechopen.100590.

While gender, menopausal status, and pregnancy all affect CSF density, their clinical significance is most likely negligible. Growing older is linked to higher block heights. The volume of CSF decreases and its specific gravity rises in elderly patients. Furthermore, older people's nerve roots are probably more susceptible to local anesthetics. In the lateral position, males are slightly more headup due to their wider shoulders in relation to their hips, while females are the opposite. Nevertheless, it's unclear if males and females genuinely have less cephalad spread in the lateral position. Spinal abnormalities like scoliosis can complicate needle insertion, but if the patient is turned supine, the impact on the spread of the local anesthetic is minimal. Nonetheless, kyphosis in a supine patient may interfere with a hyperbaric solution's ability to spread. Increases in intra-abdominal pressure (possibly), changes in the lumbar lordosis during pregnancy, the volume and density of CSF, twin pregnancies compared to singletons, and a progesterone-mediated increase in neuronal s all contribute to the spread of local anesthetic.

8.8.1.3. Procedure Factors

The patient's positioning is crucial during this time, especially in the first few minutes, as the local anesthetic's spread within the subarachnoid space seems to stop 20 to 25 minutes after injection. The spread of hyperbaric bupivacaine is not always increased by a head-down tilt, even though a 10-degree head-up tilt can lessen the spread of hyperbaric solutions without compromising hemodynamics. Hip flexion combined with the Trendelenburg position flattens the lumbar lordosis and promotes the hyperbaric solution's cephalad spread. Using a small amount of hyperbaric local anesthetic while the patient sits for up to half an hour can result in a "saddle block," which numbs only the sacral nerve roots. Patients receiving hypobaric solutions while seated experience a greater extent of block height.

Block quality may be impacted by the particular type of needle used and the orifice's orientation. Greater spread is produced with cephalad alignment of the Whitacre orifice, but not with Sprotte needles, when using hypobaric solutions. The dispersion of hyperbaric solutions does not seem to be impacted by the needle's orifice orientation. Using a Whitacre needle instead of a Quincke needle results in a more pronounced unilateral block when the needle orifice is directed to one side (and hyperbaric anesthetic is used). With hyperbaric solutions, block height is independent of injection level. The block height with isobaric solutions typically increases with increasing injection cephalad. Block height has not always been demonstrated to be influenced by injection rate or barbotage (repeated aspiration and reinjection of CSF) of isobaric and hyperbaric solutions. The block height is increased by injecting saline or a local anesthetic into the epidural space following a spinal anesthetic.

8.8.2. Duration of the Block

The main factors influencing duration are dosage, the inherent characteristics of the local anesthetic (which influence removal from the subarachnoid space), and the use of additives, if any. Compared to isobaric solutions, hyperbaric solutions act for a shorter period of time (Table 8.3).

Table 8.3. *Continuous Spinal Anesthesia*

Technique	Regimens at Authors' Institutions
CSA for labor analgesia[a]	Continuous infusion:
	– 0.1% ropivacaine or 0.0625–0.1% bupivacaine with 2 μg/ml of fentanyl at 2 ml/h
	– Provider/patient controlled top ups, 1–2 ml every 15 min up to three doses per hour
	Intermittent bolus:
	– 2 ml of 0.1% ropivacaine or 0.0625–0.1% bupivacaine with 15 μg of fentanyl every 2 h
CSA for cesarean delivery	– Initial dose of 5–7.5 mg of 0.5% isobaric bupivacaine or 0.75% hyperbaric bupivacaine
	– Titrate dose to desired level with 2.5 mg incremental blouses every 3–5 min

CSA, continuous spinal anesthesia.
[a]Standard epidural catheters (with Flat Filter) have up to 1 ml of dead space; priming of catheter to fill a catheter's dead space is required on first bolus dose.

Source: Veličković I, Pujic B, Baysinger CW and Baysinger CL (2017) Continuous Spinal Anesthesia for Obstetric Anesthesia and Analgesia. Front. Med. 4:133. doi: 10.3389/fmed.2017.00133.

8.8.3. Pharmacology

Local anesthetic and clinical effects are mediated by drug uptake, distribution, and elimination within the CSF. The pKa (dissociation ionization constant), lipid solubility, and protein binding of the local anesthetic solution, in turn, influence these variables. Instead of their pharmacologic composition (i.e., amide or ester), local anesthetics are typically categorized based on how long they last. The type (location, ambulatory) and anticipated duration of the surgery influence the selection and dosage of the local anesthetic.

8.8.3.1. Short- and Intermediate-Acting Local Anesthetics

One of the first spinal anesthetics is procaine, an ester local anesthetic. It is not widely used due to a higher failure rate than lidocaine, noticeably more nausea, and a longer recovery period. Ultra-short-acting chloroprocaine is quickly metabolized by pseudocholinesterase with negligible effects on the fetus or the systemic circulation. Due to its dependable, brief duration of spinal anesthesia and quicker recovery time compared to procaine, lidocaine, and bupivacaine, preservative-free chloroprocaine is of interest in ambulatory surgery. While transient neurologic symptoms (TNS) are possible, they happen much less frequently (0–6%) than lidocaine (14%).

Articaine is a commonly used ester for dental nerve blocks that is metabolized by nonspecific cholinesteraseases. Spinal anesthesia has not been treated with it. Lidocaine is a fast-acting, intermediate-duration local anesthetic that is hydrophilic and comparatively poorly protein bound. Intrathecal lidocaine has become less common due to a correlation with both TNS (explained later, under "Complications") and permanent nerve damage. An amide local anesthetic with an intermediate half-life is prilocaine. It can be applied in the context of ambulatory surgery and is infrequently linked to TNS. Methemoglobinemia can occur from prilocaine in large doses (>600 mg; not recommended for spinal anesthesia). Despite being an amide local anesthetic, mepivacaine's incidence of TNS following hyperbaric treatment was comparable to lidocaine's. TNS are less common when the preparation is isobaric.

8.8.3.2. Long-Acting Local Anesthetics

Tetracaine is an ester that comes in two packaging options: an isobaric 1 percent solution or niphanoid crystals. For abdominal and perineal surgery, a 0–5% hyperbaric preparation can be made. Tetracaine alone may not always last the full recommended duration, so it is typically combined with a vasoconstrictor additive. While these combinations can produce anesthesia for up to five hours, TNS has been linked specifically to the addition of phenylephrine. Due to its relatively high pKa, bupivacaine is a highly protein-bound amide with a slow onset and a 2.5–3 hour half-life of action. For ambulatory procedures, bupivacaine doses as low as 4 to 5 mg are utilized. Rarely is bupivacaine linked to TNS.

Levobupivacaine is the pure S(–) enantiomer of racemic bupivacaine. Although levobupivacaine potency appears to be slightly less than bupivacaine, the majority of clinical studies using identical doses of levobupivacaine and bupivacaine have found no significant difference in clinical efficacy for spinal anesthesia. Levobupivacaine is less cardiotoxic than bupivacaine, but this is only a theoretical risk in spinal anesthesia.

Another strong protein-bound amide local anesthetic is ropivacaine. It is less potent than bupivacaine, but it has the same pKa (8.1), a slow onset, and a long duration of action. Less cardiotoxicity and increased motorsensory block differentiation, leading to less motor block, were noted benefits of spinal ropivacaine. Ropivacaine causes somewhat less motor block and an earlier rate of recovery when administered at a dose comparable to bupivacaine.

8.8.3.3. Spinal Additives

Numerous drugs have the potential to either extend the duration of sensory and motor blockade or directly relieve pain by acting on the spinal cord and nerve roots. When these medications are taken together, it is frequently possible to reduce the amount of local anesthetic used, which has the benefit of sparing the motor block and accelerating recovery time while maintaining the same level of analgesia. The combination of cerebral opioid receptor activation following CSF transport, peripheral and central systemic effects following vascular uptake, and direct activation of the spinal cord dorsal horn opioid receptor makes opioids added to the CSF complex. Each site's effect is contingent upon the opioid's physicochemical characteristics, specifically its lipid solubility, as well as the dosage that is administered. The onset and duration of action of highly lipid-soluble drugs, like fentanyl and sufentanil, are quicker than that of more hydrophilic opioids. Increased lipid solubility also causes fast absorption into fatty tissue and blood vessels, which has an impact on the body as a whole. Therefore, compared to hydrophilic opioids like (preservative-free) morphine, which exhibit greater spread, the spread of lipophilic opioids within the CSF is more constrained.

As a result, hydrophilic opioids have a more frequent risk of late respiratory depression. The extent of neural tissue and vascular uptake also affects the potency of intrathecal opioids. For example, the relative intrathecal to intravenous potency of morphine is 200:1 to 300:1, whereas for fentanyl and sufentanil, it is only 10:1 to 20:1. Other side effects of intrathecal opioids are discussed under "Complications."

Hydrophilic Opioids

Morphine without preservatives is popular because it can relieve pain for up to 24 hours. For cesarean deliveries, 100 μg provides adequate analgesia with negligible side effects. It is unclear what the optimal dosage is for major orthopedic surgery, but doses of 300 μg or higher increase side effects without improving analgesia. When providing epidural local anesthetic-based analgesia, spinal opioids alone are frequently used as a straightforward substitute. 500 μg or more may be used for thoracotomies or major abdominal surgery. Nevertheless, the ideal dosage is still unknown. Diamorphine is a lipid-soluble prodrug that is more rapidly excreted from the CSF and crosses the dura than morphine. It is transformed into the μ-agonists morphine and 6-monoacetyl morphine, which have comparatively long half-lives. Hydromorphone has no advantages over morphine and is not frequently used for spinal analgesia. Furthermore, there aren't many data. Meperidine is a moderately soluble opioid that also possesses some local anesthetic effects. Though it is rarely used, it has been used as the only intrathecal anesthetic in both general and obstetric surgery. We don't know the neurotoxicity profile.

Lipophilic Opioids

Fentanyl and sufentanil are used frequently in obstetrics for labor analgesia and cesarean delivery as discussed elsewhere. Fentanyl is useful in ambulatory surgery because of its rapid onset time of 10 to 20 minutes and relatively short duration of 4 to 6 hours.

8.8.3.4. Vasoconstrictors

When combined with local anesthetics, epinephrine and phenylephrine prolong sensory and motor blockade. The α_1- adrenergic-mediated vasoconstriction reduces systemic local anesthetic uptake and epinephrine may also enhance analgesia via a direct α_2-adrenergic-mediated effect.

Epinephrine can prolong the effects of spinal anesthesia caused by lidocaine, bupivacaine, and tetracaine. Strong vasoconstrictive action may jeopardize the spinal cord's blood supply, despite the lack of human data to support the theory. Although it is linked to TNS, phenylephrine prolongs the effects of both lidocaine and tetracaine on spinal anesthesia.

8.8.3.5. α_2-Agonists

In the dorsal horn of the spinal cord, intrathecal clonidine, dexmedetomidine, and epinephrine all act on prejunctional and postjunctional α_2-adrenergic receptors. Clonidine enhances analgesia and extends sensory and motor blockade by about an hour. It probably results in less retention of urine than morphine, but it can cause hypotension (not related to dosage) and sedation that lasts for up to eight hours. Dexmedetomidine can prolong motor and sensory block without compromising hemodynamics, and it is roughly ten times more selective for α_2-receptors than clonidine.

8.8.3.6. Other Drugs

The benefits of intrathecal neostigmine are limited by bradycardia, nausea, vomiting, and, at higher doses, weakness in the lower extremities. However, it prolongs motor and sensory blockade and lowers the need for postoperative analgesics. Midazolam also seems to be safe and increases sensory and motor block without causing any negative side effects. Clinical utility for intrathecal ketamine, adenosine, tramadol, magnesium, and nonsteroidal anti-inflammatory drugs is unlikely. (Covino et al., 1999)

8.8.4. Technique

The technique can be classified into a series of steps: preparation, position, projection, and puncture (i.e., the four Ps).

8.8.4.1. Preparation

Risks must be documented and informed consent must be obtained. Standard monitoring is required, intravenous access needs to be secured, and resuscitation equipment needs to be on hand. The needle diameter and tip shape are the two most crucial aspects of a spinal needle.

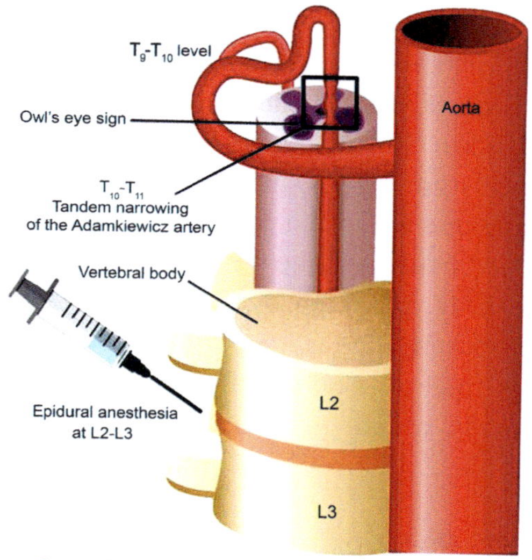

Figure 8.9. *Case study: The cartoon figure depicts the spatial relationship between the epidural anesthesia site and the spinal cord infarction site. The infarction location is a little far from the epidural anesthesia location, thus the epidural anesthesia itself as the possible cause of the spinal cord infarction is less likely.*

Source: Hsu J-L, Chin S-C, Cheng M-H, Wu Y-R, Ro A, Ro L-S. Postpartum Spinal Cord Infarction: A Case Report and Review of the Literature. Medicines. 2022; 9(11):54. https://doi.org/10.3390/medicines9110054.

Needle tip shapes cause the dura to be either cut (Pitkin and Quincke-Babcock) or spread (Sprotte and Whitacre). The conical, pencil-point tips of the needles in the latter group improve tactile perception but, more significantly, lower the risk of post-dural puncture headache. With a 29-G needle, the incidence of post-dural puncture headache drops from 40% with a 22-G needle to less than 2%. This is due to the use of smaller needles. However, 29-G needles have a higher failure rate; therefore, pencil-point needles weighing 25 G, 26 G, or 27 G are likely the best options (Figure 8.9).

The use of strict aseptic techniques is crucial. The oral commensal *Streptococcus viridans* is one of the most frequent organisms that cause postspinal bacterial meningitis, underscoring the need for mask use. The best way to clean your back is to use a mixture of alcohol and chlorhexidine. Because chlorhexidine is neurotoxic, it must be allowed to dry completely before skin piercing. According to current consensus guidelines, neuraxial blocks should only be done while the patient is awake unless both the doctor and the patient determine that the benefits outweigh the risks. If a needle is placed close to nerve tissue, a patient may not be able to recognize warning signs of pain or paresthesia due to general anesthesia or heavy sedation.

8.8.4.2. Position

Lateral decubitus and sitting are the two main patient positions. Seldom is the prone position employed. It's unclear whether one position is better than another. In addition to being more comfortable, the lateral decubitus position makes it easier to administer sedative medication if necessary. To "open up" the vertebral spaces, patients are positioned with their backs parallel to the operating table, their thighs flexed onto the abdomen, and their necks flexed to allow the forehead to be as close to the knees as possible. In order to maximize the spread of a hypobaric, isobaric, or hyperbaric solution to the surgical site, the patient should be positioned. Placing the patient in a seated position may facilitate midline identification, particularly in cases where scoliosis or obesity make it challenging to examine midline anatomy. By flexing the patient's arms and neck over a pillow, releasing tension in the shoulders, and encouraging the patient to "push out" their lower back to widen the lumbar vertebral spaces, an assistant assists in keeping the patient in a vertical plane. It's possible that sitting increases the risk of hypotension.

8.8.4.3. Projection and Puncture

Needless insertion above L1-L2 is not advised because this is the level at which the spinal cord ends. The line that is drawn between the two iliac crests is known as the intercristal line. This correlates to the level of the L4 vertebral body or the L4-L5 interspace, albeit with varying degrees of reliability. Following the selection of the proper space (typically L3-L4, L2-L3, or L4-L5), local anesthetic is infused, and an introducer is inserted through the skin, subcutaneous tissue, and supraspinous ligament to reach the interspinous ligament at a slight cephalad angle of 10 to 15 degrees. The needle is inserted slowly, with its bevel parallel to the midline, until the characteristic shift in resistance through the ligamentum flavum and dura is noticed. There is frequently a slight "click" or "pop" sound as the dura passes through. After removing the stylet, the needle hub should show clear CSF. If the CSF is not flowing, there's a chance the needle is blocked; try rotating the needle 90 degrees at a time until CSF starts to appear. It is recommended to advance the needle a few millimeters and recheck if CSF is not visible in any quadrant. The needle should be removed and the insertion procedure should be repeated if CSF has not yet appeared. Inserting the needle off the midline is a common cause of failure. An anesthetic dose is injected at a rate of about 0.2 mL/sec after

CSF is freely obtained. CSF can be aspirated into the syringe and reinjected into the subarachnoid space to confirm the location once the injection is finished.

The paramedian technique might be particularly helpful when the interspinous ligament has diffuse calcification. A skin wheal is elevated in relation to the matching spinous process by 1 cm caudad and 1 cm lateral. In a cephalomedial plane, the spinal introducer and needle are inserted 10 to 15 degrees off the sagittal plane. The needle "walked up" the lamina and was slightly redirected in a cephalad direction if it made contact with bone. Although the ligamentum flavum and dura can feel their characteristic way, this method prevents the needle from going through the supraspinous and interspinous ligaments.

8.8.4.4. Special Spinal Techniques

When spinal anesthesia is administered continuously, compared to a single-shot spinal injection, the local anesthetic can be gradually dosed, allowing for more predictable titration of the block to the proper level and improved hemodynamic stability. Patients with severe aortic stenosis or pregnant women with complex cardiac disease can benefit from this method of controlling arterial blood pressure. It can also be applied in longer cases as an alternative to the combined spinal-epidural (CSE) technique, or in situations where prior spinal surgery could impede the spread of the epidural. There are spinal microcatheters available, but there has been a connection between cauda equina syndrome and small-gauge catheters (less than 24 G in particular), most likely due to lumbosacral pooling of local anesthetic. While there are catheter-over-the-needle devices that minimize CSF leakage around the catheter, they may be more challenging to insert. These devices are also available for use with continuous spinal anesthesia. Although the terms unilateral and selective spinal anesthesia are somewhat synonymous, they both refer to small dose methods that use patient positioning and baricity to speed healing. For instance, unilateral positioning and 4–5 mg of hyperbaric bupivacaine may be sufficient for knee arthroscopy. Minimal local anesthetic doses are applied in selective spinal anesthesia with the aim of only numbing the sensory fibers in a particular area.

8.8.5. Monitoring of the Block

After the spinal anesthetic is injected, heart rate and arterial blood pressure should be watched for any subsequent sympathetic blockade, and the onset, degree, and quality of the sensory and motor blocks must be evaluated. To evaluate sensory block, the most common methods are cold feeling and pinprick, which stand for C and A-delta fibers, respectively. First usually occurs loss of sensation to cold (verified with an ethyl chloride spray, ice, or alcohol) and then loss of sensation to pinprick (verified with a needle that does not pierce the skin). Eventually, touch sensitivity is lost. Although it only accounts for lumbosacral motor fibers, the modified Bromage scale is most frequently used to measure motor block. A motor block is generally regarded as sufficient if the level of block achieved with cold or pinprick is two to three segments above the anticipated level of surgical stimulus. (Covino et al., 1999)

8.9. Epidural Anesthesia

8.9.1. Factors Affecting Epidural Block Height

8.9.1.1. Drug Factors

The two most significant drug-related variables are the injectate's volume and total mass. Generally speaking, each segment that needs to be blocked should have 1 to 2 mL of solution injected. The onset, character, and duration of analgesia and anesthesia are influenced by bicarbonate, epinephrine, and opioids; they do not affect the spread of these effects.

8.9.1.2. Patient Factors

The height of the epidural block can vary with age. For thoracic epidurals in the elderly, up to 40% less volume may be needed. This could be due to reduced local anesthetic leakage through intervertebral foramina, decreased epidural space compliance, or increased nerve sensitivity. The local anesthetic's spread in the epidural space is only affected by the patient's height extremes. Block height and weight do not have a strong correlation. Pregnant patients require less local anesthetic to achieve the same epidural spread of anesthesia, partly due to engorgement of the epidural veins brought on by elevated abdominal pressure. When positive airway pressure is maintained, a thoracic epidural block becomes taller.

8.9.1.3. Procedure Factors

The most significant procedural factor influencing the height of the epidural block is the injection level. The spread of injectate is primarily caudal in the upper cervical region, equally cephalad and caudal in the midthoracic region, and primarily cephalad in the low thoracic region. There is more cephalad than caudal spread following a lumbar epidural. According to certain research, for a given injectate volume, there may be fewer blocked segments overall in the lumbar region than in the thoracic levels. Lumbar epidural injections are influenced by the position of the patient; in the lateral decubitus position, there is a preferential spread and faster onset to the dependent side. The height of the epidural block is unaffected by sitting or supine positions. In obstetric patients, the head-down tilt position does, however, increase spread. The spread of a bolus injection does not seem to be influenced by the direction or speed of the needle bevel.

8.9.2. Pharmacology

There are three types of local anesthetics for epidural use: short-, intermediate-, and long-acting medications. Depending on the type of anesthetic used and whether any additives are used, a single bolus dose of local anesthetic can produce surgical anesthesia for up to four hours. However, the most common practice is to leave an epidural catheter in place so that analgesia or anesthesia can be maintained indefinitely.

8.9.2.1. Short-Acting and Intermediate-Acting Local Anesthetics

- **Procaine** is not commonly used because the resultant block can be unreliable and of poor quality.
- **Chloroprocaine** is available in 2% and 3% preservative-free solutions. Prior to preservative-free preparations, large volumes of chloroprocaine had been associated with deep, burning lumbar back pain. This was thought to be secondary to the ethylenediaminetetraacetic acid that chelated calcium and caused a localized hypocalcemia.
- **Articaine** is not widely used for epidural anesthesia and has not been studied extensively.
- **Lidocaine** is available in 1% and 2% solutions. Unlike spinal anesthesia, TNS is not commonly associated with epidural lidocaine.
- **Prilocaine** is available in 2% and 3% solutions. The 2% solution produces a sensory block with minimal motor block. In large doses, prilocaine is associated with methemoglobinemia.

- **Mepivacaine** is available as 1%, 1.5%, and 2% preservative-free solutions. The 2% preparation has an onset time similar to that for lidocaine of approximately 15 minutes, but a slightly longer duration (up to 200 minutes with epinephrine).

8.9.2.2. Long-Acting Local Anesthetics

The lack of consistency in block height and the potential for systemic toxicity at higher doses have made tetracaine less popular. Preservative-free solutions of bupivacaine are offered in concentrations of 0.025 percent, 0.05% percent, and 0.075 percent. Analgesia can be achieved with more diluted concentrations, such as 0–125–0–25 percent. The central nervous system and heart toxicity, as well as the possibility of motor block from higher dosages, are drawbacks.

When applied topically, levobupivacaine is less cardiotoxic and exhibits the same clinical features as bupivacaine. There is no license to use liposomal bupivacaine for epidural pain. Preservative-free preparations of ropivacaine are offered in 0.2 percent, 0.5 percent, 0.75%, and 1.0 percent concentrations. When compared to bupivacaine, it has a better safety profile because it has a higher seizure threshold and less cardiotoxicity.

8.9.2.3. Epidural Additives

Vasoconstrictors

In the epidural space, epinephrine decreases the vascular absorption of local anesthetics. The effect is limited with ropivacaine, which already has intrinsic vasoconstrictive properties, and greater with lidocaine, mepivacaine, and chloroprocaine (up to 50% prolongation). It is less with bupivacaine and levobupivacaine. The analgesic effects of epinephrine may also stem from its absorption into CSF and activation of dorsal horn α2-receptors. Compared to epinephrine, phenylephrine is less effective and used less frequently.

Opioids

Without extending motor block, opioids complement the analgesic effects of epidural local anesthetics. When used together, local anesthetic and opioid lessen their respective dose-related side effects. The side effects of opioids are dose dependent, and it seems that there is a therapeutic ceiling effect, beyond which side effects only get worse. One can also use opioids on their own. To get to the CSF and spinal cord dorsal horn, epidural opioids must pass through the dura and arachnoid membrane. Hydrophilic opioids, like morphine and hydromorphone, are found in higher concentrations in CSF than lipophilic opioids, like fentanyl and sufentanil, which partition into epidural fat. The main analgesic mechanism may be fentanyl and sufentanil's easy absorption into the systemic circulation.

Epidural morphine can be injected continuously or as a bolus, lasting up to 24 hours. A bolus analgesic dose of 2–37.5 mg is the ideal amount to reduce side effects. Hydromorphone lasts for eighteen hours and is more lipophilic than morphine but more hydrophilic than fentanyl. The half-lives of epidural fentanyl and sufentanil are only two to three hours, but they start acting more quickly. In the UK, diamorphine is readily available. In order to avoid the problems associated with ongoing local anesthetic infusions and indwelling catheters, Depodur, an extended-release liposomal formulation of morphine, is administered as a single-shot lumbar epidural dose.

α_2-Agonists

Epidural clonidine lowers the need for opioids and epidural local anesthetics while also extending sensory block more than motor block. Although clonidine has sedation, bradycardia, hypotension, and dry mouth as side effects, it may also lessen cytokine response and immune stress. Dexmedetomidine can prolong both sensory and motor block and lessen the need for an intraoperative anesthetic. It can also enhance postoperative analgesia.

Other Drugs

Although they are not frequently used, ketamine, neostigmine, midazolam, tramadol, dexamethasone, and droperidol have all been studied.

Carbonation and Bicarbonate

The pH of the solution rises with both carbonation and the addition of bicarbonate, which in turn raises the nonionized free-base proportion of the local anesthetic. Data indicate that there are no clinical benefits for carbonated solutions, despite the possibility that this could speed up the onset and quality of the block by causing faster intraneural diffusion and faster penetration of the connective tissue surrounding the nerve trunk.

8.9.3. Technique

8.9.3.1. Preparation

The same patient preparation that was previously discussed for spinal anesthesia—consent, monitoring, resuscitation tools, and intravenous access—must also be used for epidural anesthesia. Since a catheter is frequently left in place, sterility may even be more crucial than spinal anesthesia. In order to place the epidural at the proper level and select the right medications, it is necessary to comprehend the type of surgery and its duration. Depending on how severe the patient's comorbid conditions are, there will be different risks and benefits. The most often used needles are tuohy needles. They are typically 16 to 18 G in weight, with a blunt Huber needle tip that is curved 15 to 30 degrees and is marked at 1-cm intervals. This design minimizes the possibility of an unintentional dural puncture and guides the catheter cephalad. A single end hole or several side orifices close to the tip can be found on this flexible, radiopaque plastic catheter. While having multiple orifices can enhance analgesia, parturients may experience an increase in epidural vein cannulation.

8.9.3.2. Position

The epidural puncture and spinal anesthesia require the same sitting and lateral decubitus positions, and the success rates are similar. Similar to spinal anesthesia, epidurals are best administered while the patient is awake.

8.9.3.3. Projection and Puncture

The inferior angle of the scapula (corresponding to the T7 vertebral body), the root of the scapular spine (T3), the vertebra prominens (C7), and the intercristal line (corresponding to the L4-L5 interspace) are significant surface landmarks. The right thoracic space can be determined with the use of ultrasonography. There are several different needle approaches available, including the midline, paramedian, caudal, and modified paramedian (Taylor approach). For lumbar and low thoracic approaches, a midline approach—where the angle of approach is only slightly cephalad—is frequently selected. The spinous processes in the midthoracic region have a significant downward angulation, so the approach should be more cephalad. With the stylet in place, the needle should be carefully advanced through the supraspinous ligament and into the interspinous ligament, where it can be removed and the syringe attached. This technique may raise the possibility of a false loss-of-resistance, potentially as a result of interspinous ligament abnormalities.

It is customary to use air or saline (or both) in combination to identify the epidural space by looking for a loss-of-resistance. Each entails using the dominant thumb to gently press the syringe bulb intermittently (for air) or continuously (for saline) while the nondominant hand advances the needle. The ligamentum flavum is typically recognized as a more robust structure with greater resistance. When the epidural space is subsequently entered, pressure on the syringe plunger permits the solution to pass through it without encountering any obstacles. Air is probably less accurate at determining the epidural space, increases the risk of an incomplete block, and, in rare instances, can even result in venous air embolism and pneumocephalus, which can give rise to headaches. However, when air versus saline was studied, the adverse outcomes in obstetric patients remained the same. The risk of the catheter cannulating an epidural vein can also be decreased by inserting fluid through the epidural needle prior to catheter insertion. Saline, however, might make it harder to spot an unintentional dural puncture.

With the hanging-drop technique, a drop of solution such as saline is placed within the hub of the needle after the needle is placed in the ligamentum flavum. When the needle tip reaches the epidural space, the solution is "sucked in" as a result of subatmospheric pressure inside the epidural space.

In the majority of patients (80%), the lumbar midline approach results in a depth of 3–5–6 cm from the skin to the ligamentum flavum. Prior to the insertion of the needle, ultrasound can forecast this depth. Once the epidural space has been located, the depth should be recorded, the syringe taken out, and a catheter threaded gently so that 4 to 6 cm remains in the space. The risk of catheter dislodgement and insufficient analgesia may increase if the catheter is shorter than 4 cm in the epidural space. There is a higher chance of catheter malposition or complications when there is more catheter threading. A special electrically conducting catheter can be used to confirm the location of the catheter tip using the Tsui test. This causes twitches in the corresponding muscles by stimulating the spinal nerve roots with a small electrical current.

8.9.3.4. Paramedian Approach

Because the spaces are narrower and the spine's angulation is steeper in the mid-to high-thoracic region, the paramedian approach is especially helpful in this area. One to two centimeters lateral to the inferior tip of the spinous process corresponding to the vertebra above the intended interspace is where the needle should be inserted. The needle is then moved medially and cephalad to enter the epidural space after being advanced horizontally until it reaches the lamina. The Taylor method, which modifies the paramedian approach via the L5-S1 interspace, may be helpful for trauma patients who are unable to tolerate or sustain a seated posture. The needle is positioned 45 to 55 degrees medially and cephalad, 1 cm medial and 1 cm inferior to the posterior superior iliac spine. A test dose may be given prior to starting an epidural local anesthetic infusion. This is done to rule out the implantation of intrathecal or intravascular catheters.

8.10. Combined Spinal-Epidural Anesthesia

While the epidural catheter enables anesthesia or analgesia to be extended as the spinal resolves, CSE anesthesia permits the flexibility of a rapid-onset spinal block. This is especially helpful for obstetrics. Another benefit is that a small amount of intrathecal local anesthetic can be given, and if needed, the block can be extended using the epidural catheter. By compressing the dural sac and raising the block height, local anesthetic or saline alone can be inserted via the catheter into the epidural space. The latter method, known as epidural volume extension (EVE), speeds up motor recovery considerably while enabling the use of lower intrathecal local anesthetic doses. For patients at high risk, this sequential technique also offers improved hemodynamic stability.

8.10.1. Technique

Typically, the epidural needle is inserted first, and then the spinal needle is inserted at the same or a different interspace using a "needle through needle" technique using kits that are specifically designed for that purpose. Although there is a chance that the in situ epidural catheter could be sheared, the distinct needle insertion technique offers the benefit of enabling verification of the epidural catheter's functionality prior to the administration of spinal anesthesia.

8.11. Caudal Anesthesia

Pediatric anesthesia frequently uses caudal anesthesia. When upper abdominal or thoracic spread is needed in adults, caudal anesthesia can be unpredictable. Thus, it can be used in adults with the same indications as lumbar epidural anesthesia. When a lumbar anesthetic technique cannot be used due to a spinal surgery scar, or more frequently in the management of chronic pain and cancer pain, it is most helpful when sacral anesthetic spread is desired (e.g., perineal, anal, rectal procedures). The proper placement of needles can be guided by both ultrasonography and fluoroscopy.

8.11.1. Pharmacology

The local anesthetics used are similar to those described for epidural anesthesia and analgesia. In adults, approximately twice the lumbar epidural dose is required to achieve a similar block with the caudal approach.

8.11.2. Technique

Caudal anesthesia requires the same level of patient preparation as previously mentioned. It is possible to employ the knee-chest, lateral decubitus, and prone positions. Sacral hiatus identification is necessary for caudal anesthesia. Between the two sacral cornua, the sacral hiatus is covered by the sacrococcygeal ligament, which is the extension of the ligamentum flavum. After determining the location of the posterior superior iliac spines, the sacral hiatus can be roughly located by utilizing the line that separates them as one side of an equilateral triangle.

Local anesthetic is infused once the sacral hiatus has been located, and the caudal needle—or Tuohy needle, if a catheter is to be inserted—is inserted at a 45-degree angle to the sacrum. As soon as the needle enters the caudal canal, resistance to needle insertion should start to decrease. The needle is moved forward until bone, that is. the ventral plate of the sacrum's dorsal aspect) is made contact with, slightly withdrew, and then redirected to reduce the angle of insertion with respect to the skin's surface. This angle is nearly parallel to the coronal plane in male patients; in female patients, a slightly steeper angle (15 degrees) is required. The needle is only redirected so far into the caudal canal, no more than 1 to 2 cm, and loss-of-resistance is monitored to ensure entry into the epidural space. The S2 level, which is the level to which the dural sac extends in adults, is about 1 cm below the posterior superior iliac spine, and this is the level beyond which the tip should never be advanced. Progression raises the possibility of inadvertent intravascular cannulation and dural puncture. Aspirate before administering any injection. (Covino et al., 1999)

8.12. Complications

It is important to distinguish clearly between complications, which suggest a degree of harm to the patient, and the physiological effects of the neuraxial technique. Because there is always a chance of catastrophic injury, it is important to fully comprehend and acknowledge the material risks connected to neuraxial anesthesia.

8.12.1. Neurologic

Serious neurologic complications associated with neuraxial anesthesia are rare.

8.12.1.1. Paraplegia

It is estimated that the frequency is 0.1 per 10,000. Such a serious injury most likely has a complex mechanism. The spinal cord can sustain direct needle trauma, but the intrathecal injectate may be neurotoxic. When the short-acting ester local anesthetic chloroprocaine was first prepared in the early 1980s, it contained the antioxidant sodium bisulfite preservative. This combination may have led to the development of adhesive arachnoiditis, cauda equina syndrome, or permanent paresis in some patients. The preservative was later discontinued. Severe hypotension or spinal cord ischemia may also be significant contributing factors. The earlier description of anterior spinal artery syndrome included the possibility of an irreversible, painless loss of motor and sensory function while proprioception was preserved.

8.12.1.2. Cauda Equina Syndrome

Cauda equina syndrome occurs at a rate of 0.1 per 10,000 and always leaves a permanent neurologic deficit behind. The spinal cord's lumbosacral roots could be especially susceptible to direct exposure to high concentrations of local anesthetic, regardless of whether the anesthetic is injected once into a relatively highly concentrated area (e.g., 5 percent lidocaine) or extended administration of a local anesthetic via a continuous catheter (small gauge in particular, as previously mentioned).

8.12.1.3. Epidural Hematoma

If bleeding within the vertebral canal is not identified and removed quickly, it may result in ischemic compression of the spinal cord and a permanent neurologic deficit. Numerous risk factors, such as coagulopathy, age, gender, and difficulty or trauma associated with needle or catheter insertion, have been linked to the development of an epidural hematoma. Features that are frequently linked to a space occupying lesion within the vertebral canal include radicular back pain, prolonged blockade longer than the anticipated duration of the neuraxial technique, and bladder or bowel dysfunction. These conditions should immediately prompt magnetic resonance imaging. About 0.07 out of 10,000 is the rate.

8.12.1.4. Nerve Injury

According to the current consensus, neuraxial anesthesia used in adult patients for perioperative anesthesia or analgesia is linked to a higher risk of neurologic complications than neuraxial anesthesia used in obstetric, pediatric, and chronic pain settings. Additionally, epidural anesthesia, including CSE anesthesia, is linked to a higher frequency of radiculopathy or peripheral neuropathy compared with spinal anesthesia. About 0.1 out of every 10,000 people sustain a permanent nerve injury. A risk factor is experiencing paresthesia or radicular pain while the surgery is being performed.

8.12.1.5. Post–Dural Puncture Headache

This headache, which can be caused by purposeful or inadvertent puncture of the dura membrane, is rather common. By using smaller gauge, noncutting tip spinal needles and aligning the needle bevel parallel to the spine's axis, the incidence of spinal anesthesia—which is about 1%—can be reduced. In the field of obstetrics, approximately 15 percent of patients may experience an unintentional dural puncture; of these, 52 to 80 percent will experience headaches after the puncture.

As the brain sags and loses support, the loss of CSF through the dura may put strain on pain-sensitive intracranial structures. It is possible that the removal of CSF causes an uncomfortable compensatory intracerebral vasodilation in order to counteract the drop in intracranial pressure. A post-dural puncture headache is characterized by a frontal or occipital headache that is better when lying supine and gets better when standing or sitting. Nausea, vomiting, dizziness, tinnitus, diplopia, hearing loss, cortical blindness, cranial nerve palsies, and even seizures are examples of associated symptoms. After the procedure, symptoms typically appear three days later, with 66% of cases occurring within the first 48 hours. Seven days is when most cases (72 percent) resolve spontaneously; the remaining 87 percent of cases resolve within six months (Table 8.4).

Table 8.4. *Published Trials of Anesthetic Agents for Spinal Procedures*

Authors and Year	Surgical Procedure	Comparison	Findings
Laureau et al., 1999 [**66**]	Posterior instrumentation for treatment of idiopathic scoliosis	Induction via intravenous propofol (*n* = 15) vs. midazolam (*n* = 15)	Cortical somatosensory-evoked potentials did not deteriorate in either the propofol or the midazolam induction groups.
Inoue et al., 2005 [**67**]	Cervical spine surgery for unspecified pathology	Anesthetic maintenance via fentanyl and propofol (*n* = 25) vs. fentanyl and <1% sevoflurane (*n* = 25) vs. sevoflurane (*n* = 25)	Perception of pain and bucking scores following emergence- were greater for patients exposed to sevoflurane versus propofol and fentanyl and fentanyl and sevoflurane in combination.
Kurt et al., 2005 [**68**]	Unspecified spinal procedure	Anesthetic maintenance via isoflurane (*n* = 12) vs. sevoflurane (*n* = 10) vs. desflurane (*n* = 10)	Sevoflurane and isoflurane administered via volatile anesthetics were able to achieve controlled hypotension in comparison to desflurane with systolic blood pressures outside the target range of 32% and 26% for isoflurane and sevoflurane, respectively, and 44% with desflurane.

Authors and Year	Surgical Procedure	Comparison	Findings
Albertin et al., 2008 [**69**]	Lumbar spine surgery for unspecified pathology	Induction via sevoflurane (*n* = 14) or propofol (*n* = 14) as main anesthetic agents	Peripheral blood flow was greater in the propofol group before and during the hypotensive period, but had reduced blood loss and intra-operative bleeding as compared to the sevoflurane group ($p < 0.005$).
Turgut et al., 2008 [**70**]	Lumbar laminectomy	Pre-operative bolus and anesthetic maintenance via dexmedetomidine (*n* = 25) vs. fentanyl (*n* = 25) following induction via propofol as well as maintenance	Extubation and discharge times were similar between dexmedetomidine and fentanyl, but MAP values after intubation for those exposed to dexmedetomidine were higher for those exposed to fentanyl before and after extubation. Supplemental analgesia was required earlier for fentanyl group patients (34.8 +/− 1.35 min vs. 60.4 +/− 1.04 min).

Source: Nguyen A, Mandavalli A, Diaz MJ, Root KT, Patel A, Casauay J, Perisetla P, Lucke-Wold B. Neurosurgical Anesthesia: Optimizing Outcomes with Agent Selection. Biomedicines. 2023; 11(2):372. https://doi.org/10.3390/biomedicines11020372.

For post-dural puncture headaches, conservative measures include sleeping on one's back, drinking plenty of water, taking coffee, and using oral painkillers. The results of using sumatriptan can vary. The most effective treatment for post-dural puncture headache is epidural blood patch therapy, which requires just one patch and has a 90% initial improvement rate as well as a 61–75% persistent resolution of symptoms in most cases. The best time to apply a blood patch is 24 hours following a dural puncture and once the typical headache symptoms associated with the procedure have appeared. Epidural blood patching as a preventive measure is ineffective. A reasonable starting target volume for the blood patch needle is 20 mL. It is advised to insert the needle at or caudad to the level of the dural puncture. If the first epidural blood patch doesn't work, a second one can be applied 24 to 48 hours later.

8.12.1.6. Transient Neurologic Symptoms

TNS is typified by either unilateral or bilateral buttock pain that travels down the legs, or, less frequently, by isolated leg or buttock pain. The onset of symptoms happens 24 hours after the spinal anesthetic wears off and is not linked to any abnormal lab results or neurologic deficits. Either mild or severe pain can usually go away on its own in less than a week. TNS occur much less frequently with bupivacaine and are more likely following intrathecal lidocaine and mepivacaine. The phenomenon is associated with solution osmolarity, dextrose or epinephrine addition, and lidocaine concentration. TNS are less frequently linked to epidural operations. In the lithotomy position for surgery, the risk is also higher. The first line of treatment is nonsteroidal anti-inflammatory drugs (NSAIDs), but opioids might be needed in some cases.

8.12.2. Cardiovascular

8.12.2.1. Hypotension

A combination of spinal and general anesthesia, spinal puncture at or above the L2-L3 interspace, age 40 years or above, peak block height greater than or equal to T5, baseline systolic blood pressure less than 120 mm Hg, and the addition of phenylephrine to the local anesthetic increase the risk of hypotension. Additionally, body mass index (BMI), history of hypertension, chronic alcohol use, and the urgency of surgery are independently linked to hypotension. In the context of neuraxial anesthesia, nausea is frequently a sign of hypotension; other symptoms include dyspnea, vomiting, and dizziness.

8.12.2.2. Bradycardia

The mechanism has been previously discussed, but baseline heart rate of less than 60 beats per minute, age under 37, male gender, no emergency, β-adrenergic blockade, and length of surgery are all risk factors for exaggerated bradycardia.

8.12.2.3. Cardiac Arrest

The cause of sudden cardiac arrest following spinal anesthesia is unknown, and this is an uncommon occurrence. Severe bradycardia and asystole that can happen unexpectedly during well-conducted spinal anesthesia may be caused by hypoxemia and oversedation. Strangely, spinal anesthesia—rather than epidural methods—is linked to these infrequent occurrences.

8.12.3. Respiratory

Neuraxial opioids carry a dose-dependent risk of respiratory depression, which has been reported to occur approximately 3% of the time following the injection of 0.8 mg of intrathecal morphine. The rostral spread of opioids from the CSF to the brainstem's chemosensitive respiratory centers may be the cause of respiratory depression. While late respiratory depression with intrathecal morphine may happen up to 24 hours after injection, respiratory depression with lipophilic anesthetics is typically an early phenomenon that happens within the first 30 minutes (and has not been reported after 2 hours). It is advised to monitor breathing for the first twenty-four hours following intrathecal morphine administration. Patients who have sleep apnea may be particularly sensitive, so extra care needs to be taken with them. Neuraxial opioid dosages should be lowered in older patients due to their increased risk of respiratory depression. Systemic sedative coadministration raises this risk as well.

8.12.4. Infection

Meningitis caused by bacteria and epidural abscesses are uncommon but potentially fatal side effects. While oral bacteria like *S. viridans* are a common cause of infection after spinal anesthesia, staphylococcal infections resulting from organisms on the patient's skin are among the most common epidural-related infections. Risk factors include diabetes, immunocompromised conditions, concomitant systemic infections, and extended epidural (or spinal) catheter maintenance. For spinal anesthesia, the risk of a major neuraxial infection is less than 0.3 per 10,000, but the risk of infectious complications following epidural procedures may be at least twice as high. Patients undergoing childbirth have a lower risk of developing deep infections associated with epidural analgesia. When it comes to neuraxial techniques, the best antiseptic is chlorhexidine in an alcohol base.

8.12.5. Backache

There is no association between epidural analgesia and new-onset back pain up to 6 months postpartum.

8.12.6. Nausea and Vomiting

It is possible for nausea and vomiting to result from either direct exposure of the brain's chemoreceptor trigger zone to emetogenic drugs (e.g., opioids), hypotension, or hyperperistalsis in the gastrointestinal tract brought on by unopposed parasympathetic activity. Addition of phenylephrine or epinephrine to the local anesthetic, peak block height greater than or equal to T5, baseline heart rate faster than 60 beats/min, use of procaine, history of motion sickness, and development of hypotension during spinal anesthesia are risk factors for nausea or vomiting following spinal anesthesia. The greatest risk of opioid-induced nausea or vomiting is associated with intrathecal morphine, while the lowest risk is associated with sufentanil and fentanyl. Once more, the effects are based on the dosage. Lowering the dosage of morphine by less than 0 points1 mg lowers the risk without sacrificing the analgesic effect.

8.12.7. Urinary Retention

Urinary retention can occur in as many as one third of patients after neuraxial anesthesia. Local anesthetic blockade of the S2, S3, and S4 nerve roots inhibits urinary function as the detrusor muscle is weakened. Neuraxial opioids can further complicate urinary function by suppressing detrusor contractility and reducing the sensation of urge. Spontaneous return of normal bladder function is expected once the sensory level decreases to less than S2-S3. Along with male gender and age, intrathecal morphine has also been linked to urinary retention after neuraxial anesthesia.

8.12.8. Pruritus

The most frequent adverse reaction associated with intrathecal opioid administration, with rates ranging from 30% to 100%, is pruritus, which can be quite upsetting. It is independent of the kind or dosage of opioid used, though cutting back on the dosage may lessen the chance of pruritus. Treatment options include nalbuphine, a partial agonist, naltrexone, or naloxone. Propofol and ondansetron are also helpful medications.

8.12.9. Shivering

Shivering occurs up to 55% of the time and is more common with epidural than with spinal anesthesia. A possible explanation is that the relatively low temperature of the epidural injectate may have an impact on the basal sinuses, which are sensitive to temperature. Neuraxial opioids, such as meperidine and fentanyl, are added to lessen the chance of shivering. Shivering can be lessened by using a forced air warmer to warm the patient beforehand and by avoiding giving cold intravenous and epidural fluids.

8.12.10 Complications Unique to Epidural Anesthesia

8.12.10.1. Intravascular Injection

Epidural anesthesia may result in systemic toxicity induced by local anesthetic, mainly from inadvertent drug administration into an epidural vein. Vascular punctures with needles or catheters can occur up to 10% of the time. These punctures are most common in the obstetric population, when the vessels are relatively dilated. Epidural anesthesia-related seizures could occur as often as 1% of the time. In obstetrics, the risk of intravascular injection is reduced by using a single-orifice catheter rather than a multiorifice catheter or a wire-embedded polyurethane rather than a polyamide epidural catheter, advancing the catheter less than 6 cm into the epidural space, and positioning the patient in the lateral position during needle and catheter insertion. The danger of epidural vein cannulation is not decreased by the paramedian technique or by using a smaller-gauge epidural needle or catheter. Aspirating the catheter and gradually administering the local anesthetic is the best way to prevent systemic toxicity because using epinephrine mixed with local anesthetic as a test dose can be unreliable.

8.12.10.2. Subdural Injection

In human autopsies, the subdural extra-arachnoid space is easily accessed. It is a rare clinical issue that occurs with epidural anesthesia (<1%). Nonetheless, subdural local anesthetic placement needs to be taken into consideration if an epidural block is executed and a higher-than-expected block appears 15 to 30 minutes after injection. When there is a subdural block, the sympathetic block might be heightened and the motor block will be less severe than the sensory block. This is a symptomatic treatment.(Mackey, 1996) (Table 8.5).

Table 8.5. *Summary of Different and Recently Developed Techniques for Epidural Spinal Needles*

Technology	Merits	Drawbacks
Ultrasound-guided epidural needle	- Real-time and pre-procedural ultrasound guiding of the procedure is possible using ultrasound imaging of anatomical landmarks; - The depth of the EDS and the angle of the needle insertion can both be determined by ultrasound.	- Relatively expensive; - Technical complications of co-registrations of ultrasound and epidural needle for the needle to be fully automated; - Lack of measured data for force/pressure feedback
Haptic feedback-based devices	- Enclosed in portable cases; - Connect to laptops with graphic displays.	- Lack of measured data for force/pressure feedback
Epidural pressure measurement-based devices	- Monitor and record needle-inserted pressure; - Compact system.	- Different tissues are not identified through insertions; - Needs to be calibrated.

Technology	Merits	Drawbacks
FBG-based devices	- Dynamic data of force variation on the spinal needle with a high resolution.	- Require specific design of the FBGs.
OCT-based devices	- Image the tissue in front of the needle tip; - Deep learning models can be applied to automatically process the imaging data for needle localization.	- Relatively expensive.

Source: *Althobaiti M, Ali S, Hariri NG, Hameed K, Alagl Y, Alzahrani N, Alzahrani S, Al-Naib I. Recent Advances in Smart Epidural Spinal Needles. Sensors. 2023; 23(13):6065. https://doi.org/10.3390/s23136065.*

A Closer Look

Caudal Epidural Anesthesia

Caudal epidural anesthesia, often simply referred to as caudal anesthesia, is a regional anesthesia technique utilized to provide pain relief for various surgical procedures, particularly those involving the lower abdomen, pelvis, or lower extremities. It is also commonly employed as a method of pain management during labor and delivery.

This technique involves the administration of local anesthetic medication into the caudal epidural space, which is situated near the base of the spine. The caudal epidural space is accessed through the sacral hiatus, a small opening in the sacrum bone located just above the coccyx (tailbone). By injecting medication into this space, the nerves that transmit pain signals from the lower body are temporarily blocked, resulting in pain relief.

The procedure typically begins with the patient positioned either on their side or lying face down, depending on the preference of the healthcare provider and the specific needs of the patient. Using anatomical landmarks or, in some cases, ultrasound guidance, a needle is carefully inserted through the skin and into the sacral hiatus. Once the needle is correctly positioned within the caudal epidural space, the local anesthetic medication is injected.

Caudal epidural anesthesia offers several advantages. It provides effective pain relief while minimizing the need for general anesthesia, which can carry its own risks and side effects. Additionally, because the medication is administered directly to the site of the nerves responsible for transmitting pain signals, caudal anesthesia can offer targeted pain relief with fewer systemic effects compared to some other forms of anesthesia.

This technique is particularly well-suited for use in pediatric patients undergoing lower abdominal or pelvic surgeries, as well as in obstetric patients during labor and delivery. In pediatric patients, caudal anesthesia is often preferred because it can reduce the need for postoperative opioid medications, which may be associated with more side effects and complications in this population.

While caudal epidural anesthesia is generally considered safe and effective, it is not without risks. Potential complications include infection at the injection site, bleeding, nerve damage, or unintentional puncture of the dura mater, the outermost layer of the spinal cord. However, these risks can typically be minimized through careful patient selection, proper technique, and vigilant monitoring during and after the procedure.

Caudal epidural anesthesia is a valuable tool in the management of perioperative pain, particularly for surgeries and procedures involving the lower body. Its ability to provide targeted pain relief with minimal systemic effects makes it a preferred choice for many patients and healthcare providers alike.

Summary

- Spinal, epidural, and caudal anesthesia are indispensable techniques in modern anesthesia practice, providing effective pain relief and anesthesia for a wide range of surgical procedures and obstetric care.
- Spinal, epidural, and caudal blocks are collectively referred to as central neuraxial blocks. Significant technical, physiologic, and pharmacologic differences exist between the techniques, although all result in one or a combination of sympathetic, sensory, and motor blockade.
- Neuraxial blockade is widely utilized in surgery, obstetrics, acute postoperative pain management, and chronic pain relief. Single-injection spinal or epidural anesthesia is commonly used for surgery to the lower abdomen, pelvic organs (e.g., prostate), and lower limbs and for cesarean deliveries.
- The spinal cord is continuous with the medulla oblongata proximally and terminates distally in the conus medullaris as the filum terminale (fibrous extension) and the cauda equina (neural extension). This distal termination varies from L3 in infants to the lower border of L1 in adults.
- Dorsal (afferent) and ventral (efferent) nerve roots merge distal to the dorsal root ganglion to form spinal nerves. There are 31 pairs of spinal nerves (8 cervical, 12 thoracic, 5 lumbar, 5 sacral, and 1 coccygeal).
- Variations exist in the size and structure of the spinal nerve roots as well as CSF volume, both of which may contribute to variability in spinal block quality, height, and regression time.
- Blockade of the peripheral (T1-L2) and cardiac (T1-T4) sympathetic fibers as well as adrenal medullary catecholamine secretion reduces systemic vascular resistance (SVR) and, to a much lesser extent, cardiac output.
- Cardiac output is the product of heart rate and stroke volume and it is generally either maintained or slightly decreased during the onset of spinal anesthesia. Venous and arterial vasodilation reduces preload (venous return) and afterload (SVR), respectively.
- The potential rapid and significant reduction in SVR after spinal anesthesia is in theory a risk in preload dependent patients and may dangerously decrease coronary perfusion.
- The clinical effects of intrathecal local anesthetics are mediated by drug uptake and distribution within the CSF, and elimination. These variables in turn are dictated in part by the pKa (dissociation ionization constant), lipid solubility, and protein binding of the local anesthetic solution.
- Epinephrine and phenylephrine prolong sensory and motor blockade when added to local anesthetics. The α_1- adrenergic-mediated vasoconstriction reduces systemic local anesthetic uptake and epinephrine may also enhance analgesia via a direct α_2-adrenergic-mediated effect.
- Local anesthetics for epidural use may be classified into short-, intermediate-, and long-acting drugs. A single bolus dose of local anesthetic can provide surgical anesthesia

ranging from 45 minutes up to 4 hours depending on the type administered and the use of any additives.

- Opioids synergistically enhance the analgesic effects of epidural local anesthetics, without prolonging motor block. A combination of local anesthetic and opioid reduces the dose-related adverse effects of each drug independently.
- Patient preparation as previously described for spinal anesthesia must equally be applied to epidural anesthesia, namely consent, monitoring, resuscitation equipment, and intravenous access. Sterility is arguably even more important than spinal anesthesia because a catheter is often left in situ.
- CSE anesthesia allows the flexibility of a rapid onset spinal block while the epidural catheter allows anesthesia or analgesia to be extended as the spinal resolves.
- Caudal anesthesia is popular in pediatric anesthesia. In adults, caudal anesthesia is unpredictable when upper abdominal or thoracic spread is required. Therefore, its indications in adults are the same as those for lumbar epidural anesthesia.

References

1. Afshan, G., Chohan, U., Khan, F. A., et al. (2011). Appropriate length of epidural catheter in the epidural space for postoperative analgesia: Evaluation by epidurography. *Anaesthesia, 66*, 913–918.
2. American Society of Anesthesiologists Task Force on Neuraxial Opioids, Horlocker, T. T., Burton, A. W., Connis, R. T., et al. (2009). Practice guidelines for the prevention, detection, and management of respiratory depression associated with neuraxial opioid administration. *Anesthesiology, 110*, 218–230.
3. Auroy, Y., Benhamou, D., Bargues, L., et al. (2002). Major complications of regional anesthesia in France: The SOS Regional Anesthesia Hotline Service. *Anesthesiology, 97*, 1274–1280.
4. Beattie, W. S., Badner, N. H., & Choi, P. (2001). Epidural analgesia reduces postoperative myocardial infarction: A meta-analysis. *Anesthesia & Analgesia, 93*, 853–858.
5. Bell, D. N., & Leslie, K. (2007). Detection of intravascular epidural catheter placement: A review. *Anesthesia and Intensive Care, 35*, 335–341.
6. Bernards, C. M., & Hill, H. F. (1990). Morphine and alfentanil permeability through the spinal dura, arachnoid, and pia mater of dogs and monkeys. *Anesthesiology, 73*, 1214–1219.
7. Borgeat, A., Ekatodramis, G., & Schenker, C. A. (2003). Postoperative nausea and vomiting in regional anesthesia: A review. *Anesthesiology, 98*, 530–547.
8. Bromage, P. R. (1965). A comparison of the hydrochloride and carbon dioxide salts of lidocaine and prilocaine in epidural analgesia. *Acta Anesthesiologic Scandinavica Supplementum, 16*, 55–69.
9. Brull, R., McCartney, C. J. L., Chan, V. W. S., & El-Beheiry, H. (2007). Neurological complications after regional anesthesia: Contemporary estimates of risk. *Anesthesia & Analgesia, 104*, 965–974.
10. Carpenter, R. L., Hogan, Q. H., Liu, S. S., et al. (1998). Lumbosacral cerebrospinal fluid volume is the primary determinant of sensory block extent and duration during spinal anesthesia. *Anesthesiology, 89*, 24–29.

11. Casati, A., & Vinciguerra, F. (2002). Intrathecal anesthesia. *Current Opinion in Anesthesiology, 15*, 543–551.
12. Casati, A., Fanelli, G., Cappelleri, G., et al. (1998). Effects of spinal needle type on lateral distribution of 0.5% hyperbaric bupivacaine. *Anesthesia & Analgesia, 87*, 355–359.
13. Chin, K. J., Karmakar, M. K., & Peng, P. (2011). Ultrasonography of the adult thoracic and lumbar spine for central neuraxial blockade. *Anesthesiology, 114*, 1459–1485.
14. Choi, P. T., Galinski, S. E., Takeuchi, L., et al. (2003). PDPH is a common complication of neuraxial blockade in parturient: A meta-analysis of obstetrical studies. *Canadian Journal of Anesthesia, 50*, 460–469.
15. Choi, S., & Brull, R. (2009). Neuraxial techniques in obstetric and non-obstetric patients with common bleeding diatheses. *Anesthesia & Analgesia, 109*, 648–660.
16. Cook, T. M., Counsell, D., & Wildsmith, J. A. W. (2009). Royal College of Anesthetists Third National Audit Project. Major complications of central neuraxial block: Report on the Third National Audit Project of the Royal College of Anesthetists. *British Journal of Anaesthesia, 102*, 179–190.
17. Covino, B. G., Scott, D. B., & McClure, J. H. (1999). *Handbook of Epidural Anaesthesia and Analgesia*. Fribourg, Switzerland: Mediglobe.
18. Crowley, L. J., & Buggy, D. J. (2008). Shivering and neuraxial anesthesia. *Regional Anesthesia and Pain Medicine, 33*, 241–252.
19. Crystal, G. J., & Salem, M. R. (2012). The Bainbridge and the "reverse" Bainbridge reflexes: History, physiology, and clinical relevance. *Anesthesia & Analgesia, 114*, 520–532.
20. Flaatten, H., Rodt, S. A., Vamnes, J., et al. (1989). Postdural puncture headache. A comparison between 26- and 29-gauge needles in young patients. *Anaesthesia, 44*, 147–149.
21. Freise, H., & Fischer, L. G. (2009). Intestinal effects of thoracic epidural anesthesia. *Current Opinion in Anesthesiology, 22*, 644–648.
22. Goldblum, E., & Atchabahian, A. (2013). The use of 2-chloroprocaine for spinal anaesthesia. *Acta Anesthesiologic Scandinavica, 57*, 545–552.
23. Gozdemir, M., Muslu, B., Sert, H., et al. (2010). Transient neurological symptoms after spinal anesthesia with levobupivacaine 5 mg/ml or lidocaine 20 mg/ml. *Acta Anesthesiologic Scandinavica, 54*, 59–64.
24. Greene, N. M. (1981). *Physiology of Spinal Anesthesia* (3rd ed.). Baltimore: Williams & Wilkins.
25. Greene, N. M. (1985). Distribution of local anesthetic solutions within the subarachnoid space. *Anesthesia & Analgesia, 64*, 715–730.
26. Groeben, H. (2006). Epidural anesthesia and pulmonary function. *Journal of Anesthesia, 20*, 290–299.
27. Guay, J., Choi, P. T., Suresh, S., et al. (2014). Neuraxial anesthesia for the prevention of postoperative mortality and major morbidity: An overview of Cochrane Systematic Reviews. *Anesthesia & Analgesia, 119*, 716–725.
28. Gwirtz, K. H., Young, J. V., Byers, R. S., et al. (1999). The safety and efficacy of intrathecal opioid analgesia for acute postoperative pain: Seven years' experience with 5969 surgical patients at Indiana University Hospital. *Anesthesia & Analgesia, 88*, 599–604.

29. Hamber, E. A., & Viscomi, C. M. (1999). Intrathecal lipophilic opioids as adjuncts to surgical spinal anesthesia. *Regional Anesthesia and Pain Medicine, 24*, 255–263.

30. Harrington, B. E. (2004). Postdural puncture headache and the development of the epidural blood patch. *Regional Anesthesia and Pain Medicine, 29*, 136–163.

31. Hartmann, B., Junger, A., Klasen, J., et al. (2002). The incidence and risk factors for hypotension after spinal anesthesia induction: An analysis with automated data collection. *Anesthesia & Analgesia, 94*, 1521–1529.

32. Hawkins, J. L. (2010). Epidural analgesia for labor and delivery. *New England Journal of Medicine, 362*, 1503–1510.

33. Hebl, J. R. (2006). The importance and implications of aseptic techniques during regional anesthesia. *Regional Anesthesia and Pain Medicine, 31*, 311–323.

34. Hebl, J. R., Horlocker, T. T., Kopp, S. L., & Schroeder, D. R. (2010). Neuraxial blockade in patients with preexisting spinal stenosis, lumbar disk disease, or prior spine surgery: Efficacy and neurologic complications. *Anesthesia & Analgesia, 111*, 1511–1519.

35. Hilt, H., Gramm, H. J., & Link, J. (1986). Changes in intracranial pressure associated with extradural anesthesia. *British Journal of Anesthesia, 58*, 676–680.

36. Hocking, G., & Wildsmith, J. A. W. (2004). Intrathecal drug spread. *British Journal of Anaesthesia, 93*, 568–578.

37. Horlocker, T. T. (2004). What's a nice patient like you doing with a complication like this? Diagnosis, prognosis and prevention of spinal hematoma. *Canadian Journal of Anesthesia, 51*, 527–534.

38. Joshi, G. P., Bonnet, F., Shah, R., et al. (2008). The comparative effects of postoperative analgesic therapies on pulmonary outcome: Cumulative meta-analyses of randomized, controlled trials. *Anesthesia & Analgesia, 107*, 1026–1040.

39. Kim, J. T., Shim, J. K., Kim, S. H., et al. (2007). Trendelenburg position with hip flexion as a rescue strategy to increase spinal anesthetic level after spinal block. *British Journal of Anaesthesia, 98*, 396–400.

40. Kuipers, P. W., Kamphuis, E. T., van Venrooij, G. E., et al. (2004). Intrathecal opioids and lower urinary tract function: A urodynamic evaluation. *Anesthesiology, 100*, 1497–1503.

41. Leslie, K., McIlroy, D., Kasza, J., et al. (2016). Neuraxial block and postoperative epidural analgesia: Effects on outcomes in the POISE-2 trial. *British Journal of Anaesthesia, 116*, 100–112.

42. Lew, E., Yeo, S. W., & Thomas, E. (2004). Combined spinal-epidural anesthesia using epidural volume extension leads to faster motor recovery after elective cesarean delivery: A prospective, randomized, double-blind study. *Anesthesia & Analgesia, 98*, 810–814.

43. Liu, S., Kopacz, D. J., & Carpenter, R. L. (1995). Quantitative assessment of differential sensory nerve block after lidocaine spinal anesthesia. *Anesthesiology, 82*, 60–63.

44. Macfarlane, A. J. R., Prasad, G. A., Chan, V. W. S., & Brull, R. (2009). Does regional anesthesia improve outcome after total hip arthroplasty? A systematic review. *British Journal of Anesthesia, 103*, 335–345.

45. Macfarlane, A. J. R., Prasad, G. A., Chan, V. W. S., & Brull, R. (2009). Does regional anesthesia improve outcome after total knee arthroplasty? *Clinical Orthopedics and Related Research, 467*, 2379–2402.

46. Mackey, D. (1996). Physiologic effects of regional block. In D. L. Brown (Ed.), *Regional Anesthesia and Analgesia* (pp. 29–38). Philadelphia: WB Saunders.

47. Malinovsky, J. M., Renaud, G., Le Corre, P., et al. (1999). Intrathecal bupivacaine in humans: Influence of volume and baricity of solutions. *Anesthesiology, 91*, 1260–1266.

48. Marinacci, A. A. (1960). Neurological aspects of complications of spinal anesthesia, with medicolegal implications. *Bulletin of the Los Angeles Neurological Society, 25*, 170–192.

49. McDonald, S. B. (2004). Is neuraxial blockade contraindicated in the patient with aortic stenosis? *Regional Anesthesia and Pain Medicine, 29*, 496–502.

50. Meylan, N., Elia, N., Lysakowski, C., & Tramèr, M. R. (2009). Benefit and risk of intrathecal morphine without local anesthetic in patients undergoing major surgery: Meta-analysis of randomized trials. *British Journal of Anaesthesia, 102*, 156–167.

51. Mhyre, J. M., Lou, V. H., Greenfield, M., et al. (2009). A systematic review of randomized controlled trials that evaluate strategies to avoid epidural vein cannulation during obstetric epidural catheter placement. *Anesthesia & Analgesia, 108*, 1232–1242.

52. Minville, V., Asehnoune, K., Salau, S., et al. (2009). The effects of spinal anesthesia on cerebral blood flow in the very elderly. *Anesthesia & Analgesia, 108*, 1291–1294.

53. Moore, D. C., Spierdijk, J., vanKleef, J. D., et al. (1982). Chloroprocaine neurotoxicity: Four additional cases. *Anesthesia & Analgesia, 61*, 155–159.

54. Moore, J. M. (2009). Continuous spinal anesthesia. *American Journal of Therapeutics, 16*, 289–294.

55. Morison, D. H. (1995). Alkalinization of local anesthetics. *Canadian Journal of Anesthesia, 42*, 1076–1079.

56. Murphy, P. M., Stack, D., Kinirons, B., & Laffey, J. G. (2003). Optimizing the dose of intrathecal morphine in older patients undergoing hip arthroplasty. *Anesthesia & Analgesia, 97*, 1709–1715.

57. Nair, G. S., Abrishami, A., Lermitte, J., & Chung, F. (2009). Systematic review of spinal anaesthesia using bupivacaine for ambulatory knee arthroscopy. *British Journal of Anaesthesia, 102*, 307–315.

58. Neal, J. M., Barrington, M. J., Brull, R., et al. (2015). The Second ASRA Practice Advisory on Neurologic Complications Associated with Regional Anesthesia and Pain Medicine: Executive Summary 2015. *Regional Anesthesia and Pain Medicine, 40*(5), 401–430.

59. Nishimori, M., Low, J. H. S., Zheng, H., & Ballantyne, J. C. (2012). Epidural pain relief versus systemic opioid-based pain relief for abdominal aortic surgery. *Cochrane Database of Systematic Reviews, 2012*(7), CD005059.

60. Olausson, K., Magnusdottir, H., Lurje, L., et al. (1997). Anti-ischemic and anti-anginal effects of thoracic epidural anesthesia versus those of conventional medical therapy in the treatment of severe refractory unstable angina pectoris. *Circulation, 96*, 2178–2182.

61. Paech, M. J., Doherty, D. A., Christmas, T., & Wong, C. A. (2011). Epidural blood patch trial group: The volume of blood for epidural blood patch in obstetrics: A randomized, blinded clinical trial. *Anesthesia & Analgesia, 113*, 126–133.

62. Perlas, A., & Chan, V. W. S. (2005). Neuraxial anesthesia and multiple sclerosis. *Canadian Journal of Anesthesia, 52*, 454–458.

63. Rathmell, J. P., Lair, T. R., & Nauman, B. (2005). The role of intrathecal drugs in the treatment of acute pain. *Anesthesia & Analgesia, 101*(5 Suppl), S30–S43.

64. Rawal, N. (2005). Combined spinal-epidural anesthesia. *Current Opinion in Anaesthesiology, 18*, 518–521.

65. Rigler, M. L., Drasner, K., Krejcie, T. C., et al. (1991). Cauda equina syndrome after continuous spinal anesthesia. *Anesthesia & Analgesia, 72*, 275–281.

66. Sanderson, P., Read, J., Littlewood, D. G., et al. (1994). Interaction between baricity (glucose concentration) and other factors influencing intrathecal drug spread. *British Journal of Anaesthesia, 73*, 744–746.

67. Sarantopoulos, C., & Fassoulaki, A. (1994). Systemic opioids enhance the spread of sensory analgesia produced by intrathecal lidocaine. *Anesthesia & Analgesia, 79*, 94–97.

68. Schier, R., Guerra, D., Aguilar, J., et al. (2009). Epidural space identification: A meta-analysis of complications after air versus liquid as the medium for loss of resistance. *Anesthesia & Analgesia, 109*, 2012–2021.

69. Stevens, R. A., Urmey, W. F., Urquhart, B. L., & Kao, T. C. (1993). Back pain after epidural anesthesia with chloroprocaine. *Anesthesiology, 78*, 492–497.

70. Sultan, P., Gutierrez, M. C., & Carvalho, B. (2011). Neuraxial morphine and respiratory depression: Finding the right balance. *Drugs, 71*, 1807–1819.

71. Svircevic, V., van Dijk, D., Nierich, A. P., et al. (2011). Meta-analysis of thoracic epidural anesthesia versus general anesthesia for cardiac surgery. *Anesthesiology, 114*, 271–282.

72. Taivainen, T., Tuominen, M., & Rosenberg, P. H. (1990). Influence of obesity on the spread of spinal analgesia after injection of plain 0.5% bupivacaine at the L3-4 or L4-5 interspace. *British Journal of Anesthesia, 64*, 542–546.

73. Tetzlaff, J. E., O'Hara, J., Bell, G., et al. (1995). Influence of baricity on the outcome of spinal anesthesia with bupivacaine for lumbar spine surgery. *Regional Anesthesia, 20*, 533–537.

74. Tsui, B. C., Gupta, S., & Finucane, B. (1998). Confirmation of epidural catheter placement using nerve stimulation. *Canadian Journal of Anesthesia, 45*, 640–644.

75. Turnbull, D. K., & Shepherd, D. B. (2003). Post-dural puncture headache: Pathogenesis, prevention and treatment. *British Journal of Anesthesia, 91*, 718–729.

76. Urmey, W. F., Stanton, J., Bassin, P., & Sharrock, N. E. (1997). The direction of the Whitacre needle aperture affects the extent and duration of isobaric spinal anesthesia. *Anesthesia & Analgesia, 84*, 337–341.

77. Vaghadia, H., Viskari, D., Mitchell, G. W., & Berrill, A. (2001). Selective spinal anesthesia for outpatient laparoscopy. I: Characteristics of three hypobaric solutions. *Canadian Journal of Anesthesia, 48*, 256–260.

78. Van Zundert, A. A., Grouls, R. J., Korsten, H. H., & Lambert, D. H. (1996). Spinal anesthesia: Volume or concentration—What matters? *Regional Anesthesia, 21*, 112–118.

79. Visser, W. A., Lee, R. A., & Gielen, M. J. M. (2008). Factors affecting the distribution of neural blockade by local anesthetics in epidural anesthesia and a comparison of lumbar versus thoracic epidural anesthesia. *Anesthesia & Analgesia, 107*, 708–721.

80. Visser, W. A., Liem, T. H., van Egmond, J., & Gielen, M. J. (1998). Extension of sensory blockade

after thoracic epidural administration of a test dose of lidocaine at three different levels. *Anesthesia & Analgesia, 86*, 332–335.

81. Wedel, D. J., & Horlocker, T. T. (2006). Regional anesthesia in the febrile or infected patient. *Regional Anesthesia and Pain Medicine, 31*, 324–333.
82. Whiteside, J. B., & Burke, D. (2003). Comparison of ropivacaine 0.5% (in glucose 5%) with bupivacaine 0.5% (in glucose 8%) for spinal anesthesia for elective surgery. *British Journal of Anesthesia, 90*, 304–308.
83. Zaric, D., & Pace, N. L. (2009). Transient neurologic symptoms (TNS) following spinal anaesthesia with lidocaine versus other local anesthetics. *Cochrane Database of Systematic Reviews, 2009*(2), CD003006.
84. Zarzur, E. (1984). Anatomic studies of the human ligamentum flavum. *Anesthesia & Analgesia, 63*, 499–502.

Chapter

OUTPATIENT ANESTHESIA

9

Contents

Introduction

Many of the perioperative technological and pharmaceutical advancements of the last 200 years are embodied in outpatient anesthesia. Nowadays, the majority of surgeries are performed as outpatients; patients travel from their homes to a surgical facility, where they receive an operation or intervention, and then go back to recover with their loved ones. But the day of surgery and anesthesia is just one part of the outpatient surgical and anesthetic experience; the other begins much earlier and lasts much longer.

The vision for outpatient anesthesia began 100 years ago when Dr. Ralph Waters opened the first modern ambulatory surgery center (ASC) in downtown Sioux City, Iowa, "the Downtown Anesthesia Clinic." In the late 1950s and early 1960s, outpatient surgery facilities were opened in Canada and the United Kingdom to relieve waitlists for elective surgery in hospitals. In 1962, Dr. David Cohen and Dr. John Dillon opened an outpatient surgery clinic, which would be a precursor to the modern "surgicenter."

They suggested standardizing the patient pathway and flow while paying close attention to quality metrics, patient evaluation and selection, and equipment availability. They produced positive results and showed considerable savings for insurance companies and patients. Drs. Wallace Reed and John Ford founded the first contemporary American ASC, the Phoenix Surgicenter, in 1970 as the cost of inpatient surgery increased. Their main objective was to lower surgical costs for patients without sacrificing quality or safety. These locations epitomized the benefits that surgery centers and office-based surgical practices continue to offer: superior care, patient and family convenience, and financial savings for the surgical team. Important components of that convenience include promptness, efficiency in operations, and superior clinical results in terms of the patient experience.

Orientation and Directional Terms

Term	Definition	Illustration
Postanaesthesia discharge scoring system (PADSS)	Postanaesthesia discharge scoring system (PADSS) is the most commonly used tool to determine home readiness. This scoring system requires that patients have stable vital signs, can ambulate at preoperative level, and have minimal postoperative nausea and vomiting (PONV), pain and bleeding.	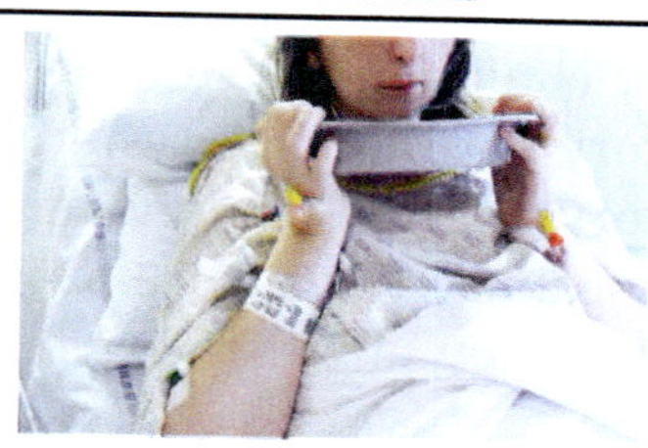
Post-anesthesia care unit (PACU)	Post-anesthesia care unit (PACU) and sometimes referred to as post-anesthesia recovery or PAR, or simply recovery, is a part of hospitals, ambulatory care centers, and other medical facilities.	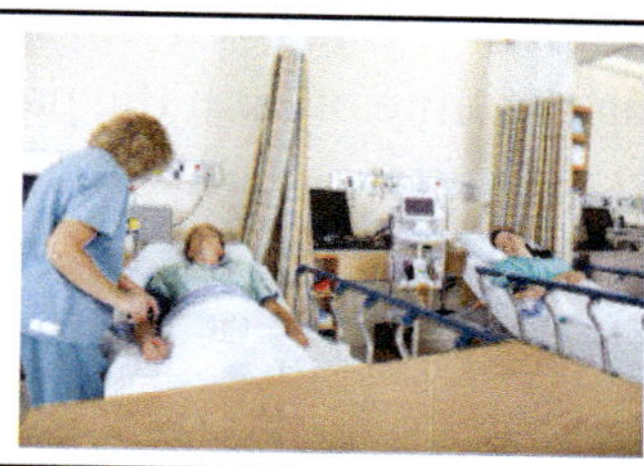
Advanced Cardiac Life Support (ACLS)	Advanced cardiac life support refers to a set of clinical guidelines established by the American Heart Association (AHA) for the urgent and emergent treatment of life-threatening cardiovascular conditions that will cause or have caused cardiac arrest, using advanced medical procedures, medications, and techniques.	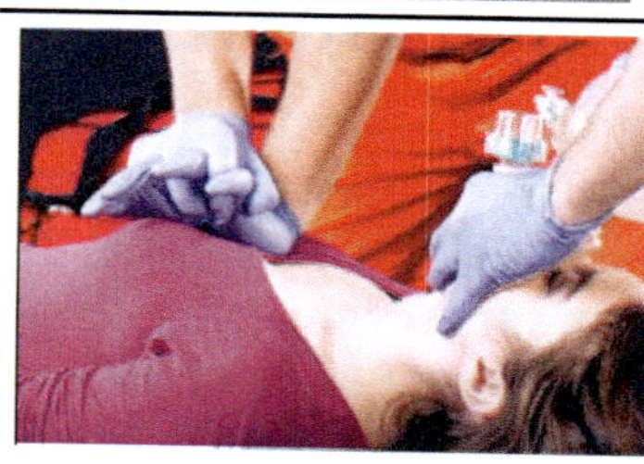
Laparoscopic cholecystectomy	Laparoscopic cholecystectomy is a minimally invasive surgical procedure for removal of a diseased gallbladder. This technique essentially has replaced the open technique for routine cholecystectomies since the early 1990s.	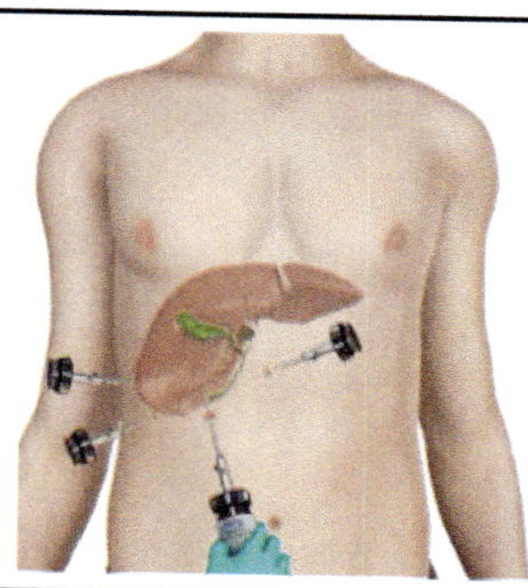
Obstructive sleep apnea	Obstructive sleep apnea is the most common sleep-related breathing disorder. People with obstructive sleep apnea repeatedly stop and start breathing while they sleep. There are several types of sleep apnea. Obstructive sleep apnea occurs when the throat muscles relax and block the airway.	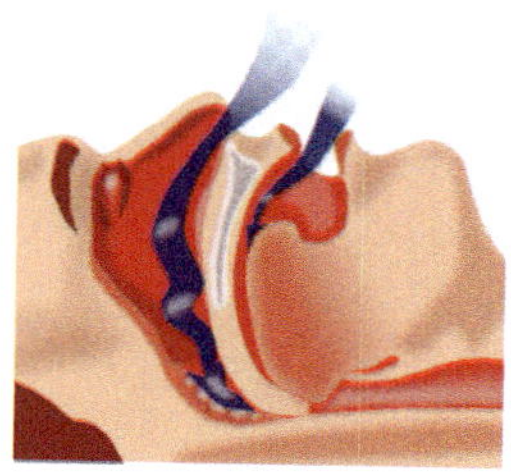

9.1. Outpatient Anesthesia is Different

The Society for Ambulatory Anesthesia (SAMBA) was established in 1985 with the goal of defining the outpatient anesthesia field. SAMBA established guidelines and standards of care, which influenced research, clinical practice, and education. Many surgeries conducted nationwide moved to the ambulatory setting as a result of advances in anesthesiology and surgery technology, and the ambulatory anesthesia provider's practice patterns quickly changed along with the shift. While not all anesthesiologists are expected to perform complex heart valve replacement surgery under anesthesia, they might be expected to perform an effective ambulatory anesthetic.

An anesthetic that is followed by a patient's discharge home is not the same as an ambulatory or outpatient anesthetic. An outpatient anesthetic procedure maximizes predictability by planning ahead and preventing even the smallest morbidities in the hours to days that follow the procedure, respecting the time of both the patient and the surgeon as valuable resources. In summary, outpatient anesthesia is patient-centered, affordable, accessible, multidisciplinary, and, at its core, a model for the "Surgical Home." (Vila et al,2008; American Society of Anesthesiologists guidelines for office-based anesthesia; American Society of Anesthesiologists Task Force on Acute Pain Management, 2012)

9.2. Outpatient Anesthesia is Patient-Centered

A minimally invasive anesthetic is necessary for ambulatory surgery, with a focus on the comfort, safety, and recovery of the patient at all times. The difficulties posed by this requirement have prompted ambulatory groups to develop creative, highly patient-centered solutions. Before performing outpatient surgery and anesthesia, it is important to evaluate the patient's expectations and the support system of their family to make sure the facility and its staff are capable of meeting those needs. The anesthesia providers and the facility's leadership should adhere to specific goals to meet the expectations of patients, families, and the medical team (Figure 9.1).

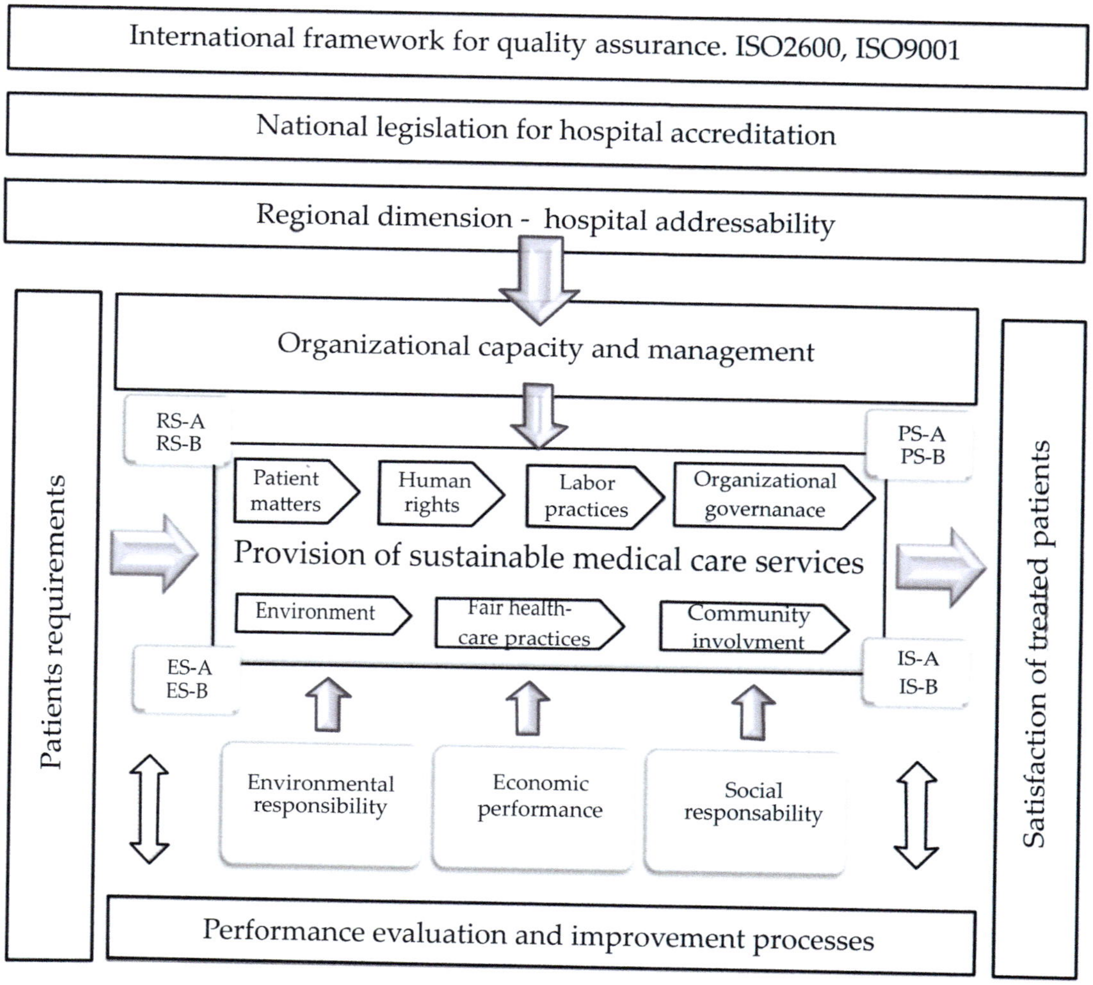

Figure 9.1. *Health Sustainability (H-S) Reference Framework: (PS–A)–Accreditation of Health System, (PS–B)–Design of Patient Centered Medical Services, (IS–A)–Medical Services Delivery, (IS–B)–Patient Transfer, (ES–A)–Institutional Outlook Leaders, (ES–B)–Satisfaction Degree Evaluation, (RS–A)–Self-Appraisal, (RS–B)–Medical Services Re-Conception. In our Model, the social area, Which Belongs To Sustainability, is Organized Following the Requirements of the Social Responsibility Standard ISO 26000*

Source: *Moldovan F, Moldovan L. Assessment of Patient Matters in Healthcare Facilities. Healthcare. 2024; 12(3):325. https://doi.org/10.3390/healthcare12030325.*

9.3. Defining the Value of Ambulatory Care

Patients can undergo outpatient surgery in a variety of settings, but it is usually characterized by a "come and go" experience on the same day. The procedures can be performed in an office, freestanding ASC, freestanding hospital outpatient department, hospital-based outpatient department, or near a hospital. Equal diversity in facility ownership is possible. Ambulatory surgical centers have a well-established safety record in both the US and Canada. Positive results in a high volume of procedures are achieved with a modicum of complications and an extremely low or even rare mortality rate thanks to accreditation and multidisciplinary oversight, well-established patient safety-related standards of care, careful patient and procedure selection, and a specialized workforce.

For patients, surgeons, and insurance companies, ambulatory surgical care offers some financial and social advantages. Significant cost savings are possible in the outpatient surgical setting, and patient satisfaction and safety are greatly improved. Between 1981 and 2011, the number of outpatient procedures increased by nearly ten times, making up between 19% and over 60% of all surgeries carried out in the US. ASCs perform surgeries faster than inpatient hospitals. New freestanding ASCs opened between 2008 and 2010, mostly in economically favorable markets with low levels of competition. ASC profitability is influenced by commercial payer rates, case volume, cost containment, and specialty billing procedures. (Vila et al., 2008; American Society of Anesthesiologists guidelines for office-based anesthesia; American Society of Anesthesiologists Task Force on Acute Pain Management, 2012)

9.4. Outpatient Selection

9.4.1. Patient

It is necessary to carefully choose, assess, and prepare patients in terms of comorbid conditions and social structure to enable successful outcomes. Selectivity helps clinicians to predict how long the admission and getting ready process, the anesthesia assessment, the surgery, and the recovery will probably take. Depending on the participating practitioners, the planned procedure, and the practice environment, there may be differences in the ideal surgical candidate. ASCs have historically been safe spaces because of careful patient and procedure selection intended to prevent unanticipated events. However, further information regarding the patient's characteristics (e.g., comorbid conditions and baseline pathophysiologic derangements) may, on rare occasions, result in shortcomings related to quality and safety.

Both intraoperative and postoperative care must be given to numerous comorbid conditions. Ignorance of comorbidities can lead to higher expenses and, more critically, perioperative morbidity. Care pathways are usually implemented by facilities to guarantee evidence-based, consistent care. Not every venue will accept the same set of patients or case types. To develop a customized treatment plan for each patient, professional societies' current guidelines should be carefully considered. The goal should be to reduce complexity and increase predictability.

9.4.2. Practitioner

Ambulatory anesthesia practitioners, like all subspecialists, possess a unique set of abilities that distinguish them from their colleagues. In addition to using broad but affordable multimodal analgesia and minimally invasive short-acting, fast-emergence anesthesia for a quick and safe recovery, an ambulatory anesthesia provider values the time of the patient and the surgeon, communicates with the team effectively, and values standardized work. The length and predictability of the operative room and post-anesthesia care unit (PACU) stays are largely determined by the specialization of the team that works in an operating suite.

9.4.2.1. Medical Direction

A facility's ability to lead is essential to its overall health. Although the specific procedures used by the different outpatient anesthesia venues vary, all sites must adhere to the same standards for patient safety, crisis preparedness, staff training, and cost control. These standards are set by the facility's leadership team. To fulfill the role of medical director and assist the site in adhering to legislative and regulatory directives, ASC and office anesthesia providers usually find that their responsibilities are expanded. Maintaining compliance necessitates an understanding of state, payer, and federal regulations regarding a wide range of topics, such as maintaining medication records, facility size limitations, emergency equipment maintenance, sterilizing systems, staff-to-patient ratios, and recovery bed availability. Anesthesia providers usually become advisors to the administrative teams that run the facility and often end up serving as the de facto medical director because they are often present for the longest periods of time at ASCs and offices. The path to becoming the medical director of an ambulatory surgery center does not have any courses or curricula. The ambulatory track at the annual meetings of the SAMBA and the American Society of Anesthesiologists (ASA) provides a network for mentorship and guidance as well as some continuing education in medical direction. The success of the facility's daily operations, as well as the safety and experience of the patients, depend on having a highly effective medical director. Under the direction of the medical director, the facility is jointly responsible for maintaining accreditation.

9.4.2.2. Multidisciplinary Leadership and Standardized Care

In healthcare delivery, unsafe, inefficient, and expensive practices are frequently the result of needless variation and a hierarchical culture that discourages openness and collaboration. Integrating published studies and guidelines with local outcome analysis is one efficient response that health care delivery teams can take. Development of the data is then necessary. When adjusting or getting rid of extra variation, algorithm-driven policies should be applied. An especially good place for this work is the ASC or office. When compared to an inpatient operating suite, it is a uniform setting with fewer providers carrying out a reduced range of procedures. Best practices and optimal results are attained when patient care decisions are made in stable clinical settings.

To maximize predictability, surgeons, facility administrators, and anesthesia providers should come to a consensus on uniform guidelines and directives for managing particular patient comorbid conditions. These guidelines and directives should then be documented into long-lasting policies and procedures for future reference. The best ways to create standard care plans are with multidisciplinary teams of doctors and nurses who analyze the literature, visit model peer sites, develop protocols with precise exclusion criteria, track the clinical outcomes of practitioners who follow the protocols and those who don't, and report the results back to the team as a whole. These kinds of guidelines differ from venue to venue and need to be reviewed often to stay up to date with the ever-changing patient care environment. Unless an alternate approach yields results that are on par with or superior to the published "best practice," it should be expected that providers will adhere to established practice guidelines or care pathways. Leadership ought to review the current practice guidelines at that point.

9.4.2.3. Ancillary Personnel

The outpatient ancillary care staff is a specialized workforce that makes a significant contribution to the facility's objectives being met. Because of the facility's relative isolation, specialized nursing and anesthesia staff members are usually trained and practiced in emergency care in the freestanding or office setting. Because ASC operating room providers are often the primary caregivers in an emergency, often for a longer period of time than a nurse in a tertiary care facility's operating room, accrediting bodies frequently require them to complete Advanced Cardiac Life Support (ACLS) and Pediatric Advanced Life Support (PALS) training.

9.4.3. Procedure

Procedure selection aims to reduce complexity to guarantee a predictable operative course and recovery, much like patient selection does. The staff, patients, and resources available to a facility may enable complex procedures. Orthopedic procedures, laparoscopic cholecystectomy, and lens and cataract operations comprise the bulk of ambulatory surgical procedures. The possibility of case delays, delayed discharge, unexpected admission, and their effects on patient satisfaction and facility efficiency should be considered when considering increased complexity. An increased risk of unexpected admission exists for patients with large body mass index (BMI), advanced age, ASA physical status III or IV, and longer surgeries lasting more than an hour.

Venous thromboembolism is more likely to occur when certain elective outpatient procedure combinations are combined. Because outpatient cholecystectomy has been specifically shown to be safe, it is often carried out as an ambulatory procedure. However, following an appendectomy, same-day discharge could present difficulties. In an ASC, emergency laparoscopic appendectomy might be possible if candidates who require less than 12 hours of postoperative observation are chosen using a predictive scoring system. However, a lot of patients require their appendectomy to be done during times when the ambulatory center is closed. Patients who fit the verified requirements for a shortened observation can spend less time in the hospital during their hospital stay or observation. Procedure selection may also be influenced by rates of postoperative complications leading to revisits. Although the postoperative morbidity and mortality profiles of same-day thyroidectomy and parathyroidectomy are good, follow-up visits may be necessary during the first week following surgery for hypocalcemia, bleeding, seroma, or hematoma. Because of the potential for acute postoperative airway compromise brought on by these complications, it is strongly advised that these cases be handled in facilities that offer inpatient care.

9.4.4. Place (Surgical Facility)

The surgical site selection is influenced by the maximization of predictability. Resources and location usually encourage or prohibit very complex procedures. For the treatment of sicker patients or more complicated procedures, nonhospital facilities' accessibility to hospital-based care must be taken into account. A particular surgery should be performed somewhere that allows for 23 hours of postoperative observation if 98% of patients can be sent home the same day after the procedure, but 2% need to stay overnight. One rare event that is used as a quality metric for outpatient surgery is a hospital transfer. In one series, hospital-based acute care encounters through the ER were almost thirty times more common than hospital transfers. Introducing more complex cases into the ambulatory setting safely is the current challenge for outpatient anesthesia.

9.4.4.1. Office-Based Anesthesia

In the past, operating rooms (ASCs) were considered less dangerous than offices for performing surgery. The freestanding ASCs' meticulous attention to the case and patient selection, along with their on-site preparation, were cited as the causes of the purported discrepancy. According to a 2014 study, anesthesia procedures performed in offices can be just as safe as those performed in hospitals or ASCs. Safety in office-based surgery is improved by facility accreditation, provider credentialing, office accreditation, appropriate procedure and patient selection, patient safety checklists, and the application of professional society guidelines.

Instead of ambulatory surgery centers or hospitals, offices are now the site of dental, plastic, and an increasing range of surgical procedures. The office space is economical, private, and practical. Office locations have clearly defined anesthetic techniques, case selection criteria, and facility requirements. Office-based procedures have typically produced excellent results. Regardless of the site of service, there is always a need for careful anesthesia care and oversight, as demonstrated by a few very public tragedies following procedures in offices. The lack of adequate reporting mechanisms in hospitals, ASCs, and office settings makes it challenging to compare the risks associated with anesthesia and surgery. To increase readiness for office-based procedures, the Institute for Safety in Office-Based Surgery has created a safety checklist. Not mistakes in patient selection, but rather insufficient monitoring is the primary cause of the majority of anesthesia-related remote-site injuries. A few things that raise the risk in an office setting are using untrained surgical or anesthesia personnel, not having the right equipment, and not having enough training for resuscitation and other emergency situations.

9.4.4.2. Simulation and Drills: Site Preparedness

Site preparation needs to be very careful in case of unforeseen emergencies. It is recommended that ASC and office staff practice common emergencies in order to improve provider and system readiness for such incidents. A publication endorsed by SAMBA offers comprehensive drill scenarios along with instructional materials to help outpatient practices evaluate and enhance their readiness and responsiveness for common emergencies. Simulations and drills, like their real-world counterparts, can be stressful. Debriefings should be held afterward, with an emphasis on potential improvements in teamwork and system design rather than individual shortcomings. Simulations can also provide light on necessary modifications to patient and procedure selection, as well as the rules and regulations that influence these decisions. (Vila et al., 2008; American Society of Anesthesiologists guidelines for office-based anesthesia; American Society of Anesthesiologists Task Force on Acute Pain Management, 2012)

9.5. The Perioperative Journey of an Ambulatory Surgical Patient

9.5.1. An Itinerary for Success

In the ambulatory context, a patient's experience doesn't end when they are released from the recovery room; it starts long before they even arrive at an ASC. A defined, distinct itinerary is required for ambulatory surgery due to the need for predictability. Although the ambulatory schematic may vary from location to location, there are typically multiple phases. Delivering high-quality ambulatory care requires an understanding of the phases of care, as well as the objectives and difficulties that come with each one.

9.5.2. Preoperative Phase: Days to Weeks before Surgery

Preliminary patient, procedure, and site selection occurs in the surgeon's office and adheres to the protocols, rules, and directives established by the medical site administration. Candidate characteristics that compromise predictability, add complexity, or pose risk during the intraoperative, postoperative, or post-discharge phases of care are identified during the preoperative screening process.

9.5.2.1. Assessing for Adequate Social Support

The patient screening questions concern social support, which includes a driver to take the patient home after surgery, an escort on the day of the procedure, and a caregiver to help with everyday living activities and postoperative care. Every patient should have an escort on site or readily available the day of surgery. Also, a driver should be available right away to take the patient home. Certain facilities demand that the patient sign a document confirming that they will have overnight care following surgery. The escort is present while the patient is being admitted and gets ready for surgery. The surgery is not scheduled if the patient cannot arrange for a driver, caregiver, or escort the night following the procedure. While some patients may find these requirements burdensome, early detection of patients in need of these resources lowers patient risk and lowers the possibility of surgical case cancellation on the day of surgery. Patients who only received a small dose of local anesthesia and no additional medications related to anesthesia are the only ones who may be released on their own.

9.5.2.2. Evaluation and Testing: Before the Day of Surgery

In order to prevent cancellations on the day of surgery and to guarantee that the best care setting is chosen, outpatient centers create procedures for patient screening. Surgeons determine whether a patient is a candidate for outpatient surgery; however, medical conditions that affect intraoperative care and recovery may prevent a patient from being an outpatient. The initial preoperative evaluation is guided by the preliminary clinical history provided at the time of surgical evaluation and may be supplemented by patient-completed health assessment forms. A form for the preoperative surgical evaluation can be filled out on the spot to determine the relevant health status. When the form is filled out, it offers a medical history review, a social support identification, and a systems review. After that, the form and the case booking are sent to the anesthesia department of the surgical facility. Based on the type of surgery and the comorbid condition of the patient, a licensed practitioner from the group (physician, advanced practice nurse, certified registered nurse anesthetist [CRNA], or anesthesiology assistant) reviews the forms and decides whether a follow-up phone call is necessary. An initial assessment of anesthesia is conducted along with a review of the state of medical conditions.

Testing ought to be evidence-based and economical. Although preoperative testing has no effect on postoperative outcomes, it is overused in patients undergoing low-risk ambulatory surgery. These results have also been validated in non-cardiac elective surgery by a systematic review. The cost of providing care has decreased in ASCs and office settings, but routine preoperative evaluation for low-risk outpatient surgery is still expensive. Preoperative evaluations were performed on 53% of Medicare beneficiaries having cataract surgery in 2011. In comparison to the previous 11 months, this cohort's health care expenses increased by $12.4 million in the month before the cataract surgery. Routine testing prior to cataract surgery did not improve safety. However, not all ambulatory procedures have the minimal anesthetic exposure and favorable risk profile of cataract surgery. A patient's eligibility for particular outpatient procedures and the environment in which they are carried out should be ascertained through preoperative screening (Figure 9.2).

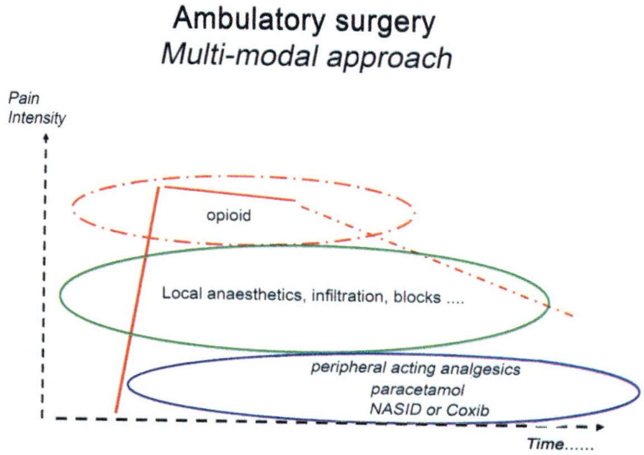

Figure 9.2. *The journey of managing an ambulatory surgical patient.*

Source: *Jakobsson JG. Pain Management in Ambulatory Surgery—A Review. Pharmaceuticals. 2014; 7(8):850-865. https://doi.org/10.3390/ph7080850.*

In order to adjust risk and stabilize an existing medical condition, published guidelines indicate a move away from routine testing and toward risk stratification-driven targeted testing. Current research on important subjects in risk assessment and management for patients undergoing ambulatory surgery is provided by a 2014 review. Effective ambulatory anesthesia groups reduce last-minute cancellations, delayed discharge, unexpected admission, and patient dissatisfaction by using screening paradigms in accordance with guidelines and communicating with patients prior to the day of surgery. This review covers a number of significant clinical issues that should prompt additional conversation prior to the day of surgery. (Vila et al., 2008; American Society of Anesthesiologists guidelines for office-based anesthesia; American Society of Anesthesiologists Task Force on Acute Pain Management, 2012)

9.5.2.3. Cardiovascular Risk Assessment

An algorithm for the perioperative cardiovascular evaluation and care of patients with coronary artery disease undergoing noncardiac surgery is provided by the 2014 American College of Cardiology/American Heart Association (ACC/AHA) guidelines. Given that perioperative cardiac complications are uncommon following most ambulatory surgery procedures, the guidelines recommend that a patient show a functional capacity of at least four metabolic equivalent (MET) values for activities, such as the ability to climb two flights of stairs without experiencing any symptoms. Major adverse cardiac events are contingent upon the surgical technique and the individual patient. Before surgery, the guidelines advise determining combined risk using one of two risk-calculating techniques. High-risk patients are identified using the revised cardiac risk index or the surgical risk calculator of the National Surgical Quality Improvement Program.

Patients with a risky profile may attempt ambulatory procedures after thorough evaluation and risk stratification, provided that medical status issues have been appropriately identified and treated. The chance of perioperative complications is higher in certain important traits. Patients who have these associated characteristics might not be good candidates for ambulatory surgery and need to undergo a thorough evaluation. The guidelines state that patients undergoing intermediate- or high-risk procedures who have a history of known coronary heart disease, significant arrhythmia, peripheral arterial disease, or cerebrovascular disease are the only ones who should have a preoperative resting 12-lead ECG. It is best to complete such a risk assessment well in advance of the surgery date. (Vila et al., 2008; American Society of Anesthesiologists guidelines for office-based anesthesia; American Society of Anesthesiologists Task Force on Acute Pain Management, 2012)

9.5.2.4. Obstructive Sleep Apnea

The physiology of the patient as well as the preoperative and postoperative care are impacted by obstructive sleep apnea (OSA). Sympathetic neuron activation by OSA causes hypertension and cardiovascular abnormalities, which can result in perioperative morbidity or even death. The majority of patients have undiagnosed OSA, which raises the risk of death, difficult intubation, bleeding, myocardial infarction, perioperative respiratory events, and cerebrovascular events. Establishing this diagnosis is essential prior to ambulatory surgery.

Patients with established OSA, regardless of severity or CPAP therapy compliance, did not experience any unexpected admissions or delayed discharges in an ambulatory surgical cohort, indicating appropriate patient selection and monitoring. Preoperatively identifying patients with OSA may help with preparation and risk assessment, or it may facilitate referral to a hospital environment. Regarding the perioperative care of patients with OSA, the ASA and SAMBA have updated their respective guidelines. Using a validated screening tool like the STOP-BANG questionnaire, patients can be screened during the surgical evaluation or over the phone. No particular screening instrument is advised by the ASA. A comprehensive preoperative evaluation determines which patients are at risk and whether coexisting conditions are adequately treated. Before surgery, patients with known or suspected OSA should, at the very least, be screened systematically by a licensed practitioner (physician, registered nurse [RN], CRNA, or anesthesiology assistant) over the phone.

The evaluation verifies whether an OSA diagnosis is present or not, whether CPAP therapy is being followed, whether a CPAP machine and mask are in place, and whether related comorbid conditions are under control. Suitability may depend on the kind of surgery, the facility's capacity to manage complications from undiagnosed or uncontrolled OSA and its comorbid conditions, and its ability to reduce opioid exposure through local or regional anesthetic procedures. If this higher degree of care cannot be given, management should be transferred to a hospital (Tables 9.1 and 9.2).

Table 9.1. *Dindo-Clavien Classification of Complications*

Grade I	Any deviation from the normal postoperative course without the need for pharmacological treatment or surgical, endoscopic and radiological interventions. Permitted therapeutic regimens include: drugs as antiemetics, antipyretics, analgetics, diuretics and electrolytes and physiotherapy. This grade also includes wound infections opened at the bedside.
Grade II	Pharmacological treatment required with other medications than the permitted complications of grade I; including blood transfusions and total parenteral nutrition.
Grade III	Requiring surgical, endoscopic or radiological intervention
IIIa	Intervention not under general anesthesia
IIIb	Intervention under general anesthesia
Grade IV	Life-threatening complication (including CNS complications)* requiring ICU-management
IVa	Single organ dysfunction (including dialysis)
IVb	Multiorgan dysfunction
Grade V	Death of a patient

ICU, intensive care unit; CNS, central nervous system.

Source: Arens P, Hardt J, Angrick JC, Olze H and Coordes A (2022) Modified dindo-clavien system for registration of perioperative complications in children undergoing adenotonsillectomy. Front. Pediatr. 10:1049942. doi: 10.3389/fped.2022.1049942.

Table 9.2. *Postoperative Complications and Associated Hospital Costs in a Study*

Postoperative complications	Number	Hospital costs (USD) Median (IQR) Minimum: Maximum	*p*-value
Patients without complications	17 (27.4%)	30,946.9 (23,910.8–46,828.1) [16,672.5:106,850.5]	0.151[a]
Patients with any complication	45 (72.6%)	40,717.8 (27,358.0–59,834.3) [19,148.4:214,377.7]	
Number of complications per patient			
Count of complications	2 (1–3) [1:6]	–	*Not applicable*
1–3	38 (84.4%)	35,765.2 (26,306.5–54,004.5) [191,48.4:129,568.3]	0.015*[b]
≥4	7 (15.6%)	51,327.0 (49,201.5–140,980.6) [40,553.7:214,377.7]†	
CVD grade of complication			
I, II	39 (86.7%)	37,341.4 (26,462.1–51,327.0) [19,148.4:129,568.3]	0.007*[c]
III, IV	6 (13.3%)	109,051.3 (47,149.2–159,329.9) [40,992.4:214,377.7]†	

Note: Data are presented as n (%) or median (interquartile range), [minimum : maximum]. CVD, Clavien–Dindo classification system.
[a]Mann–Whitney U-statistic = 291.0;
[b]Kruskal–Wallis one-way analysis of variance on ranks, H(2) = 8.404;
[c]Kruskal–Wallis one-way analysis of variance on ranks, H(2) = 10.007.
**p < 0.0167, Bonferroni's adjustment.*
†p < 0.05 vs other two levels, Dunn's all pairwise multiple comparison procedure.

Source: Weinberg L, Ratnasekara V, Tran AT, Kaldas P, Neal-Williams T, D'Silva MR, Hua J, Yip S, Lloyd-Donald P, Fletcher L, Ma R, Perini MV, Nikfarjam M and Lee D (2022) The Association of Postoperative Complications and Hospital Costs Following Distal Pancreatectomy. Front. Surg. 9:890518. doi: 10.3389/fsurg.2022.890518.

9.5.2.5. Diabetes Mellitus

A hemoglobin A_{1c} (HbA_{1c}) of more than 7 percent is linked to unfavorable perioperative outcomes, but there is no HbA1c value that prevents a patient from undergoing outpatient surgery. The particular ambulatory procedure is relevant because poor glucose control may be a sign of other organ system dysfunction, such as cardiovascular and renal comorbid conditions. Preventing hypoglycemia while perioperatively maintaining basal physiologic insulin levels is the fundamental idea on the day of surgery. It is important to understand the level of preoperative baseline blood glucose control, end-organ dysfunction brought on by hyperglycemia, and the current course of therapy. Before the day of the procedure, this information is gathered. Practical knowledge on perioperative management of the diabetic patient in the ambulatory setting is provided by a SAMBA consensus statement.

9.5.2.6. Chronic Pain

For optimal treatment planning, patients with opioid dependence, chronic pain, severe uncontrolled postsurgical pain in the past, or who are on buprenorphine or methadone therapy should be identified well in advance of the surgery date. For patients who may develop a tolerance or intolerance to pain therapy, or for those who are currently receiving care from a pain physician, a formal plan for postoperative pain control and follow-up should be established, as pain and nausea are frequently the cause of delayed discharge and unexpected admission.

Patients who are opioid-dependent may need to increase their baseline opioid dosage by 100–200 percent after surgery if neural blockade is not used. Certain surgeons or surgical facilities might not be qualified to perform such "uptitration" It may not be appropriate to use regional anesthesia for certain procedures or patients. Preoperative planning and screening can lower unexpected admissions, discharge delays, and ER visits related to pain.

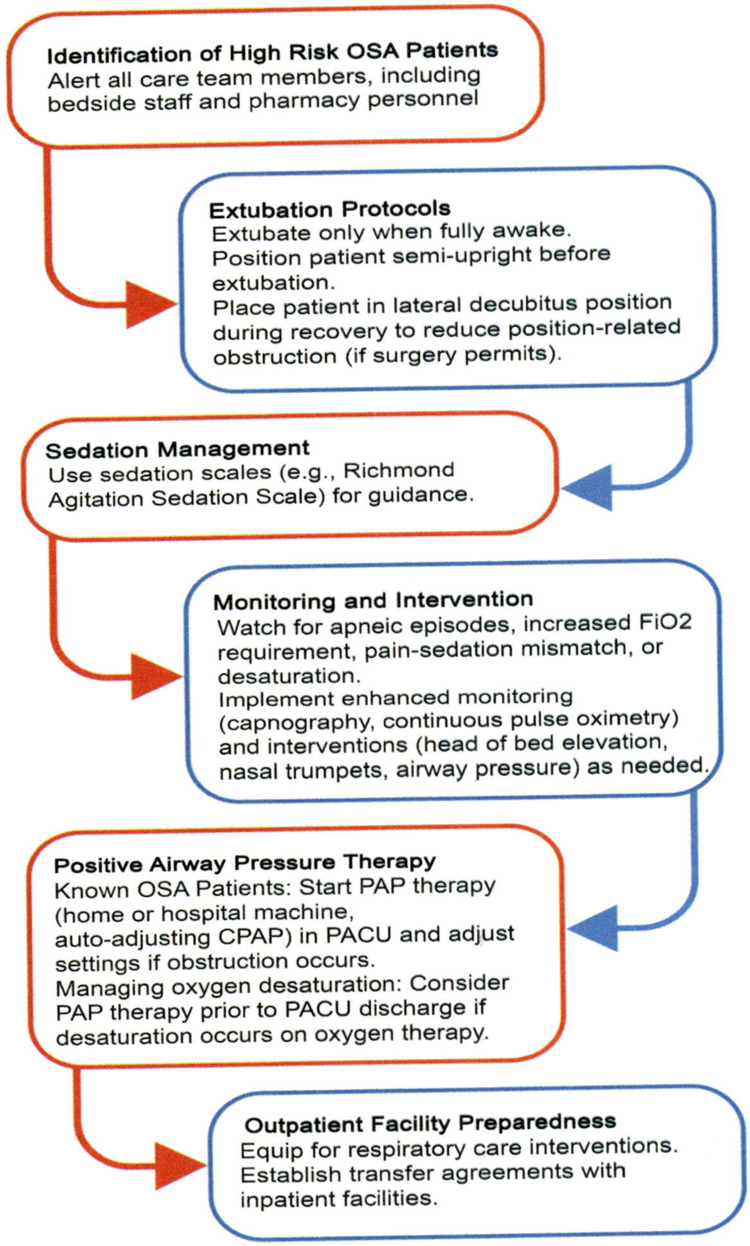

Figure 9.3. *OSA Recovery roadmap: guidelines for the OR and PACU. abbreviations: OR, operating room; PACU, postoperative anesthesia care unit; PAP, positive airway pressure; FiO2, fraction of inhaled oxygen.*

Source: Chaudhry RA, Zarmer L, West K, Chung F. Obstructive Sleep Apnea and Risk of Postoperative Complications after Non-Cardiac Surgery. Journal of Clinical Medicine. 2024; 13(9):2538. https://doi.org/10.3390/jcm13092538.

Prior to surgery, patients with chronic pain might not have had much faith in their ability to return home right away. Prior to surgery, such anxiety or expectation should be noted and dealt with through treatment planning, patient education, and potentially hospital-based care (American Society of Anesthesiologists Task Force on Perioperative Management of patients with obstructive sleep apnea, 2014) (Figure 9.3).

9.5.3. Preoperative Phase: Day(s) Before Surgery

The patient's appointment with the facility is confirmed once preoperative evaluation, assessment, and preparation are finished and the results reviewed. Information about a ride and escort is also confirmed at that point. A preoperative phone call, made a few days prior to surgery, verifies the time of arrival, restates instructions for medication and oral intake, addresses any concerns the patient may have, and confirms that the escort, ride, and postoperative caregiver will be available. A designated facility employee verifies the information regarding the arrival time and requirement for an escort and ride within 24 hours of the surgery. These steps lessen the amount of resources needed to care for a patient who has been abandoned, as well as the delay and cancellation of cases.

The anesthesia team has plenty of time to conduct a preliminary evaluation of the patient's candidacy in the days or weeks leading up to the procedure. It is possible that the anesthesia provider won't be allocated to the case until the day prior. After assignment, the last preparations get under way. The day before surgery, health assessment forms are available for the patient's anesthesia provider to review. In order to add more instructions or treatments, a timely review helps identify errors or omissions in treatment planning. Even if it were possible to prepare at the last minute, it would not be feasible if the chart review was postponed until the next morning.

9.5.4. Preoperative Phase: Day of Surgery

9.5.4.1. The Anesthesia Preoperative Assessment

A preoperative review of the patient's medical and social history as well as a physical examination by an anesthesiologist are deemed necessary by the American Society of Anesthesiologists (ASA) and the Center for Medicaid Services (CMS). It is impossible to shortchange the process of taking a thorough history because increasingly complex procedures and patients are being admitted to the outpatient setting. Anesthesia professionals frequently find important health changes in their patients that may have an impact on their long-term and postoperative outcomes. Thorough evaluation of a patient's medical status is important because it has a correlation with unexpected admission and delayed discharge. With little time commitment, a quick motivational interview and advice on preventive health concerns, like quitting smoking, from anesthesia professionals can also be beneficial.

The difficult decision of whether to proceed with surgery for a patient who is not feeling well on a daily basis presents a challenge to the anesthesia provider. Essentially, the decision revolves around whether there is an increased risk to the patient. The anesthesia provider asks this premature question when patients become critically ill, when the preoperative preadmission evaluation is lacking, or when patients do not follow prior recommendations for crucial consultation, testing, or therapy. If not, does the added complexity jeopardize the predictability of the procedure and the anesthetic effects?

9.5.4.2. Acute Pulmonary Conditions

If a patient has received enough therapy to reach the best possible state of health (e.g., surgery should be carried out in a hospital setting where respiratory therapy services are ideal if the patient has pulmonary hypertension, is still symptomatic (e.g., wheezing at rest, a bedside forced expiratory time of less than 6 seconds, inability to climb stairs due to dyspnea, medication review by the primary physician, and no additional therapy is thought to be necessary). If pediatric intensivists and respiratory therapists with pediatric expertise are easily accessible, complicated pediatric airway surgery may be scheduled in a hospital rather than a freestanding center. Because of the possibility of respiratory complications during the perioperative period, an acute upper respiratory infection (URI) that is current or recent may be sufficient justification for delaying a case. Patients with URI may experience coughing, stridor, laryngospasm, desaturation, and supraglottic edema when under general anesthesia, especially if endotracheal intubation has been done. Though these patients may experience fewer issues if supraglottic airway devices are used.

If the procedure can be carried out safely without endotracheal intubation, the patient has no additional cardiac or pulmonary issues, and the patient has a mild URI that has occurred recently or in the past, then elective surgery can proceed. Asthma, chronic obstructive pulmonary disease (COPD), or congenital heart disease), and the surgical procedure won't affect the airway. If more than a local anesthetic is needed, severe, functionally impairing active, or recent pulmonary symptoms call for closer examination and possibly postponement of elective surgery. Even in that case, it might be preferable for the patient to start with primary care rather than a procedure that could further impair function or everyday activities while they recover.

9.5.4.3. Hypertension

After surgery, patients with medication-dependent hypertension are up to 50% more likely to experience unfavorable cardiovascular outcomes in the 30 days following the procedure. Angiotensin-converting enzyme (ACE) inhibitors lower blood pressure, but they also raise the risk of severe hypotension following the induction of general anesthesia. This conclusion has been questioned by others. Postoperative morbidity and death rates rise in patients who suffer hypotension following the induction of anesthesia. Even for a brief 24-hour period, the decision to forego antihypertensive medication prior to surgery may result in an increase in arterial blood pressure. The neurohumoral response to surgical stimuli can be profound, leading to postoperative lability and difficult-to-treat hypertension in an at-risk population, even though sedation and general anesthesia can lower arterial blood pressure.

It is best to postpone elective ambulatory surgery if there are any of the following conditions: new-onset angina, chronic unstable angina, new cardiac arrhythmia, signs of decompensated congestive heart failure, or recent percutaneous coronary stenting or angioplasty. Surgery should not be cancelled based on a predetermined arterial blood pressure reading, but severe preoperative hypertension should prompt a multidisciplinary discussion. When making decisions about whether to postpone surgery or manage intraoperatively, the patient's baseline arterial blood pressure range is a useful guide. The ambulatory procedure is rescheduled and the patient is transferred to acute care if there are signs of a hypertensive emergency.

9.5.4.4. The Difficult Airway

The ambulatory setting poses a significant challenge when dealing with a "difficult" airway. It is important to determine if the patient has a history of difficult breathing well in advance of the surgery by talking with them beforehand or by looking over their health questionnaire. To lower risk on the day of surgery, a preoperative airway assessment is necessary. Every case should be ready for thorough airway management in a facility. The unexpected nature of the occult lingual tonsil is what distinguishes it. The equipment needed to fully utilize the ASA's challenging airway algorithm should be readily available and routinely tested for functionality for this reason, among many others. In the event that a patient with a known difficult airway is given regional or neuraxial anesthesia, the surgeon and the patient should discuss the possibility of insufficient anesthesia prior to surgery to make sure everyone is aware of the potential risks associated with "a touch of sedation." While the patient is awake, endotracheal intubation (i.e., which might entail a modest dosage of preoperative medication) might be the safest choice in spite of the apparent workflow delay.

9.5.4.5. Pregnancy Testing

Some facilities require pregnancy tests for all women of childbearing age, and others offer it only to those women who say they may be pregnant. In one study, mandating that all women undergo pregnancy testing resulted in a cost of over $3000 per positive test, a particularly troubling price in view of an unknown level of benefit. A separate study found that the cost per positive result was $1,005 with an unknown benefit of not performing elective surgery on a pregnant woman. Some providers screen patients during preoperative evaluation: "Is there any chance you could be pregnant today?" A "yes" response triggers a test, and a "no" response triggers a statement of confirmation and further counseling: "If there is any chance, we should confirm to make sure we do not unknowingly expose a developing fetus to anesthesia."

9.5.4.6. Preoperative Medications

Numerous nonpharmacologic methods of anxiolysis, such as aromatherapy or listening to their favorite music, can be helpful for anxious patients. The perioperative experience of the anxious or catastrophizing patient may also be enhanced by the administration of 1200 mg of gabapentin or short-acting benzodiazepines. Preoperative administration of nonsteroidal anti-inflammatory drugs (NSAIDs) and acetaminophen, gabapentin, or pregabalin starts preventive analgesia so that serum concentrations are therapeutic prior to surgical stimuli, potentially lowering postoperative opioid requirements, opioid-related side effects, and secondary hyperalgesia (Table 9.3).

Preoperative dexamethasone administration may also enhance the patient's physical, mental, and pain management following surgery. Transdermal scopolamine can be applied prior to surgery in high-risk patients to help reduce postoperative nausea and vomiting (PONV). In adults, scopolamine patches can prevent postoperative nausea and vomiting just as well as droperidol or ondansetron.

(Vila et al., 2008; American Society of Anesthesiologists guidelines for office-based anesthesia; American Society of Anesthesiologists Task Force on Acute Pain Management, 2012)

Table 9.3. *Anxiolysis: Clinical Studies on Cognitive Behavioral Therapy (CBT), Guided Imagery Relaxation and Hypnosis in Preoperative Anxiety*

References	Title	Intervention	Control	Population	Surgery	Type of study	Conclusion
Dao et al. (45)	Randomized controlled trial of brief cognitive behavioral intervention for depression and anxiety symptoms preoperatively in patients undergoing coronary artery bypass graft surgery	CBT	Standard pre-operative care	100	Coronary artery bypass graft surgery	RCT	CBT targeting preoperative depression and anxiety is both feasible and acceptable for patients undergoing CABG surgery.
Gade et al. (46)	The Impact of a preoperative cognitive behavioral therapy (CBT) on dysfunctional eating behaviors, affective symptoms and body weight 1 year after bariatric surgery: a randomized controlled trial	CBT	Nutritional support and education	80	Bariatric Surgery	RCT	The 10-week CBT intervention showed beneficial effects preoperatively.
Cassin et al. (47)	A pilot randomized controlled trial of telephone-based cognitive behavioral therapy for preoperative bariatric surgery patients	CBT	Standard pre-operative care	47	bariatric surgery	RCT	Tele-CBT holds promise as a brief intervention for improving eating psychopathology and depression in bariatric surgery candidates.
Rajeswari et al. (48)	Effectiveness of cognitive behavioral play therapy and audiovisual distraction for management of preoperative anxiety in children	I—CBT II—audiovisual	Tell-show-do technique	45 children	dental	RCT	Active distraction with cognitive behavioral play therapy is found to be more effective in reducing the preoperative anxiety in children compared to audiovisual distraction and tell-show-do technique.
Birch et al. (49)	No effect of cognitive behavioral patient education for patients with pain catastrophizing before total knee arthroplasty: a randomized controlled trial	CBT	Standard pre-operative care	60	Total knee arthroplasty	RCT	We found no difference in the primary outcome measure, VAS during activity, between the 2 groups but both groups had large reductions over time.
Felix et al. (50)	Guided imagery relaxation therapy on preoperative anxiety: a randomized clinical trial	Guided imagery relaxation	Standard care	24	Video-laparoscopic bariatric surgery	RCT	Guided imagery relaxation therapy is an effective nursing intervention for the reduction of state anxiety and blood cortisol levels in the preoperative period in patients undergoing video-laparoscopic bariatric surgery.
Vagnoli et al. (51)	Relaxation-guided imagery reduces perioperative anxiety and pain in children: a randomized study	Guided imagery relaxation	Standard care	60 children	Minor surgery	RCT	Relaxation-guided imagery reduces preoperative anxiety and postoperative pain in children.
Halpin et al. (52)	Guided imagery in cardiac surgery.	Guided imagery relaxation	Without guided imagery	711	Cardiac surgery	RCT	The guided imagery patient group experienced significantly decreased LOS compared to the control group, thereby lowering hospital costs.
Charette et al. (53)	Guided imagery for adolescent post-spinal fusion pain management: a pilot study	Guided imagery relaxation	Standard care	40	Orthopedic surgery for adolescent idiopathic scoliosis (spinal fusion)	RCT	Addition of a guided imagery and relaxation exercise DVD for home use was more effective than standard care alone for postoperative pain.
Kekecs et al. (54)	Effects of patient education and therapeutic suggestions on cataract surgery patients: a randomized controlled clinical trial	Guided imagery relaxation	Standard care	84	Cataract surgery	RCT	Preoperative information combined with positive suggestions and anxiety management techniques might reduce patient anxiety in the perioperative period of cataract surgery.

References	Title	Intervention	Control	Population	Surgery	Type of study	Conclusion
Manyande et al. (55)	Preoperative rehearsal of active coping imagery influences subjective and hormonal responses to abdominal surgery	Imagery intervention	Control received background information about the hospital	51	Abdominal surgery patients	RCT	State-anxiety was similar in each group, but imagery patients experienced less postoperative pain than did the controls, were less distressed by it, felt that they coped with it better, and requested less analgesia. Hormone levels measured in peripheral venous blood did not differ on the afternoon of admission, before preparation. Cortisol levels were, however, lower in imagery patients than in controls immediately before and after surgery. Noradrenaline levels were greater on these occasions in imagery patients than controls.
Amraoui et al. (56)	Effects of a hypnosis session before general anesthesia on postoperative outcomes in patients who underwent minor breast cancer surgery: the HYPNOSEIN randomized clinical trial	Hypnosis	Standard care	150 women	Minor breast cancer surgery	RCT	No benefit of hypnosis was found on postoperative breast pain; however, hypnosis seems to have other benefits regarding fatigue, anxiety, and patient satisfaction.
Saadat et al. (57)	Hypnosis reduces preoperative anxiety in adult patients.	Hypnosis	Standard care	50	Ambulatory surgical	RCT	Patients in the hypnosis group were significantly less anxious post-intervention as compared with patients in the attention-control group and the control group.
Duparc-Alegria et al. (58)	Assessment of a short hypnosis in a pediatric operating room in reducing postoperative pain and anxiety: a randomized study	Hypnosis	Standard care	120 children	Major orthopedic surgery.	RCT	This randomized study on a short hypnosis session performed in the operating room prior to a major surgery showed no difference in postoperative anxiety and pain levels. The decrease in anxiety and pain levels may be due to the addition of nurse pre-operative interviews and optimisation in communication in the operating room.
Hermes et al. (59)	Evaluation of intraoperative standardized hypnosis with the state-trait anxiety inventory.	Hypnosis	Standard care	50	Dental surgery	RCT	Hypnosis reduces intraoperative anxiety of oral and maxillofacial patients significantly.
Calipel et al. (60)	Premedication in children: hypnosis vs. midazolam.	Hypnosis	Oral midazolam	50 children	Mixed surgery	RCT	Hypnosis seems effective as premedication in children scheduled for surgery.
Huet et al. (61)	Hypnosis and dental anesthesia in children: a prospective controlled study	Hypnosis	Standard care	30 children	Dental surgery	RCT	Hypnosis may be effective in reducing anxiety and pain in children receiving dental anesthesia.
Ashton et al. (62)	Self-hypnosis reduces anxiety following coronary artery bypass surgery. A prospective, randomized trial	Self-hypnosis	No therapy	32	Coronary artery bypass surgery	RCT	This study demonstrates the beneficial effects self-hypnosis relaxation techniques on patients undergoing coronary artery bypass surgery.
Schnur et al. (63)	Hypnosis decreases presurgical distress in excisional breast biopsy patients	Hypnosis	Presurgery attention control session	90 Women	Excisional breast biopsy	RCT	The study results indicate that a brief pre-surgery hypnosis intervention can be an effective means of controlling pre-surgical distress in women awaiting diagnostic breast cancer surgery.

Source: Wang R, Huang X, Wang Y and Akbari M (2022) Non-pharmacologic Approaches in Preoperative Anxiety, a Comprehensive Review. Front. Public Health 10:854673. doi: 10.3389/fpubh.2022.854673.

9.5.5. Intraoperative Phase: Anesthesia Techniques

The general objectives of outpatient anesthesia, as stated by Drs. Ralph Waters, Wallace Reed, and John Ford many years ago, remain the same: convenience, low cost, patient safety, and care that is in line with the objectives of both the patient and the surgeon. As a result, the anesthetic methods used should be selected with safety in mind as well as to reduce or eliminate pain, nausea, vomiting, and prolonged cognitive impairment following surgery. The choice of anesthetic methods facilitates a prompt recovery. However, efficiency shouldn't endanger patients' safety or compromise their level of comfort or satisfaction. Remifentanil, for instance, promotes dependable and quick recovery; however, patients undergoing invasive surgery or with a history of chronic pain should not use it due to the possibility of hyperalgesia.

The choice between sedation, general anesthesia, and regional anesthesia is influenced by a number of variables, including the patient's characteristics, expectations, positioning, surgical anatomy and technique, surgeon preference, anesthesia provider preference, and policies or facility guidelines that reduce risk or prioritize efficiency. While there isn't a single optimal anesthetic method for all patients, standardizing care could lead to better results. Treatment pathways necessitate patient selection, education, and possibly a number of pathway detours for customized care within the framework of standardization. Patients with comorbid conditions, psychological issues, or other needs that prevent them from following the usually chosen pathway may not be eligible for care. There's a thin ethical line between maintaining the effectiveness of outpatient centers and preventing patients from receiving care. Any deviation from the "typical" pathway ought to be noted beforehand and factored into the daily schedule or the overall strategy for staffing and using operating rooms.

9.5.5.1. Sedation

Sedation administered by an anesthesia provider is referred to as monitored anesthesia care (MAC) in anesthesia billing. When a patient's condition changes during surgery, titrated sedation and ongoing monitoring are frequently used to transition the patient in and out of general anesthesia. This procedure should only be used by medical professionals with anesthesia privileges. Therefore, sedation or general anesthesia administered by a MAC or anesthesia provider is not the same as other forms of light sedation administered by non-anesthesia staff.

Deep sleep (i.e., in between moderate sedation and general anesthesia) is selected when regional or general anesthesia is deemed too time-consuming or invasive for the patient or procedure. Deep sedation carries a risk of catastrophic consequences comparable to or greater than that of general anesthesia, with operating room fires and oversedation being two such risks. Due to the potential for hypoventilation and hypoxemia during deep sedation, caution and monitoring are essential. The potential need for oxygen supplementation must be taken into account when deciding between general anesthesia and deep sedation. Increased levels of supplemental oxygen may be necessary if the procedure will be so uncomfortable that the patient must be mostly unconscious. If deep sedation is used without a secured airway during electrocautery and surgery close to the airway, there is a chance that the accumulated oxygen under the surgical drapes will catch fire. Safer delivery of supplemental oxygen is made possible by closed systems general anesthesia. A history of uncontrolled GORD, difficult endotracheal intubation or ventilation, or a history of OSA may pose difficulties or conflicts.

9.5.5.2. Regional Anesthesia

Patients and the facility may benefit from regional anesthesia, either by itself or in combination with general anesthesia or sedation. An expert in regional anesthesia, the modern ambulatory anesthesia provider learns and applies newly discovered techniques while modifying tried-and-true methods. When compared to general anesthesia, regional nerve blocks in a preoperative area reduce overall anesthesia time without increasing turnover time for patients undergoing orthopedic procedures. It is possible to shorten the PACU discharge period and improve the patient's quality of life during the first postoperative phase. Peripheral nerve blocks were used more frequently by practitioners during ambulatory ankle arthroscopy procedures between 1994 and 2006, rising from 6% to 26%. When used in conjunction with safe post-discharge protocols, regional catheterization can lessen postoperative pain and enhance recovery in the days following surgery. Regional anesthesia techniques have revolutionized hernia and breast surgery. Paravertebral regional block decreases opioid exposure, PONV, urinary retention, and pain scores as compared to general or neuraxial anesthetics. Multilevel paravertebral blocks combined with total intravenous anesthesia for breast tumor resection were reliable and improved postoperative analgesia, enhanced quality of recovery, and expedited PACU discharge compared with inhaled anesthetics or opioid-based general anesthesia. Paravertebral block for patients undergoing mastectomy may decrease the incidence of chronic postsurgical chest wall pain and tumor recurrence or metastasis. The serratus anterior plane block and pectoral nerve blocks (pecs I and II) are novel interfascial plane blocks for breast surgery analgesia.

9.5.5.3. Central Neuraxial Anesthesia

After lower extremity, gynecologic, and abdominal surgery, as well as for patients with chronic respiratory diseases, neuraxial blockade has been shown to decrease the incidence of PONV and pain, with or without sedation. When used in an ambulatory setting, a brief "speed spinal" has significant benefits. For shorter procedures like knee arthroscopy and inguinal hernia repair, spinal doses of lidocaine, mepivacaine, and 2-chloroprocaine offer excellent anesthesia. Low-dose bupivacaine for the spine (e.g., 4mg with 20μg fentanyl) is a fast-acting, efficient treatment that quickly resolves transurethral procedures in elderly male patients without postponing discharge. 7.5 mg of 0.5 percent hyperbaric ropivacaine is sufficient for anesthesia during an outpatient knee arthroscopy, but it takes up to 2.5 hours to fully wear off and up to 3 hours to discharge, which is significantly longer than it does with 2-chloroprocaine.

9.5.5.4. General Anesthesia

Certain patient-procedure combinations, particularly those involving airway surgery, carry a risk due to the natural airway. Risk factors related to the patient and the procedure should be taken into consideration when deciding whether to provide general anesthesia with or without endotracheal intubation. Compared to deep sedation or regional anesthesia, general anesthesia carries a higher risk of postoperative nausea and vomiting (PDNV), airway injury, postoperative hypothermia, postoperative cognitive dysfunction, and delayed discharge. However, for procedures requiring peritoneal insufflation or neuromuscular blockade, general anesthesia might be required. It may be necessary to administer a general anesthetic because certain patients refuse regional anesthesia or have medical conditions that preclude it.

General anesthesia can be accomplished through total intravenous techniques, combined maintenance with volatile anesthesia and intravenous drugs, or solely with volatile anesthetics. Nitrous oxide may be an adjunct to general anesthesia. Limiting duration of nitrous oxide exposure has been shown to reduce the risk of PONV.

With volatile anesthetic or total intravenous anesthesia, perioperative morbidity is rare. The postoperative risk of nausea and vomiting following general anesthesia is further decreased by low-dose propofol infusions, multimodal analgesia, and antiemetic techniques.

9.5.6. Postoperative Phase: Beginning of Recovery

Patients are moved to the recuperation stage of care as soon as they awaken from anesthesia. Before a patient is transferred, a standard sign-out procedure for communication from the operating room to the recovery room should be established. The timing of a patient's transfer from the operating room to recovery may depend on the type of anesthetic used, the patient's coexisting medical conditions, the procedure, and the staff's availability in the recovery room. For instance, a pediatric patient who is otherwise healthy but still under deep anesthesia may regularly be under sufficient observation by a skilled pediatric nurse. If pediatric (or less-than-healthy) patients are awake and able to maintain their airway prior to exiting the operating room, a less experienced postanesthetic nurse might be able to provide them with better care.

The recovery process is divided into three stages: early, intermediate, and late. Phase I of the early recovery lasts until anesthesia wears off or surgically induced abnormalities in motor function and protective reflexes go away. When patients meet these requirements and their pain and nausea are under control, they are moved to phase II recovery. Certain patients can be admitted directly to phase II if they meet these requirements before they even leave the operating room. Table 9.4 describes the modified Aldrete criteria and White criteria, which offer scoring systems for assessing phase II readiness. Phase III takes place at home as the patient returns to their preoperative physiologic state, while Phase II lasts until the discharge requirements are satisfied.

The anesthesia provider orally communicates to the responsible recovery nurse the patient's medical history, current state, and any other pertinent clinical information upon arrival at the designated recovery setting. Since poor communication can lead to avoidable medical errors and unfavorable outcomes, handoff forms or checklists can help patients remember critical patient and perioperative information. (Vila et al., 2008; American Society of Anesthesiologists guidelines for office-based anesthesia; American Society of Anesthesiologists Task Force on Acute Pain Management, 2012)

9.5.6.1. Fast-Tracking: Phase I Bypass

Certain patients are moved straight from the operating room to phase II of recovery, skipping the initial phase and possibly the PACU. Fast-tracking is appropriate for patients with stable cardiopulmonary indices, sufficient analgesia, and no need for airway support. In addition to improving the experience for the patient and family by quickly reuniting patients with their loved ones, fast-tracking may lower outpatient facility costs, contingent on personnel management procedures. Even under general anesthesia, fast-tracking is possible thanks to the use of multimodal analgesia and preventative measures to lower PONV. Important preoperative patient characteristics, such as age greater than 60, ASA physical status score less than 3, and nongeneral surgery, may be used to predict the success of fast-tracking. Using well-defined phase II criteria and fast-track anesthetic techniques does not increase the incidence of immediate postoperative complications. Nursing workload reductions and potential cost savings may be negligible if patient selection is off because the workload is transferred from the PACU to the phase II recovery area.

9.5.6.2. Multimodal Analgesia and Systematic Pain Management

Pain is an unpleasant, subjective, and highly individual experience. For this reason, a multifaceted approach to pain assessment is necessary. It's important to distinguish between pain following surgery and possible chronic pain, anxiety, or even emotional distress. Through risk assessment and treatment planning, a systematic approach to pain management aims to effectively manage pain, reduce side effects, and avoid postoperative and postdischarge patient discomfort. A few professionals support the three Is: intervene, implement, and identify. Understanding the elements that influence the pain experience—the surgical injury mechanism, the patient's characteristics, and the range of multimodal pain therapy—is necessary to identify patients who are at risk. The American Society of Pain Management's practice guidelines for acute pain management advocate for tailored treatment that puts effectiveness and few side effects first. Patient satisfaction may be impacted by counseling patients prior to surgery about the possibility of pain following surgery and the steps that will be taken to minimize it.

Effective analgesia is made possible by implementing a multimodal pain plan that minimizes side effects and spares opioids. One such plan includes regional anesthesia. During preoperative regional anesthesia procedures, the amount of opioids exposed is decreased by intradermal local anesthesia.

PONV may be reduced if opioids are not given prior to the postoperative phase. Preoperative and intraoperative opioid use are linked to increased postoperative sedation and opioid requirements. Both single-shot and continuous peripheral neural blockades decreased the amount of opioids used, enhanced patient comfort, sped up recovery, raised patient satisfaction, and decreased the incidence of adverse events. In addition to reducing pain, multimodal analgesia promotes high patient satisfaction and quick throughput, or "fast-tracking." Preoperative COX-2 inhibitors, intraoperative β-adrenergic blockers, magnesium, pregabalin and gabapentin, subanesthetic-dose ketamine, magnesium, dexamethasone, methylprednisolone, dexmedetomidine, and intravenous lidocaine infusion are all supported by numerous studies as ways to lessen the need for postoperative opioids, relieve acute postoperative pain, and shorten the period of time until discharge. Since there are so many non-opioid analgesics on the market, ambulatory surgical patients who run the risk of experiencing procedural pain can take at least one of these medications. Declining pain scores during recovery are predictive of length of stay in the PACU.

The ambulatory anesthesia provider must act quickly and effectively when multimodal analgesia is insufficient. In order to evaluate the possibility of neural blockade, more nonopioids are given following a multidimensional assessment of pain. In cases of severe uncontrolled postoperative pain, opioids may be warranted; however, it is important to take into account the possibility of delayed discharge due to PONV and other opioid-related adverse events. Nonpharmacologic methods of treating pain ought to be included as well.

Table 9.4. *Clinical Studies on the Efficacy of Aromatherapy and Massage in Preoperative Anxiety*

References	Title	Intervention	Control	Population	Surgery	Type of study	Conclusion
Stanley et al. (121)	Randomized prospective placebo-controlled study of the effects of lavender aromatherapy on preoperative anxiety in cataract surgery patients	Lavender aromatherap	Grape seed oil	75	Cataract surgery	RCT	Lavender aromatherapy reduced anxiety in preoperative cataract surgery patients.
Jaruzel et al. (122)	Aromatherapy for preoperative anxiety: a pilot study	Lavender Aromatherap	Standard pre-operative care	75 Women	Breast surgery	Observational	Use of aromatherapy is beneficial in reducing anxiety experienced by females undergoing breast surgery.
Genc and Saritas (123)	The effects of lavender oil on the anxiety and vital signs of benign prostatic hyperplasia patients in preoperative period	Lavender Aromatherap	Standard pre-operative care	110 Men	BPH surgery	Quasi-experimental	The findings showed that lavender oil inhalation reduced anxiety levels and had effects on the vital signs of BPH patients in their preoperative period.
Ayik and Özden (124)	The effects of preoperative aromatherapy massage on anxiety and sleep quality of colorectal surgery patients: A randomized controlled study	Lavender Aromatherap massage	Standard pre-operative care	80	Colorectal surgery patients	RCT	Aromatherapy massage with lavender oil increased the sleep quality and reduced the level of anxiety in patients with colorectal surgery in the preoperative period.
Bozkurt and Vural (125)	Effect of lavender oil inhalation on reducing presurgical anxiety in orthognathic surgery patients	Lavender aromatherap	No oil	90	Orthognathic surgery	RCT	The results of this study suggested that 1 h of pre-surgical inhalation of 0.1-mL and 0.3-mL lavender oil diffusions in 120 mL of water did not have an anxiolytic effect on patients undergoing orthognathic surgery.
Muzzarelli et al. (126)	Aromatherapy and reducing preprocedural anxiety: a controlled prospective study. Gastroenterology nursing	Lavender aromatherap	Inert oil (placebo)	118	Colonoscopy or esophagogas troduodeno scopy	RCT	This study did not show aromatherapy to be effective based on statistical analysis, patients did generally report the lavender scent to be pleasant.
Akhlaghi et al. (127)	Citrus aurantium blossom and preoperative anxiety	Citrus aurantium Aromatherapy	Saline solution (placebo)	60	Minor operation	RCT	Citrus aurantium blossom may be effective in terms of reduction in preoperative anxiety before minor operation.
Dagli et al. (128)	The effects of aromatherapy using rose oil (Rosa damascena Mill.) on preoperative anxiety: a prospective randomized clinical trial	Rose oil aromatherapy	Standard care	99	Septorhinoplasty/ rhinoplasty	RCT	The application of rose oil aromatherapy by inhalation reduced the scores of preoperative anxiety of patients undergoing septorhinoplasty/rhinoplasty.
Fazlollahpour-Rokni et al. (110)	The effect of inhalation aromatherapy with rose essential oil on the anxiety of patients undergoing coronary artery bypass graft surgery	Rose oil Aromatherapy	Standard care	66	Coronary artery bypass graft surgery	RCT	Inhalation aromatherapy with rose essential oil could not significantly reduce anxiety in CABG patients.
References	**Title**	**Intervention**	**Control**	**Population**	**Surgery**	**Type of study**	**Conclusion**
Kim et al. (129)	The effect of 1, 8-cineole inhalation on preoperative anxiety: a randomized clinical trial.	Limonene, 1,8-cineole, or eucalyptus oil, Aromatherapy	Almond oil (placebo)	62	Selective nerve root block (SNRB).	RCT	Inhalation of 1,8-cineole may be used to relieve anxiety before, during, and after various operations, in addition to SNRB.
Pasyar et al. (130)	The effect of bergamot orange essence on anxiety, salivary cortisol, and alpha amylase in patients prior to laparoscopic cholecystectomy: a controlled trial	Bergamot orange Aromatherapy	Grape seed oil (placebo)	60	Laparoscopic cholecystectomy	RCT	Bergamot orange essence decreased anxiety and salivary alpha amylase level.
Li et al. (131)	Benefits of hand massage on anxiety in preoperative outpatient: a quasi-experimental study with pre-and post-tests.	Massage	Rest	138	Mixed surgery	Quasi-experimental	After receiving a 15-min non-therapeutic hand massage, patients experienced reduced anxiety levels and increased satisfaction.
Farahani et al. (132)	Effects of extremity massage on preoperative anxiety: a three-arm randomized controlled clinical trial on phacoemulsification candidates.	Massage	Placebo	90 Women	Phacoemul sification cataract surgery	RCT	Application of hand or foot massage seems to be effective in managing anxiety in patients waiting for phacoemulsification cataract surgery.
Brand et al. (133)	The effect of hand massage on preoperative anxiety in ambulatory surgery patients	Massage	Customary nursing care	86	Ambulatory surgery	Quasi-experimental	Hand massage reduces anxiety for patients awaiting ambulatory surgery and outpatient procedures
Mohammadpourhodki et al. (134)	Evaluating the effect of massage based on slow stroke back massage on the anxiety of candidates for cataract surgery.	Massage	Standard care	60	Cataract surgery.	Quasi-experimental	Slow-stroke-back massage, significantly reduces anxiety in patients who are candidates for cataract surgery.
Peng et al. (135)	Effects of massage on the anxiety of patients receiving percutaneous coronary intervention	Massage	Standard care	117	Percutaneous coronary intervention	RCT	Massage treatments reduced the emergency response and level of anxiety of cardiovascular patients before PCI. The post-intervention blood pressure, heart rate, and pain score of the intervention group were significantly better than those of the control group
Rosen et al. (136)	Massage for perioperative pain and anxiety in placement of vascular access devices	Massage	Usual care with structured attention	60	Surgical placement of vascular access devices	RCT	Massage therapy participants had a statistically significant, greater reduction in anxiety after the first intervention compared with individuals receiving structured attention.
McRee et al. (137)	Using massage and music therapy to improve postoperative outcomes	I-massage with music therapy II- massage only III- music therapy only	Standard care	52	Mixed surgery	Quasi-experimental	Ostoperative anxiety levels were significantly lower and postoperative prolactin levels were significantly higher for all groups.

Source: Wang R, Huang X, Wang Y and Akbari M (2022) Non-pharmacologic Approaches in Preoperative Anxiety, a Comprehensive Review. Front. Public Health 10:854673. doi: 10.3389/fpubh.2022.854673.

9.5.6.3. Postoperative Nausea and Vomiting

There is unquestionably a connection between pain, opioid-based painkillers, and nausea and vomiting. Patients rank the prevention of PONV as being on par with the treatment and prevention of pain. The objectives of perioperative medicine and ambulatory anesthesia care are incompatible with PONV and PDNV because they impede the recovery of everyday function following surgery. PONV frequently lowers the standard of recovery, causes delays in discharge, and can result in an unforeseen admission.

Apfel's scoring system is used to direct prophylaxis against PONV. It is predictive of PONV in the PACU and the first 24 hours after discharge, but the scoring system is a poor predictor of nausea and vomiting 24 to 72 hours after discharge (PDNV). PONV occurs in up to 74% of untreated at-risk outpatients, and PDNV in up to 33%. The treatment of PONV begins preoperatively when baseline risk is assessed and multimodal analgesia and PONV prophylaxis are planned and implemented. For most patients, guideline-driven multimodal management reduces the incidence of PONV early in the discharge period. A regimen of both intravenous dexamethasone 8 mg and ondansetron 4 mg intraoperatively, followed by oral tablets of 8 mg ondansetron at discharge and on postoperative days 1 and 2, virtually eliminates early and late PONV/PDNV in many patients including those in the highest risk categories. Recent metaanalysis and guidelines, however, support an equivalent reduction in the incidence of PONV with a 4-mg to 5-mg dose of dexamethasone. Despite triple prophylaxis with dexamethasone, ondansetron, and scopolamine, and omitting anesthetic triggers, a small residual group of patients still experiences significant PONV. Intravenous hydration has been shown to occasionally lower the frequency of both PONV and pain. Adequate hydration and dual prophylaxis (dexamethasone and ondansetron) can reduce the risk of PONV in the majority of otherwise healthy pediatric patients by up to 80%. Even when administered intraoperatively, ondansetron is less effective when used repeatedly in the PACU for nausea and vomiting in adults than a small intravenous dose of promethazine (6 points and 25 mg).

9.5.7. Postoperative Phase: Discharging Patients Home

9.5.7.1. Patient Assessment

The majority of patients will recover at home, and recovery may last several days after discharge. A doctor or other designated health care provider evaluates the patient's preparedness for return home prior to discharge. The postanesthesia discharge scoring system (PADSS) is one validated scoring system that makes use of standardized criteria. When compared to arbitrary PACU time requirements, the application of such criteria has been linked to shorter lengths of stay in the unit. One hour following surgery, the majority of children are safely discharged from the PACU when the criteria in the pediatric PADSS are followed. Practice guidelines further distinguish between necessary and superfluous discharge criteria.

9.5.7.2. Patient Instructions

An excellent outcome from ambulatory surgery depends on patient preparation and education. A long time in advance of the procedure, the patient, as well as the friends and family who will serve as primary caregivers, get ready. Legal action may be a possibility if adverse events occur after ambulatory anesthesia discharge. Patients undergoing regional anesthesia may avoid further harm or the need for emergency care if they follow clear and concise instructions. The administration of crutches or other immobilization devices, the timing of analgesic and antiemetic therapy, and the care of the insensate limb are all covered in the instructions. It is possible to enhance patient readiness and lessen resource-consuming misunderstandings in the recovery room by starting this kind of preoperative education and training early on. Further guidelines advise the patient not to drive, drink alcohol, operate heavy machinery, or make important life or financial decisions after receiving any degree of anesthesia or sedation. The escort or caregiver must be physically and mentally capable of helping the patient, identifying when assistance is required, facilitating communication with medical professionals, and obtaining emergency care if necessary. Regular reviews and modifications of criteria and adherence to discharge criteria are necessary (Figure 9.4).

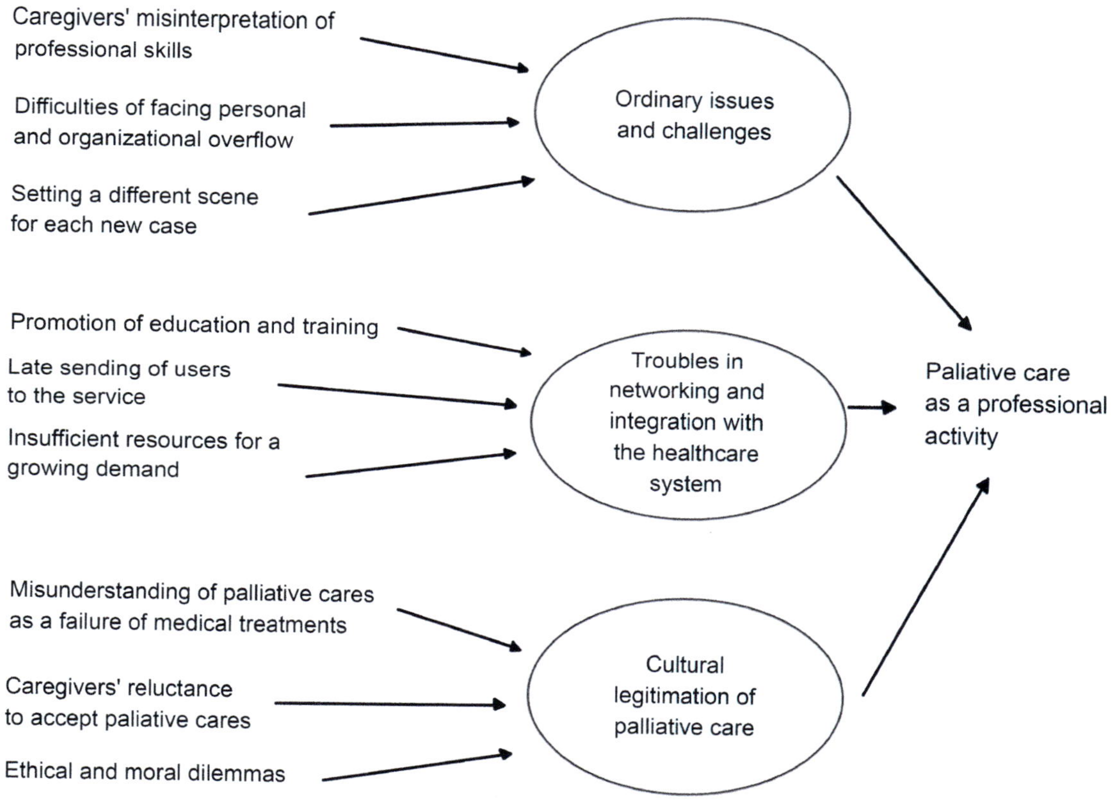

Figure 9.4. *Themes in caregiver activity.*

Source: Rossi P, Crippa M, Scaccabarozzi G. The Relationship between Practitioners and Caregivers during a Treatment of Palliative Care: A Grounded Theory of a Challenging Collaborative Process. International Journal of Environmental Research and Public Health. 2021; 18(15):8081. https://doi.org/10.3390/ijerph18158081.

9.5.7.3. PACU Management

In a busy ambulatory surgery center or office, the availability of anesthesia staff to handle airway or cardiopulmonary emergencies may be restricted in the absence of advance planning. In the event that a patient becomes medically unstable or is unable to maintain an airway, an anesthesia provider should be on call at all times. The PACU frequently serves as the last venue for post-discharge care review and patient education. Particular instructions on how to address queries or concerns with the ambulatory care team should be provided to caregivers. An ambulatory care facility may decide to have a hotline or answering service for round-the-clock support and guidance for patients and caregivers.

9.5.7.4. Patient Transfer or 23-Hour Observation

A patient is moved to a hospital or short-stay unit for ongoing monitoring or care if their condition does not meet the requirements for discharge. Generally speaking, admission to observation units is less expensive than hospital stays or ER visits. A clear management plan should be in place for patient transfers at procedural sites. A thorough physician-to-physician hand-off is provided by the ASC, outlining the patient's medical history, surgical course, present condition, concerns, and needs upon transfer. The right level of care should be determined by the clinical status for planned or unexpected 23-hour observation. The patient ought to be moved to a hospital-based facility if the observation unit's capacity for care and monitoring is inadequate. In a busy medical facility, the amount of time it takes to get a patient access to a bed may be reduced by quickly determining whether admission or transfer is necessary. Transfer delays may lead to higher morbidity and higher expenses since recovery resources will need to be used more frequently.

(Vila et al., 2008; American Society of Anesthesiologists guidelines for office-based anesthesia; American Society of Anesthesiologists Task Force on Acute Pain Management, 2012)

9.5.8. Postoperative Phase: Postdischarge Issues

The post-discharge phase (phase III) creates challenges for the patient and ambulatory clinicians. After discharge many patients suffer moderate to severe pain, cognitive impairment, and PDNV. They may take several days to return to normal activity. The demands of the recovering patient and the strain on the caregivers can swiftly outweigh the convenience of returning home following a procedure. Patients might need more time to recover than previously thought. Caregiver burden rises in response to both increased pain and longer recovery times. Patients' and caregivers' daily lives may be emotionally and physically disrupted by informal caregiving. These results may be similar to research on caregiver burden in conditions of chronic illness.

Regarding the patient's mental and physical well-being, their stay in the hospital, and the provision of care following outpatient surgery, numerous significant themes have been found. Patients should have ongoing access to reeducation and redirection, as suggested by a 2012 study that found a 25% accuracy rate for information retention and interpretation of information given in a preoperative educational session in healthy volunteers. Because of this, a hotline or answering service maintains the multidisciplinary team approach; anesthetists shouldn't prioritize surgical wound drainage, and surgeons are usually unable to troubleshoot peripheral nerve catheters. Many studies have evaluated the quality of recovery during the first postoperative week of treatment. Two months after abdominal surgery, 33 percent of patients had suboptimal recovery, despite being discharged from the hospital within 24 hours of the procedure. Three weeks following surgery, patients who were older, experienced complications, had a low baseline health-related quality of life, or engaged in a high baseline level of physical activity, had a lower likelihood of returning to preoperative levels.

9.5.8.1. Postdischarge Nausea and Vomiting

A validated prediction model for PDNV up to 48 hours after ambulatory surgery uses several components: operating room time,

PONV history, use of ondansetron, and pain during days 3 to 7 to predict PDNV 3 to 7 days after discharge. Patients at risk should receive triple therapy (dexamethasone, ondansetron, scopolamine), continuous regional anesthesia when appropriate, robust nonopioid analgesic treatment, and additional rescue drugs in the event triple therapy is insufficient. Although newer, long-acting drugs have entered clinical practice, traditional and less expensive options appear equally efficacious.

9.5.8.2. Postdischarge Pain

Effective multimodal pain management can address two of the main post-discharge concerns, as pain is one of the determinants of post-stroke neuropathy (PDNV). Peripheral neural blockade helps to minimize the need for opioids by providing analgesia continuously. Clinical access should be available 24/7, and patients receiving continuous blocks should be contacted every day. The painful area that the peripheral nerve catheter treats should be disclosed to the patients. Should the patient self-administer a bolus every hour for saphenous-mediated, medial ankle pain, the sciatic nerve catheter's pump reservoir can be rapidly emptied in the case of ankle surgery. Visual reference materials are provided as a result. The materials show which parts of the operated extremity are best treated with a demand dose of local anesthetic administered by the patient, and which areas are treated with an oral analgesic dose. We recommend avoiding combination tablets (e.g, codeine and acetaminophen, hydrocodone and acetaminophen). Without excessive or subtherapeutic exposure to acetaminophen, "uptitration" or discontinuation of opioids via telephone directive is made possible by tramadol or small-dose oxycodone. Acetaminophen may be given continuously if needed, with the FDA's 3g daily limit acknowledged.

9.5.8.3. Nerve Injury or Motor Deficits

In the days following surgery, follow-up correspondence from the anesthesia group or an ASC delegate should confirm that neural blockade has completely resolved. The patient's attending surgeon and anesthesiologist are alerted for evaluation and treatment in the event of ongoing sensory or motor impairments. After orthopedic surgery, iatrogenic injuries can occasionally complicate a doctor's evaluation of the injury's etiology.

9.5.9. Outcomes

A patient may or may not be aware that they were readmitted following surgery due to severe, uncontrollable postoperative pain, nausea, and vomiting, depending on the ambulatory anesthesia provider. The anesthesia provider might not be aware of the patient's ongoing acute pain in the days or weeks after her discharge or her ongoing severe pain six months later if there is no follow-up. Given this result, would the anesthesiologist be more inclined to employ different methods in similar cases in the future? Results from ambulatory surgery encompass what happens after the patient is released from the hospital and sometimes even weeks or months following the procedure. Potential improvements in preoperative and intraoperative management, as well as postoperative and post-discharge care, require evaluation of the healing process. Events like post-disordered breathing (PDNV), chronic moderate to severe pain, regional anesthetic failure or complication, ER visits, cognitive dysfunction, and dissatisfied service should be regularly monitored by an ambulatory anesthesia group. In some industries, including health care, the use of outcome measurement data to standardize care has successfully improved safety and service delivery. A well-established principle of evidence-based medicine is to use historical patient outcomes to inform treatment decisions. Data should be gathered via anesthesia information systems on the day of surgery, merged with follow-up data from phone calls made after discharge, and compared across different practice settings, peer institutions, and individual practitioners using the numerous outcome databases. (Vila et al., 2008; American Society of Anesthesiologists guidelines for office-based anesthesia; American Society of Anesthesiologists Task Force on Acute Pain Management, 2012).

A Closer Look

Ambulatory Surgery

Ambulatory surgery, also known as outpatient surgery or same-day surgery, is a medical procedure performed on a patient who is admitted and discharged from a medical facility on the same day. This surgical approach has become increasingly popular due to advancements in medical technology, anesthesia techniques, and the desire to reduce healthcare costs and improve patient convenience. Ambulatory surgery encompasses a wide range of procedures across various medical specialties, including orthopedics, ophthalmology, dermatology, and gastroenterology, among others. Common ambulatory surgeries include cataract removal, hernia repair, tonsillectomy, and arthroscopic knee surgery. The process of ambulatory surgery typically begins with preoperative assessment and preparation, where the patient undergoes a thorough evaluation to ensure they are suitable for same-day discharge. This assessment involves reviewing the patient's medical history, performing necessary tests, and providing education about the procedure and postoperative care. Once cleared for surgery, the patient arrives at the outpatient facility on the day of the procedure and undergoes the necessary preoperative procedures, including administration of anesthesia.

Ambulatory surgery facilities are specially designed to accommodate the unique needs of outpatient procedures, with streamlined workflows and efficient patient care processes. These facilities are equipped with state-of-the-art surgical suites, recovery areas, and amenities to ensure patient comfort and safety. The surgical team, consisting of surgeons, nurses, anesthesiologists, and other healthcare professionals, collaborates closely to deliver high-quality care throughout the entire surgical experience. One of the key advantages of ambulatory surgery is its cost-effectiveness compared to traditional inpatient procedures. By avoiding overnight hospital stays, patients can significantly reduce their healthcare expenses while still receiving the necessary medical treatment. Additionally, ambulatory surgery offers greater flexibility and convenience for patients, allowing them to undergo procedures without disrupting their daily routines or spending extended periods away from home. Despite its benefits, ambulatory surgery may not be suitable for all patients or procedures. Certain medical conditions, such as complex surgeries or underlying health issues, may necessitate inpatient care for proper monitoring and management of postoperative complications. Additionally, patients with limited access to transportation or inadequate support at home may face challenges with same-day discharge following surgery.

Ambulatory surgery represents a significant advancement in modern healthcare, offering patients a safe, efficient, and cost-effective alternative to traditional inpatient procedures. With the careful patient selection, meticulous preoperative planning, and comprehensive postoperative care, ambulatory surgery continues to play a crucial role in meeting the evolving needs of patients and healthcare systems worldwide. (Vila et al., 2008; American Society of Anesthesiologists guidelines for office-based anesthesia; American Society of Anesthesiologists Task Force on Acute Pain Management, 2012)

Summary

- Ambulatory surgery requires a minimally invasive anesthetic with maximal emphasis on patient safety, comfort, and recovery. The challenges inherent to this requirement have led to innovative and highly patient-centered methods by ambulatory groups.
- An ambulatory anesthesia provider appreciates the value of standardized work, effectively communicates with the team, values the patient's and surgeon's time, employs broad but cost-effective multimodal analgesia, and administers minimally invasive short-acting, fast-emergence anesthesia for a rapid and safe recovery.
- The ancillary care staff in the outpatient setting is a specialized workforce that contributes substantively to the achievement of the facility's goals. Specialized nursing and anesthesia personnel typically are trained and rehearsed in emergency care in the freestanding or office setting because of the facility's relative isolation.
- In an ambulatory surgical cohort, patients with established OSA, regardless of severity or compliance with continuous positive airway pressure (CPAP) therapy, had no unanticipated admissions or delayed discharges, suggesting good patient selection and monitoring.
- Patients with chronic pain, opioid dependence, or a history of severe uncontrolled postsurgical pain or who are receiving buprenorphine or methadone therapy are best identified well in advance of the day of surgery for proper treatment planning.
- The ASA and Center for Medicaid Services (CMS) have determined that a preoperative review of the patient's medical and social history and a physical examination by an anesthesia provider are necessary.
- Monitored anesthesia care (MAC), a term of anesthesia billing describes sedation by an anesthesia provider. Titrated sedation and continuous monitoring often transition the patient in and out of general anesthesia, as required by changes in patient or surgical conditions.
- Regional anesthesia techniques have revolutionized hernia and breast surgery. Paravertebral regional block decreases opioid exposure, PONV, urinary retention, and pain scores as compared to general or neuraxial anesthetics.
- Neuraxial blockade, with or without sedation, has been reported to reduce the incidence of PONV and pain after lower extremity, gynecologic, and abdominal surgery and for patients with chronic respiratory disease.
- The natural airway creates a potential risk for some patient-procedure combinations, especially those involving surgery in the airway. The decision to provide general anesthesia with or without endotracheal intubation should be determined by patient and procedure-related risk factors.
- In the event a patient's condition has not met discharge criteria, the patient is transferred to a hospital facility or short-stay unit for continued observation or treatment. Admission to observation units typically costs less than emergency room visits or hospital admission.
- The ambulatory anesthesia provider may or may not be aware of a patient's readmission after surgery for severe, uncontrolled, postoperative pain, nausea and vomiting.

References

1. Abbass, I. M., Krause, T. M., Virani, S. S., et al. (2015). Revisiting the economic efficiencies of observation units. *Managed Care, 24*(3), 46–52.
2. Abdallah, F. W., Morgan, P. J., Cil, T., et al. (2014). Ultrasound-guided multilevel paravertebral blocks and total intravenous anesthesia improve the quality of recovery after ambulatory breast tumor resection. *Anesthesiology, 120*(3), 703–713.
3. Agarwala, A. V., Firth, P. G., Albrecht, M. A., et al. (2015). An electronic checklist improves transfer and retention of critical information at intraoperative handoff of care. *Anesthesia & Analgesia, 120*(1), 96–104.
4. Ahmad, J., Ho, O. A., Carman, W. W., et al. (2014). Assessing patient safety in Canadian ambulatory surgery facilities: A national survey. *Plastic Surgery, 22*(1), 34–38.
5. Aldrete, J. A. (1995). The post-anesthetic recovery score revisited. *Journal of Clinical Anesthesia, 7*, 89–91.
6. American Association for Accreditation of Ambulatory Facilities. (2014). Medicare standards and checklist for accreditation of ambulatory surgery facilities, version 6.5. Retrieved from: http://www.aaaasf.org/standards.html (accessed on 29 July 2024).
7. American Society of Anesthesiologists Task Force on Acute Pain Management. (2012). Practice guidelines for acute pain management in the perioperative setting: An updated report by the American society of anesthesiologist's task force on acute pain management. *Anesthesiology, 116*(2), 248–273.
8. American Society of Anesthesiologists Task Force on Perioperative Management of Patients with Obstructive Sleep Apnea. (2014). Practice guidelines for the perioperative management of patients with obstructive sleep apnea: An updated report by the American society of anesthesiologist's task force on perioperative management of patients with obstructive sleep apnea. *Anesthesiology, 120*(2), 268–286.
9. Andreae, M. H., & Andreae, D. A. (2012). Local anesthetics and regional anesthesia for preventing chronic pain after surgery. *Cochrane Database of Systematic Reviews, 2012*(10), CD007105.
10. Angioli, R., De Cicco Nardone, C., Plotti, F., et al. (2014). Use of music to reduce anxiety during office hysteroscopy: Prospective randomized trial. *Journal of Minimally Invasive Gynecology, 21*(3), 454–459.
11. Angst, M. S., & Clark, J. C. (2006). Opioid-induced hyperalgesia: A qualitative systematic review. *Anesthesiology, 104*, 570–587.
12. Apfel, C. C. (2012). Who is at risk for post discharge nausea and vomiting after ambulatory surgery? *Anesthesiology, 117*, 475–486.
13. Apfel, C. C., Korttila, K., Abdalla, M., et al. (2004). A factorial trial of six interventions for the prevention of postoperative nausea and vomiting. *New England Journal of Medicine, 350*(24), 2441–2451.
14. Apfel, C. C., Laara, E., Koivuranta, M., et al. (1999). A simplified risk score for predicting postoperative nausea and vomiting: Conclusions from cross-validations between two centers. *Anesthesiology, 91*, 693–700.

15. Apfelbaum, J. L., Hagberg, C. A., Caplan, R. A., et al. (2013). Practice guidelines for management of the difficult airway: An updated report by the American society of anesthesiologists task force on management of the difficult airway. *Anesthesiology, 118*(2), 251–270.

16. Apfelbaum, J. L., Lichtor, J. L., Lane, B. S., et al. (1996). Awakening, clinical recovery, and psychomotor effects after desflurane and propofol anesthesia. *Anesthesia & Analgesia, 83*, 721–725.

17. Apfelbaum, J., Silverstein, J., Chung, F., et al. (2013). Practice guidelines for postanesthetic care: An updated report by the American Society of Anesthesiologists Task Force on Postanesthetic Care. *Anesthesiology, 118*, 291–307.

18. Bashandy, G. M., & Abbas, D. N. (2015). Pectoral nerves I and II blocks in multimodal analgesia for breast cancer surgery: A randomized clinical trial. *Regional Anesthesia and Pain Medicine, 40*(1), 68–74.

19. Bennarroch-Gampel, J., Sheffield, K. M., Duncan, C. B., et al. (2012). Preoperative laboratory testing in patients undergoing elective, low-risk ambulatory surgery. *Annals of Surgery, 256*(3), 518–528.

20. Berkow, L. C., Greenberg, R. S., Kan, K. H., et al. (2009). Need for emergency surgical airway reduced by a comprehensive difficult airway program. *Anesthesia & Analgesia, 109*(6), 1860–1869.

21. Berwick, D. M. (1992). The clinical process and the quality process. *Quality Management in Health Care, 1*, 1–8.

22. Best, M. J., Buller, L. T., & Miranda, A. (2015). United States trends in ankle arthroscopy: Analysis of the national survey of ambulatory surgery and national hospital discharge survey. *Foot & Ankle Specialist, 8*(4), 266–272.

23. Bhananker, S. M., Posner, K. L., Cheney, F. W., et al. (2006). Injury and liability associated with monitored anesthesia care: A closed claims analysis. *Anesthesiology, 104*, 228–234.

24. Bilimoria, K. Y., Liu, Y., Paruch, J. L., et al. (2013). Development and evaluation of the universal ACS NSQIP surgical risk calculator: A decision aid and informed consent tool for patients and surgeons. *Journal of the American College of Surgeons, 217*(5), 833–842.

25. Bingham, A. E., Fur, R., Horn, J. L., et al. (2012). Continuous peripheral nerve block compared with single-injection peripheral nerve block: A systematic review and meta-analysis of randomized controlled trials. *Regional Anesthesia & Pain Medicine, 37*(6), 583–594.

26. Bouzinac, A., Brenier, G., Dao, M., & Delbas, A. (2015). Bilateral association of pecs I block and serratus plane block for postoperative analgesia after double modified radical mastectomy. *Minerva Anesthesiologic, 81*(5), 589–590.

27. Brotman, D. J., Bakhru, M., Saber, W., et al. (2007). Discontinuation of antiplatelet therapy prior to low-risk noncardiac surgery in patients with drug eluting stents: A retrospective cohort study. *Journal of Hospital Medicine, 2*, 378–384.

28. Brown, E. C., & Kros, J. (2010). Reducing room turnaround time at a regional hospital. *Quality Management in Health Care, 19*(1), 90–100.

29. Bryson, G. L., Gomez, C. P., & Jee, R. M., et al. (2012). Unplanned admission after day surgery: A historical cohort study in patients with obstructive sleep apnea. *Canadian Journal of Anesthesia, 59*(9), 842–851.

30. Bryson, G. L., Mercer, C., & Varpio, L. (2014). Patient and caregiver experience following ambulatory surgery: Qualitative analysis in a cohort of patients 65 yr. and older. *Canadian Journal of Anesthesia, 61*(11), 986–994.

31. Butz, S. (Ed.). (2015). *Perioperative Drill-Based Crisis Management*. Cambridge, England: Cambridge University Press.

32. Candiotti, K. A., Kovac, A. L., Melson, T. I., et al. (2008). A randomized, double-blind study to evaluate the efficacy and safety of three different doses of palonosetron versus placebo in preventing postoperative nausea and vomiting. *Anesthesia & Analgesia, 107*, 445–451.

33. Cappelleri, G., Aldegheri, G., Danelli, G., et al. (2005). Spinal anesthesia with hyperbaric levobupivacaine and ropivacaine for outpatient knee arthroscopy: A prospective, randomized, double-blind study. *Anesthesia & Analgesia, 101*, 77–82.

34. Carlhed, R., & Bojestig, M. (2009). Improved clinical outcome after acute myocardial infarction in hospitals participating in a Swedish quality improvement initiative. *Circulation: Cardiovascular Quality and Outcomes, 2*(3), 458–464.

35. Carli, F., Kehlet, H., Baldini, G., et al. (2011). Evidence basis for regional anesthesia in multidisciplinary fast-track surgical care pathways. *Regional Anesthesia & Pain Medicine, 36*, 63–72.

36. Carmosino, M. J., Friesen, R. H., & Doran, A. (2007). Perioperative complications in children with pulmonary hypertension undergoing noncardiac surgery or cardiac catheterization. *Anesthesia & Analgesia, 104*, 521–527.

37. Casati, A., Danelli, G., Berti, M., et al. (2006). Intrathecal 2-chloroprocaine for lower limb outpatient surgery: A prospective, randomized, double-blind, clinical evaluation. *Anesthesia & Analgesia, 103*, 234–238.

38. Chanthong, P., Abrishami, A., Wong, J., et al. (2009). Systematic review of questionnaires of measuring patient satisfaction in ambulatory anesthesia. *Anesthesiology, 110*(5), 1061–1067.

39. Chen, C. L., Lin, G. A., Bardach, N. S., et al. (2015). Preoperative medical testing in Medicare patients undergoing cataract surgery. *New England Journal of Medicine, 372*(16), 1530–1538.

40. Chen, L., Tang, J., White, P. F., et al. (1998). The effect of location of transcutaneous electrical nerve stimulation on postoperative opioid analgesic requirement: Acupoint versus nonacupoint stimulation. *Anesthesia & Analgesia, 87*, 1129–1134.

41. Chin, K. J., & Chee, V. W. (2006). Laryngeal edema associated with the ProSeal laryngeal mask airway in upper respiratory tract infections. *Canadian Journal of Anesthesia, 53*(4), 389–392.

42. Chung, F. (1995). Recovery pattern and home-readiness after ambulatory surgery. *Anesthesia & Analgesia, 80*(5), 896–902.

43. Chung, F., & Mezei, G. (1999). Factors contributing to a prolonged stay after ambulatory surgery. *Anesthesia & Analgesia, 89*, 1352–1359.

44. Chung, F., Kayumov, L., Sinclair, D. R., et al. (2005). What is the driving performance of ambulatory surgical patients after general anesthesia? *Anesthesiology, 103*(5), 951–956.

45. Chung, F., Subramanyam, R., Liao, P., et al. (2012). High STOP-Bang score indicates a high probability of obstructive sleep apnoea. *British Journal of Anesthesia, 108*, 768–775.

46. Chung, F., Yegneswaran, B., Herrera, F., et al. (2008). Patients with difficult intubation may need referral to sleep clinics. *Anesthesia & Analgesia, 107*, 915–920.

47. Chung, S., Yuan, H., & Chung, F. (2008). A systematic review of obstructive sleep apnea and its implications for anesthesiologists. *Anesthesia & Analgesia, 107*, 1543–1563.

48. Clarke, H., Kirkham, K. R., Orser, B. A., et al. (2013). Gabapentin reduces preoperative anxiety and pain catastrophizing in highly anxious patients prior to major surgery: A blinded randomized placebo-controlled trial. *Canadian Journal of Anesthesia, 60*(5), 432–442.

49. Coley, K. C., Williams, B. A., DaPos, S. V., et al. (2002). Retrospective evaluation of unanticipated admissions and readmissions after same day surgery and associated costs. *Journal of Clinical Anesthesia, 14*(5), 349–353.

50. Collard, V., Mistraletti, G., Taqi, A., et al. (2007). Intraoperative esmolol infusion in the absence of opioids spares postoperative fentanyl in patients undergoing ambulatory laparoscopic cholecystectomy. *Anesthesia & Analgesia, 105*(5), 1255–1262.

51. Coloma, M., Chiu, J. W., & White, P. F. (2001). The use of esmolol as an alternative to remifentanil during desflurane anesthesia for fast-track outpatient gynecologic laparoscopic surgery. *Anesthesia & Analgesia, 92*, 352–357.

52. Colson, P., Saussine, M., Seguin, J. R., et al. (1992). Hemodynamic effects of anesthesia in patients chronically treated with angiotensin-converting enzyme inhibitors. *Anesthesia & Analgesia, 74*, 805–808.

53. Committee on Standards and Practice Parameters, Apfelbaum, J. L., Connis, R. T., Nickinovich, D. G., et al. (2012). Practice advisory for paranesthesia evaluation: An updated report by the American Society of Anesthesiologists Task Force on Preanesthesia Evaluation. *Anesthesiology, 116*(3), 522–538.

54. Cook, T. M., Woodall, N., & Frerk, C. (2011). Major complications of airway management in the UK: Results of the Fourth National Audit Project of the Royal College of Anesthetists and the Difficult Airway Society. Part 1: Anesthesia. *British Journal of Anesthesia, 106*(5), 617–631.

55. Coriat, P., Richer, C., Douraki, T., et al. (1994). Influence of chronic angiotensin-converting enzyme inhibition on anesthetic induction. *Anesthesiology, 81*, 299–307.

56. De Oliveira, G. S., Agarwal, D., & Benzon, H. T. (2012). Perioperative single dose ketorolac to prevent postoperative pain: A meta-analysis of randomized trials. *Anesthesia & Analgesia, 114*, 424–433.

57. De Oliveira, G. S., Almeida, M. D., & Benzon, H. T., et al. (2011). Perioperative single dose systemic dexamethasone for postoperative pain. *Anesthesiology, 115*, 575–588.

58. De Oliveira, G. S., Castro-Alves, L. J., Ahmad, S., et al. (2013). Dexamethasone to prevent postoperative nausea and vomiting: An updated meta-analysis of randomized controlled trials. *Anesthesia & Analgesia, 116*(1), 58–74.

59. De Oliveira, G. S., Fitzgerald, P., Streicher, L. F., et al. (2012). Systemic lidocaine to improve postoperative quality of recovery after ambulatory laparoscopic surgery. *Anesthesia & Analgesia, 115*(2), 262–267.

60. Dickerson, D. M. (2014). Acute pain management. *Anesthesiology Clinics, 32*(2), 495–504.

61. Dincer, H. E., & O'Neill, W. (2006). Deleterious effects of sleep-disordered breathing on the heart and vascular system. *Respiration, 73*, 124–130.

62. Dwyer, T., Drexler, M., Chan, V. W., et al. (2015). Neurological complications related to elective orthopedic surgery: Part 2: Common hip and knee procedures. *Regional Anesthesia and Pain Medicine, 40*(5), 443–454.

63. Dwyer, T., Henry, P. D., Cholvisudhi, P., et al. (2015). Neurological complications related to elective orthopedic surgery: Part 1: Common shoulder and elbow procedures. *Regional Anesthesia and Pain Medicine, 40*(5), 455–466.

64. Dzwonczyk, R., Weaver, T. E., Puente, E. G., & Bergese, S. D. (2012). Postoperative nausea and vomiting prophylaxis from an economic point of view. *American Journal of Therapeutics, 19*(1), 11–15.

65. Eid, H. (2009). Paravertebral block: An overview. *Current Anesthesia & Critical Care, 20*, 65–70.

66. Eijkemans, M. J., van Houdenhoven, M., Nguyen, T., et al. (2010). Predicting the unpredictable: A new prediction model for operating room times using individual characteristics and the surgeon's estimate. *Anesthesiology, 112*, 41–49.

67. el-Ganzouri, A. R., McCarthy, R. J., Tuman, K. J., et al. (1996). Preoperative airway assessment: Predictive value of a multivariate risk index. *Anesthesia & Analgesia, 82*, 1197–1204.

68. Engelman, E., Salengros, J., & Barvais, L. (2008). How much does pharmacologic prophylaxis reduce postoperative vomiting in children? *Anesthesiology, 109*, 1023–1035.

69. Evron, S., & Ezri, T. (2009). Organizational prerequisites for anesthesia outside the operating room. *Current Opinion in Anesthesiology, 22*, 514–518.

70. Exadaktylos, A. K., Buggy, D. J., Moriarty, D. C., et al. (2006). Can anesthetic technique for primary breast cancer surgery affect recurrence or metastasis? *Anesthesiology, 105*, 660–664.

71. Fleisher, L. A., Fleischmann, K. E., Auerbach, A. D., et al. (2014). 2014 ACC/AHA guideline on perioperative cardiovascular evaluation and management of patients undergoing noncardiac surgery: A report of the American college of cardiology/American heart association task force on practice guidelines. *Circulation, 130*(24), e278–e333.

72. Fleisher, L. A., Pasternak, L. R., & Lyles, A. (2007). A novel index of elevated risk of inpatient hospital admission immediately following outpatient surgery. *Archives of Surgery, 142*(3), 263–268.

73. Fleisher, L. A., Pasternak, L. R., Herbert, R., & Anderson, G. F. (2004). Inpatient hospital admission and death after outpatient surgery in elderly patients: Importance of patient and system characteristics and location of care. *Archives of Surgery, 139*(1), 67–72.

74. Fong, R., & Sweitzer, B. J. (2014). Preoperative optimization of patients undergoing ambulatory surgery. *Current Anesthesiology Reports, 4*, 303–315.

75. Ford, M. K., Beattie, W. S., & Wijeysundera, D. N. (2010). Prediction of perioperative cardiac complications and mortality by the revised cardiac risk index: A systematic review. *Annals of Internal Medicine, 152*, 26–35.

76. Fox, J. P., Vashi, A. A., Ross, J. S., et al. (2014). Hospital-based, acute care after ambulatory surgery center discharge. *Surgery, 155*(5), 743–753.

77. Fredman, B., Nathanson, M. H., Smith, I., et al. (1995). Sevoflurane for outpatient anesthesia: A comparison with propofol. *Anesthesia & Analgesia, 81*, 823–828.

78. Fung, D., Cohen, M. M., Stewart, S., et al. (2005). What determines patient satisfaction with cataract care under topical local anesthesia and monitored sedation in a community hospital setting? *Anesthesia & Analgesia, 100*, 1644–1650.

79. Gan, J., Sloan, F., Dear, G., et al. (2001). How much are patients willing to pay to avoid postoperative nausea and vomiting? *Anesthesia & Analgesia, 92*, 393–400.

80. Gan, T. J., Diemunsch, P., Habib, A. S., et al. (2014). Consensus guidelines for the management of postoperative nausea and vomiting. *Anesthesia & Analgesia, 118*(1), 85–113.

81. Gerbershagen, H. J., Aduckathil, S., van Wijck, A. J., et al. (2013). Pain intensity on the first day after surgery: A prospective cohort study comparing 179 surgical procedures. *Anesthesiology, 118*(4), 934–944.

82. Greenland, K. B. (2012). Difficult airway management in an ambulatory surgical center? *Current Opinion in Anesthesiology, 25*(6), 659–664.

83. Grisel, J., & Arjmand, E. (2009). Comparing quality at an ambulatory surgery center and a hospital-based facility: Preliminary findings. *Otolaryngology–Head and Neck Surgery, 141*(6), 701–709.

84. Gupta, A., Stierer, T., Zuckerman, R., et al. (2004). Comparison of recovery profile after ambulatory anesthesia with propofol, isoflurane, sevoflurane, and desflurane: A systematic review. *Anesthesia & Analgesia, 98*(3), 632–641.

85. Gupta, A., Wu, C. L., Elkassabany, N., et al. (2003). Does the routine prophylactic use of antiemetics affect the incidence of post-discharge nausea and vomiting following ambulatory surgery? A systematic review of randomized controlled trials. *Anesthesiology, 99*, 488–495.

86. Gurusamy, K., Junnarkar, S., Farouk, M., et al. (2008). Meta-analysis of randomized controlled trials on the safety and effectiveness of day laparoscopic cholecystectomy. *British Journal of Surgery, 95*(2), 161–168.

87. Habib, A. S., Reuveni, J., Taguchi, A., et al. (2007). A comparison of ondansetron with promethazine for treating postoperative nausea and vomiting in patients who received prophylaxis with ondansetron: A retrospective database analysis. *Anesthesia & Analgesia, 104*, 548–551.

88. Hadzic, A., Alris, J., Kerimoglu, B., et al. (2004). A comparison of infraclavicular nerve block versus general anesthesia for hand and wrist day-case surgeries. *Anesthesiology, 101*, 127–132.

89. Hadzic, A., Kerimoglu, B., Loreio, D., et al. (2006). Paravertebral blocks provide superior same-day recovery over general anesthesia for patients undergoing inguinal hernia repair. *Anesthesia & Analgesia, 102*, 1076–1081.

90. Hadzic, A., Williams, B. A., Karaca, P. E., et al. (2005). For outpatient rotator cuff surgery, nerve block anesthesia provides superior same-day recovery over general anesthesia. *Anesthesiology, 102*, 1001–1007.

91. Hanna, M. N. (2012). Does patient perception of pain control affect patient satisfaction across surgical units? *Journal of Medical Quality, 27*, 411–416.

92. Hernandez, A. F., Whellan, D. J., Stroud, S., et al. (2004). Outcomes in heart failure patients after major noncardiac surgery. *Journal of the American College of Cardiology, 44*, 1446–1453.

93. Hole, J., Hirsch, M., Ball, E., & Meads, C. (2015). Music as an aid for postoperative recovery in adults: A systematic review and meta-analysis. *The Lancet, 386*(10004), 1659–1671.

94. Hutzler, L., Kraemer, K., Palmer, N., et al. (2014). Cost benefit analysis of same day pregnancy tests in elective orthopedic surgery. *Bulletin of the Hospital for Joint Diseases, 72*(2), 164–166.

95. Hwang, J. Y., Na, H. S., Jeon, Y. T., et al. (2010). I.V. infusion of magnesium sulphate during spinal anesthesia improves postoperative analgesia. *British Journal of Anesthesia, 104*(1), 89–93.

96. Idvall, E., Berg, K., Unosson, M., et al. (2009). Assessment of recovery after day surgery using a modified version of quality of recovery-40. *Acta Anesthesiologic Scandinavica, 53*(5), 673–677.

97. Ilfeld, B. M. (2011). Continuous peripheral nerve blocks in the hospital and at home. *Anesthesiology Clinics, 29*(2), 193–211.

98. Ilfeld, B. M. (2011). Continuous peripheral nerve blocks: A review of the published evidence. *Anesthesia & Analgesia, 113*(4), 904–925.

99. Ilfeld, B. M., Morey, T. E., & Enneking, F. K. (2002). Continuous infraclavicular brachial plexus block for post-operative pain control at home: A randomized, double-blinded, placebo-controlled study. *Anesthesiology, 96*, 1297–1304.

100. Iohom, G., Abdalla, H., O'Brien, J., et al. (2006). The associations between severity of early post-operative pain, chronic post-surgical pain, and plasma concentration of stable nitric oxide products after breast surgery. *Anesthesia & Analgesia, 103*, 995–1000.

101. Ip, H. Y., & Chung, F. (2009). Escort accompanying discharge after ambulatory surgery: A necessity or a luxury? *Current Opinion in Anesthesiology, 22*, 748–754.

102. Ip, H. Y., Abrishami, A., Peng, P. W., et al. (2009). Predictors of postoperative pain and analgesic consumption: A qualitative systematic review. *Anesthesiology, 111*, 657–677.

103. Jamtvedt, G., Young, J. M., Kristoffersen, D. T., et al. (2006). Audit and feedback: Effects on professional practice and health care outcomes. *Cochrane Database of Systematic Reviews, 2006*(2), CD000259.

104. Johansson, T., Fritsch, G., Flamm, M., et al. (2013). Effectiveness of non-cardiac preoperative testing in non-cardiac elective surgery: A systematic review. *British Journal of Anaesthesia, 110*(6), 926–939.

105. Joshi, G. P., Ankichetty, S. P., Gan, T. J., et al. (2012). Society for Ambulatory Anesthesia Consensus statement on preoperative selection of adult patients with obstructive sleep apnea scheduled for ambulatory surgery. *Anesthesia & Analgesia, 115*, 1060–1068.

106. Joshi, G. P., Chung, F., Vann, M. A., et al. (2010). Society for Ambulatory Anesthesia consensus statement on perioperative blood glucose management in diabetic patients undergoing ambulatory surgery. *Anesthesia & Analgesia, 111*, 1378–1387.

107. Kahn, R. L., Stanton, M. A., Tong-Ngork, S., et al. (2008). One-year experience with day-of-surgery pregnancy testing before elective orthopedic procedures. *Anesthesia & Analgesia, 106*, 1127–1131.

108. Kaye, A. D., Baluch, A., Kaye, A. J., et al. (2008). Pharmacology of cyclooxygenase-2 inhibitors and preemptive analgesia in acute pain management. *Current Opinion in Anesthesiology, 21*, 439–445.

109. Keay, L., Lindsley, K., Tielsch, J., et al. (2012). Routine preoperative medical testing for cataract surgery. *Cochrane Database of Systematic Reviews, 14*(3), CD007293.

110. Kessler, J., Marhofer, P., Hopkins, P. M., & Hollmann, M. W. (2015). Peripheral regional anesthesia and outcome: Lessons learned from the last 10 years. *British Journal of Anesthesia, 114*(5), 728–745.

111. Keyes, G. R., Singer, R., Iverson, R. E., et al. (2008). Mortality in outpatient surgery. *Plastic and Reconstructive Surgery, 122*, 245–250.

112. Khadim, M., Gans, I., Baldwin, K., et al. (2016). Do surgical times and efficiency differ between inpatient and ambulatory surgery centers that are both hospitals owned? *Journal of Pediatric Orthopedics, 36*(4), 423–428.

113. Kheterpal, S., O'Reilly, M., Englesbe, M. J., et al. (2009). Preoperative and intraoperative predictors of cardiac adverse events after general, vascular, and urological surgery. *Anesthesiology, 110*, 58–66.

114. Kim, S. H., Stoicea, N., Soghomonyan, S., & Bergese, S. D. (2014). Intraoperative use of remifentanil and opioid-induced hyperalgesia/acute opioid tolerance: Systematic review. *Frontiers in Pharmacology, 5*, 108.

115. Kim, S. Y., Song, J. W., Park, B., et al. (2011). Pregabalin reduces post-operative pain after mastectomy: A double-blind randomized, placebo-controlled study. *Acta Anesthesiologic Scandinavica, 55*(3), 290–296.

116. Klein, S. M., Pietrobon, R., Nielsen, K. C., et al. (2002). Peripheral nerve blockade with long-acting local anesthetics: A survey of the Society for Ambulatory Anesthesia. *Anesthesia & Analgesia, 94*, 71–76.

117. Kodeih, M. G., Al-Alami, A. A., Atiyeh, B. S., & Kanazi, G. E. (2009). Combined spinal epidural anesthesia in an asthmatic patient undergoing abdominoplasty. *Plastic and Reconstructive Surgery, 123*(3), e118–e120.

118. Kolodzi, K., & Apfel, C. C. (2009). Nausea and vomiting after office-based anesthesia. *Current Opinion in Anesthesiology, 22*, 532–538.

119. Korhonen, A. M., Valanne, J. V., Jokela, R. M., et al. (2004). A comparison of selective spinal anesthesia with hyperbaric bupivacaine and general anesthesia with desflurane for outpatient knee arthroscopy. *Anesthesia & Analgesia, 99*, 1668–1673.

120. Lacasse, M. A., Roy, J. D., Forget, J., et al. (2011). Comparison of bupivacaine and 2-chloroprocaine for spinal anesthesia for outpatient surgery: A double-blind randomized trial. *Canadian Journal of Anesthesia, 58*, 384–391.

121. Laffel, G., & Blumenthal, D. (1989). The case for using industrial quality management science in health care organizations. *JAMA, 262*(20), 2869–2873.

122. Lai, H. C., Lai, H. C., Wang, K. Y., et al. (2007). Severe pulmonary hypertension complicates postoperative outcome of noncardiac surgery. *British Journal of Anesthesia, 99*, 184–190.

123. Laskowski, K., Stirling, A., McKay, W. P., et al. (2011). A systematic review of intravenous ketamine for postoperative analgesia. *Canadian Journal of Anesthesia, 58*, 911–923.

124. Leape, L., Berwick, D., & Clancy, C. (2009). Transforming healthcare: A safety imperative. *Quality & Safety in Health Care, 18*, 424–428.

125. Lee, A., Gin, T., Lau, A. S., et al. (2005). A comparison of patients' and health care professionals' preferences for symptoms during immediate postoperative recovery and the management of postoperative nausea and vomiting. *Anesthesia & Analgesia, 100*, 87–93.

126. Lee, T. H., Marcantonio, E. R., Mangione, C. M., et al. (1999). Derivation and prospective validation of a simple index for prediction of cardiac risk of major noncardiac surgery. *Circulation, 100*, 1043–1049.

127. Lefrancois, M., Lefevre, J. H., Chafai, N., et al. (2015). Management of acute appendicitis in ambulatory surgery: Is it possible? How to select patients? *Annals of Surgery, 261*(6), 1167–1172.

128. Lenart, M. J., Wong, K., Gupta, R. K., et al. (2012). The impact of peripheral nerve techniques on hospital stays following major orthopedic surgery. *Pain Medicine, 13*(6), 828–834.

129. Lentschener, C., Tostivint, P., White, P. F., et al. (2007). Opioid-induced sedation in the post anesthesia care unit does not insure adequate pain relief: A case-control study. *Anesthesia & Analgesia, 105*, 1143–1147.

130. Li, G., Warner, M., Lang, B. H., et al. (2009). Epidemiology of anesthesia-related mortality in the United States, 1999–2005. *Anesthesiology, 110*(4), 759–765.

131. Lichtor, J. L., & Glass, P. S. (2008). We're tired of waiting. *Anesthesia & Analgesia, 107*(2), 353–355.

132. Licker, M., Schweizer, A., & Ellenberger, C. (2007). Perioperative medical management of patients with COPD. *International Journal of Chronic Obstructive Pulmonary Disease, 2*(4), 493–515.

133. Liu, S. S., Strodtbeck, W. M., Richman, J. M., et al. (2005). A comparison of regional versus general anesthesia for ambulatory anesthesia: A meta-analysis of randomized controlled trials. *Anesthesia & Analgesia, 101*(6), 1634–1642.

134. Lubarsky, D. A. (1996). Fast-track in the post anesthesia care unit: Unlimited possibilities. *Journal of Clinical Anesthesia, 8*, 70–72.

135. Macario, A. (2009). Truth in scheduling: Is it possible to accurately predict how long a surgical case will last? *Anesthesia & Analgesia, 108*(3), 681–685.

136. Macario, A., Weinger, M., Carney, S., & Kim, A. (1999). Which clinical anesthesia outcomes are important to avoid? The perspective of patients. *Anesthesia & Analgesia, 89*(3), 652–658.

137. Macario, A., Weinger, M., Truong, P., & Lee, M. (1999). Which clinical anesthesia outcomes are both common and important to avoid? The perspective of a panel of expert anesthesiologists. *Anesthesia & Analgesia, 88*(5), 1085–1091.

138. Maharaj, C. H., Kallam, S. R., & Malik, A. (2005). Preoperative intravenous fluid therapy decreases postoperative nausea and pain in high-risk patients. *Anesthesia & Analgesia, 100*, 675–682.

139. Manohar, A., Cheung, K., Wu, C. L., et al. (2014). Burden incurred by patients and their caregivers after outpatient surgery: A prospective observational study. *Clinical Orthopedics and Related Research, 473*(5), 1416–1426.

140. Mariano, E. R., Chu, L. F., Peinado, C. F., et al. (2009). Anesthesia-controlled time and turnover time for ambulatory upper extremity surgery performed with regional versus general anesthesia. *Journal of Clinical Anesthesia, 21*, 253–257.

141. Mattila, K., Kontinen, V. K., Kalso, E., et al. (2010). Dexamethasone decreases oxycodone consumption following osteotomy of the first metatarsal bone: A randomized controlled trial in day surgery. *Acta Anesthesiologic Scandinavica, 54*, 268–276.

142. Meltron, M., Nielsen, K., Tucker, M., et al. (2014). Long-acting serotonin antagonist (palonosetron) and the NK-1 receptor antagonists. *Anesthesiology Clinics, 32*(2), 505–516.

143. Memtsoudis, S., Liu, S. S., Ma, Y., et al. (2011). Perioperative pulmonary outcomes in patients with sleep apnea after noncardiac surgery. *Anesthesia & Analgesia, 112*(1), 113–121.

144. Menachemi, N., Chukmaitov, A., Brown, L. S., et al. (2007). Quality of care differs by patient characteristics: Outcome disparities after ambulatory surgical procedures. *American Journal of Medical Quality, 22*(6), 395–401.

145. Metzner, J., & Kent, C. D. (2012). Ambulatory surgery: Is the liability risk lower? *Current Opinion in Anesthesiology, 25*, 654–658.

146. Metzner, J., Posner, K. L., & Domino, K. B. (2009). The risk and safety of anesthesia at remote locations: The US closed claims analysis. *Current Opinion in Anesthesiology, 22*, 502–508.

147. Milby, A., Bohmer, A., Gerbershagen, M. U., et al. (2014). Quality of post-operative patient handover in the post-anesthesia care unit: A prospective analysis. *Acta Anesthesiologic Scandinavica, 58*(2), 192–197.

148. Moncel, J. B., Nardi, N., Wodey, E., et al. (2015). Evaluation of the pediatric post anesthesia discharge scoring system in an ambulatory surgery unit. *Pediatric Anesthesia, 25*(6), 636–641.

149. Munnich, E. L., & Parente, S. T. (2014). Procedures take less time at ambulatory surgery centers, keeping costs down and ability to keep demand up. *Health Affairs, 33*(5), 764–769.

150. Murphy, G. S., Szokol, J. W., Greenberg, S. B., et al. (2011). Preoperative dexamethasone enhances quality of recovery after laparoscopic cholecystectomy: Effect on in-hospital and post discharge recovery outcomes. *Anesthesiology, 1114*(4), 882–890.

151. Naja, Z., & Lonnqvist, P. A. (2001). Somatic paravertebral nerve blockade. Incidence of failed block and complications. *Anesthesia, 56*, 1181–1201.

152. Neal, J. M., Barrington, M. J., Brull, R., et al. (2015). The second ASRA practice advisory on neurologic complications associated with regional anesthesia and pain medicine: Executive summary. *Regional Anesthesia & Pain Medicine, 40*(5), 401–430.

153. Ni, C. H., Hou, W. H., Kao, C. C., et al. (2013). The anxiolytic effect of aromatherapy on patients awaiting ambulatory surgery: A randomized controlled trial. *Evidence-Based Complementary and Alternative Medicine, 2013*, 927419.

154. Norman, P. H., Daley, M. D., & Lindsey, R. W. (2001). Preemptive analgesic effects of ketorolac in ankle fracture surgery. *Anesthesiology, 94*(4), 599–603.

155. O'Donnell, B. D., & Iohom, G. (2008). Regional anesthesia techniques for ambulatory orthopedic surgery. *Current Opinion in Anesthesiology, 21*(6), 723–728.

156. Odom-Forren, J., Jalota, L., Moser, D. K., et al. (2013). Incidence and predictors of post discharge nausea and vomiting in a 7-day population. *Journal of Clinical Anesthesia, 25*(7), 551–559.

157. Ong, C. K., Seymour, R. A., Lirk, P., et al. (2010). Combining paracetamol (acetaminophen) with nonsteroidal anti-inflammatory drugs: A qualitative systematic review of analgesic efficacy for acute postoperative pain. *Anesthesia & Analgesia, 110*(4), 1170–1179.

158. Orosco, R. K., Lin, H. W., Bhattacharyya, N., et al. (2015). Ambulatory thyroidectomy: A multistate study of revisits and complications. *Otolaryngology—Head and Neck Surgery, 152*(6), 1017–1023.

159. Outpatient quality reporting slated. (2007). *OR Manager, 23*(9), 5.

160. Ovassapian, A., Glassenberg, R., Randel, G. I., et al. (2002). The unexpected difficult airway and lingual tonsil hyperplasia: A case series and a review of the literature. *Anesthesiology, 97*(1), 124–132.

161. Pan, P. H., Lee, S. C., & Harris, L. C. (2008). Antiemetic prophylaxis for post-discharge nausea and vomiting and impact on functional quality of living during recovery in patients with high emetic risks: A prospective, randomized, double-blind comparison of two prophylactic antiemetic regimens. *Anesthesia & Analgesia, 107*, 429–438.

162. Pavlin, D. J., Chen, C., Peñaloza, D. A., et al. (2002). Pain as a factor complicating recovery and discharge after ambulatory surgery. *Anesthesia & Analgesia, 95*(3), 627–634.

163. Pavlin, D. J., Rapp, S. E., Polissar, N. L., et al. (1998). Factors affecting discharge time in adult outpatients. *Anesthesia & Analgesia, 87*, 816–826.

164. Pavlin, J. D., Horvarth, K. D., Pavlin, E. G., et al. (2003). Preincisional treatment to prevent pain after ambulatory hernia surgery. *Anesthesia & Analgesia, 97*, 1627–1632.

165. Pawlowski, J., Orr, K., Kim, K. M., et al. (2012). Anesthetic and recovery profiles of lidocaine versus mepivacaine for spinal anesthesia in patients undergoing outpatient orthopedic arthroscopic procedures. *Journal of Clinical Anesthesia, 24*(2), 109–115.

166. Peyton, P. J., & Wu, C. Y. (2014). Nitrous oxide-related postoperative nausea and vomiting depends on duration of exposure. *Anesthesiology, 120*, 1137–1145.

167. Reich, D. L., Hossain, S., Krol, M., et al. (2005). Predictors of hypotension after induction of general anesthesia. *Anesthesia & Analgesia, 101*, 622–628.

168. Roh, Y. H., Gong, H. S., Kim, J. H., et al. (2014). Factors associated with postoperative nausea and vomiting in patients undergoing an ambulatory hand surgery. *Clinical Orthopedics and Related Research, 6*(3), 273–278.

169. Romundstad, L., Breivik, H., Roald, H., et al. (2006). Methylprednisolone reduces pain, emesis, and fatigue after breast augmentation surgery: A single-dose, randomized, parallel-group study with methylprednisolone 125 mg, parecoxib 40 mg, and placebo. *Anesthesia & Analgesia, 102*(2), 418–425.

170. Rosen, M. A., Salas, E., Wilson, K. A., et al. (2008). Measuring team performance in simulation-based training: Adopting best practices for healthcare. *Simulation in Healthcare, 3*(1), 33–41.

171. Ryu, J. H., Kang, M. H., Park, K. S., et al. (2008). Effects of magnesium sulphate on intraoperative anesthetic requirements and postoperative analgesia in gynecology patients receiving total intravenous anesthesia. *British Journal of Anesthesia, 100*(3), 397–403.

172. Saad, A. N., Parina, R., Chang, D., et al. (2014). Risk of adverse outcomes when plastic surgery procedures are combined. *Plastic and Reconstructive Surgery, 134*(6), 1415–1422.

173. Salas, E., Wilson, K. A., Burke, C. S., et al. (2005). Using simulation-based training to improve patient safety: What does it take? *Joint Commission Journal on Quality and Patient Safety, 31*(7), 363–371.

174. Salman, N., Uzun, S., Coskun, F., et al. (2009). Dexmedetomidine as a substitute for remifentanil in ambulatory gynecologic laparoscopic surgery. *Saudi Medical Journal, 30*(2), 117–122.

175. Sandberg, E. H., Sharma, R., & Sandberg, W. S. (2012). Deficits in retention for verbally presented medical information. *Anesthesiology, 117*, 772–779.

176. Sarin, P., Philip, B. K., Mitani, A., et al. (2012). Specialized ambulatory anesthesia teams contribute to decreased ambulatory surgery recovery room length of stay. *Ochsner Journal, 12*(2), 94–100.

177. Schwenkglenks, M., Gerbershagen, H. J., Taylor, R. S., et al. (2014). Correlates of satisfaction with pain treatment in the acute postoperative period: Results from the international PAIN OUT registry. *Pain, 155*, 1401–1411.

178. Scuderi, P. E., James, R. L., Harris, L., et al. (2000). Multimodal antiemetic management prevents early postoperative vomiting after outpatient laparoscopy. *Anesthesia & Analgesia, 91*, 1408–1414.

179. Shapiro, F. E., Punwani, N., Rosenberg, N. M., et al. (2014). Office-based anesthesia: Safety and outcomes. *Anesthesia & Analgesia, 119*(2), 276–285.

180. Singh, M., Liao, P., Kobah, S., et al. (2013). Proportion of surgical patients with undiagnosed obstructive sleep apnoea. *British Journal of Anesthesia, 110*, 629–636.

181. Siyam, M. A., & Benhamou, D. (2002). Difficult endotracheal intubation in patients with sleep apnea syndrome. *Anesthesia & Analgesia, 95*, 1098–1102.

182. Smith, K. N., & Kopacz, D. J. (2004). Spinal 2-chloroprocaine: A dose-ranging study and the effect of added epinephrine. *Anesthesia & Analgesia, 98*, 81–88.

183. Song, D., Chung, F., Ronayne, M., et al. (2004). Fast tracking (bypassing the PACU) does not reduce nursing workload after ambulatory surgery. *British Journal of Anaesthesia, 93*, 768–774.

184. Spear, S. (2004). Learning to lead at Toyota. *Harvard Business Review, 82*(5), 78–86.

185. Spencer, F. C. (2000). Human error in hospitals and industrial accidents: Current concepts. *Journal of the American College of Surgeons, 191*(4), 410–418.

186. Suskind, A. M., Zhang, Y., Dunn, R. L., et al. (2015). Understanding the diffusion of ambulatory surgery centers. *Surgical Innovation, 22*(3), 257–265.

187. Suzuki, M. (2009). Role of N-methyl-D-aspartate receptor antagonists in postoperative pain management. *Current Opinion in Anesthesiology, 22*(5), 618–622.

188. Swenson, J. D., Bay, N., Loose, E., et al. (2002). Outpatient management of continuous peripheral nerve catheters placed using ultrasound guidance: An experience in 620 patients. *Anesthesia & Analgesia, 103*, 1436–1443.

189. Tait, A. R., & Malviya, S. (2005). Anesthesia for the child with an upper respiratory tract infection: Still a dilemma? *Anesthesia & Analgesia, 100*, 59–65.

190. Tait, A. R., Burke, C., Voepel-Lewis, T., et al. (2007). Glycopyrrolate does not reduce the incidence of perioperative adverse events in children with upper respiratory tract infections. *Anesthesia & Analgesia, 104*, 265–270.

191. Tait, A. R., Malviya, S., Voepel-Lewis, T., et al. (2001). Risk factors for perioperative adverse respiratory events in children with upper respiratory tract infections. *Anesthesiology, 95*, 299–306.

192. Tait, A. R., Pandit, U. A., Voepel-Lewis, T., et al. (1998). Use of the laryngeal mask airway in

children with upper respiratory tract infections: A comparison with endotracheal intubation. *Anesthesia & Analgesia, 86*, 706–711.

193. Turan, A., White, P. F., Karamanlioglu, B., et al. (2007). Premedication with gabapentin: The effect on tourniquet pain and quality of intravenous regional anesthesia. *Anesthesia & Analgesia, 104*(1), 97–101.
194. Twersky, R. S., Sapozhnikova, S., & Toure, B. (2008). Risk factors associated with fast-track ineligibility after monitored anesthesia care in ambulatory surgery patients. *Anesthesia & Analgesia, 106*, 1421–1426.
195. Uhlig, P. (2009). Interview with a quality leader: Paul Uhlig on transforming healthcare. Interviewed by Jason Trevor Fogg. *Journal of Healthcare Quality, 31*(3), 5–9.
196. Urman, R. D., & Desai, S. (2012). History of ambulatory anesthesia. *Current Opinion in Anesthesiology, 25*(6), 641–647.
197. Urman, R. D., Sarin, P., Mitani, A., et al. (2012). Presence of anesthesia resident trainees in day surgery unit has mixed effects on operating room efficiency measures. *Ochsner Journal, 12*(1), 25–29.
198. Van Klei, W. A., Moons, K. G., Rutten, C. L., et al. (2002). The effect of outpatient preoperative evaluation of hospital inpatients on cancellation of surgery and length of hospital stays. *Anesthesia & Analgesia, 94*, 644–649.
199. Veljkovic, A., Dwyer, T., Lau, J. T., et al. (2015). Neurological complications related to elective orthopedic surgery: Part 3: Common foot and ankle procedures. *Regional Anesthesia & Pain Medicine, 40*(5), 431–432.
200. Vila, H. Jr., Desai, M. S., & Miguel, R. V. (2008). Office-based anesthesia. In R. S. Twersky & B. K. Philip (Eds.), *Handbook of Ambulatory Anesthesia* (pp. 283–324). New York: Springer Science & Business Media.
201. Vila, H. Jr., Soto, R., Cantor, A. B., & Mackey, D. (2003). Comparative outcomes analysis of procedures performed in physicians' offices and ambulatory surgery centers. *Archives of Surgery, 138*(9), 991–995.
202. Viscomi, C. M., Friend, A., Parker, C., et al. (2009). Ketamine as an adjuvant in lidocaine intravenous regional anesthesia: A randomized, double-blind, systematic control trial. *Regional Anesthesia & Pain Medicine, 34*, 130–133.
203. Visser, K., Hassingk, E. A., Bonsel, G. J., et al. (2001). Randomized controlled trial of total intravenous anesthesia with propofol versus inhalation anesthesia with isoflurane-nitrous oxide: Postoperative nausea with vomiting and economic analysis. *Anesthesiology, 95*, 616–626.
204. Warner, D. O. (2009). American Society of Anesthesiologists Smoking Cessation Initiative Task Force. Feasibility of tobacco interventions in anesthesiology practices: A pilot study. *Anesthesiology, 110*(6), 1223–1228.
205. Waters, R. M. (1919). The downtown anesthesia clinic. *American Journal of Surgery, 33*(7), 71–77.
206. Watson, J. C., & Huntoon, M. A. (2015). Neurologic evaluation and management of perioperative nerve injury. *Regional Anesthesia & Pain Medicine, 40*(5), 491–501.
207. Wax, D. B., Porter, S. B., Lin, H. M., et al. (2010). Association of paranesthesia hypertension with adverse outcomes. *Journal of Cardiothoracic and Vascular Anesthesia, 24*, 927–930.

208. Whippey, A., Kostandoff, G., Paul, J., et al. (2013). Predictors of unanticipated admission following ambulatory surgery: A retrospective case-control study. *Canadian Journal of Anesthesia, 60*(7), 675–683.

209. Whitaker, D. K., Booth, H., Clyburn, P., et al. (2013). Guidelines: Immediate post anesthesia recovery. *Anaesthesia, 68*, 288–297.

210. White, P. F. (2004). Prevention of postoperative nausea and vomiting: A multimodal solution to a persistent problem. *New England Journal of Medicine, 350*, 2511–2512.

211. White, P. F. (2005). Changing role of COX-2 inhibitors in the perioperative period. Is parecoxib really the answer? *Anesthesia & Analgesia, 100*, 1306–1308.

212. White, P. F. (2005). The changing role of nonopioid analgesic techniques in the management of postoperative pain. *Anesthesia & Analgesia, 101*(Suppl 5), S5–S22.

213. White, P. F., & Eng, M. (2007). Fast-track anesthetic techniques for ambulatory surgery. *Current Opinion in Anesthesiology, 20*, 545–557.

214. White, P. F., & Song, D. (1999). New criteria for fast-tracking after outpatient anesthesia: A comparison with the modified Aldrete's scoring system. *Anesthesia & Analgesia, 88*(5), 1069–1072.

215. White, P. F., Kehlet, H., Neal, J. M., et al. (2007). The role of the anesthesiologist in fast-track surgery: From multimodal analgesia to perioperative medical care. *Anesthesia & Analgesia, 104*, 1380–1396.

216. White, P. F., O'Hara, J. F., Roberson, C. R., et al. (2008). The impact of current antiemetic practices on patient outcomes: A prospective study on high-risk patients. *Anesthesia & Analgesia, 107*, 452–458.

217. White, P. F., Sacan, O., Nuangchamnong, N., et al. (2008). The relationship between patient risk factors and early versus late postoperative emetic symptoms. *Anesthesia & Analgesia, 107*, 459–463.

218. White, P. F., Tang, J., & Song, D. (2007). Transdermal scopolamine: An alternative to ondansetron and droperidol for the prevention of postoperative and post discharge emetic symptoms. *Anesthesia & Analgesia, 104*, 92–96.

219. White, P. F., Tang, J., Wender, R. H., et al. (2011). The effects of oral ibuprofen and celecoxib in preventing pain, improving recovery outcomes and patient satisfaction after ambulatory surgery. *Anesthesia & Analgesia, 112*(2), 323–329.

220. White, P. F., Wang, B., Tang, J., et al. (2003). The effect of intraoperative use of esmolol and nicardipine on recovery after ambulatory surgery. *Anesthesia & Analgesia, 97*, 1633–1638.

221. Woods, B. D., & Sladen, R. N. (2009). Perioperative considerations for the patient with asthma and bronchospasm. *British Journal of Anaesthesia, 103*(Suppl 1), i57–i65.

222. Wu, C. L., Berenholtz, S. M., & Provonost, P. J. (2002). Systematic review and analysis of post-discharge symptoms after outpatient surgery. *Anesthesiology, 96*, 994–1003.

223. Wulf, H., Hampl, K., & Steinfeldt, T. (2013). Speed spinal anesthesia revisited: New drugs and their clinical effects. *Current Opinion in Anesthesiology, 26*(5), 613–620.

224. Yabroff, K. R., & Kim, Y. (2009). Time costs associated with informal caregiving for cancer survivors. *Cancer, 115*(Suppl 18), 4362–4373.

225. Yoos, J. R., & Kopacz, D. J. (2005). Spinal 2-chloroprocaine for surgery: An initial 10-month experience. *Anesthesia & Analgesia, 100*, 553–558.

226. Zhao, J., Chung, F., Hanna, D. B., et al. (2004). Dose-response relationship between opioid use and adverse effect after ambulatory surgery related events. *Pain Medicine, 28*(1), 35–46.

227. Zohar, E., Noga, Y., Rislick, U., et al. (2007). Intrathecal anesthesia for elderly patients undergoing short transurethral procedures: A dose-finding study. *Anesthesia & Analgesia, 104*(3), 552–554.

Chapter

ANESTHESIA FOR TRAUMA

10

Contents

Introduction

Anesthesia for trauma plays a critical role in the management of patients with injuries resulting from accidents, falls, or other traumatic events. These patients often present with a range of injuries that require urgent medical intervention, necessitating prompt and effective anesthesia to facilitate emergent surgical procedures and diagnostic interventions.

The primary goals of anesthesia in trauma cases are to ensure rapid induction of anesthesia, stabilize vital signs, and provide adequate pain control while minimizing the risk of further injury. Trauma patients may present with various physiological derangements, including hypovolemia, hypoxia, and altered mental status, necessitating a multidisciplinary approach involving anesthesia providers, trauma surgeons, and other healthcare professionals.

In many trauma scenarios, rapid sequence induction (RSI) of anesthesia is employed to achieve swift and secure airway management while minimizing the risk of aspiration and maintaining cervical spine immobilization. This technique involves the administration of induction agents and neuromuscular blocking agents in rapid succession, followed by endotracheal intubation to secure the airway and support ventilation.

Additionally, regional anesthesia techniques, such as nerve blocks and local infiltration, may be utilized to provide targeted pain relief and facilitate procedural anesthesia while minimizing the need for systemic sedation or general anesthesia. The choice of anesthesia technique in trauma cases depends on factors such as the nature and severity of injuries, hemodynamic stability, and the urgency of surgical intervention, with the primary focus on ensuring patient safety and optimizing outcomes in the acute trauma setting.

Approximately 5 million deaths, or 9% of all deaths globally, are attributed to injuries, making them the leading cause of death worldwide. In 2013, trauma was a factor in about 192,900 deaths, resulting in over $400 billion in medical expenses and lost productivity in the US, according to the Centers for Disease Control and Prevention (CDC). With 31.9% of deaths in the 1–9 age group, 40.5% in the 10–24 age group, and 27.1% in the 25–44 age group, trauma is the most common cause of death for people in the 1–44 age group. Because trauma accounts for more than 30% of years of potential life lost in individuals under 65, younger age groups are disproportionately affected by the relative burden of disease associated with trauma.

As the quality of care for patients with severe injuries has improved over the past few decades, mortality trends have also continued to decline. Severe injury patients receive emergency care at trauma centers that have been approved and independently validated based on stringent standards set by the American College of Surgeons. Level I trauma centers are the most specialized and can provide specialized multidisciplinary care around-the-clock. When compared to non-trauma centers, the overall mortality risk is reduced by 25% when trauma care is provided at Level I trauma centers. Particularly when it comes to the acute resuscitation and treatment of patients with severe injuries, anesthesia providers are indispensable.

Orientation and Directional Terms

Term	Definition	Illustration
Rapid sequence induction (RSI)	Rapid sequence induction (RSI) is a set of actions during induction of anaesthesia in unfasted patients or patients at risk of aspiration/regurgitation of gastric contents. The purpose of RSI is to secure the airway quickly and safely while actively reducing the risk of aspiration.	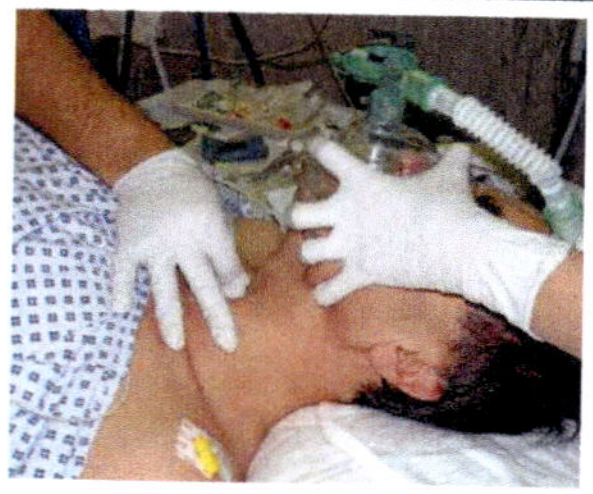
Blood pressure	Blood pressure is the pressure of circulating blood against the walls of blood vessels. Most of this pressure results from the heart pumping blood through the circulatory system. When used without qualification, the term "blood pressure" refers to the pressure in a brachial artery, where it is most commonly measured.	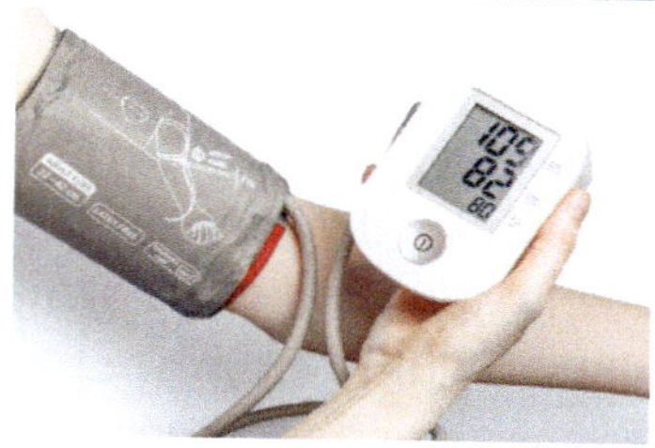
Glasgow Coma Scale (GCS)	Glasgow Coma Scale (GCS) is a system to "score" or measure how conscious you are. It does that by giving numbered scores for how awake you are, your level of awareness and how you respond to basic instructions.	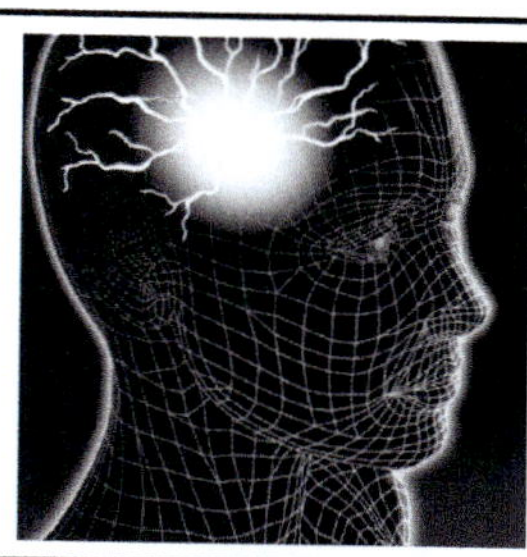
Advanced Trauma Life Support (ATLS)	Advanced trauma life support is a training program for medical providers in the management of acute trauma cases, developed by the American College of Surgeons. Similar programs exist for immediate care providers such as paramedics.	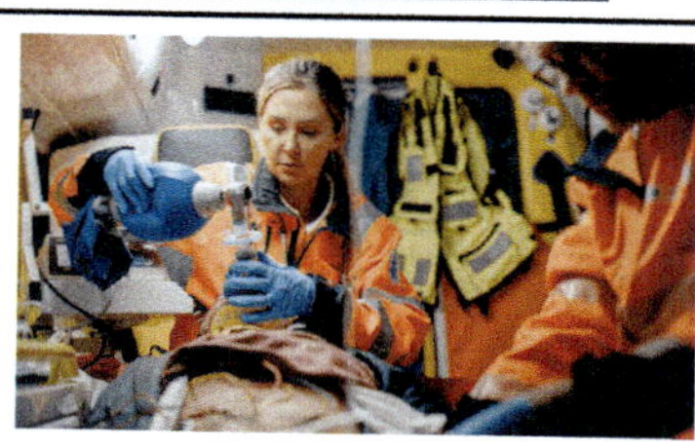
Systolic blood pressure(SBP)	Systolic blood pressure is the maximal pressure within the artery during ventricular systole, diastolic blood pressure is the lowest pressure in the vessel just before the next systole, and pulse pressure is the difference between the systolic and diastolic values.	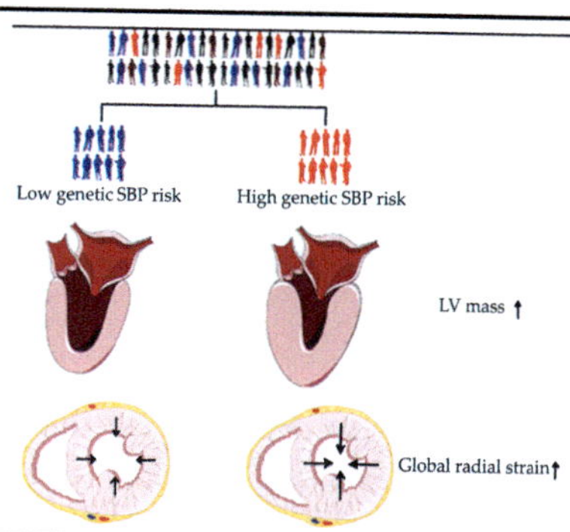

10.1. Physiology in Trauma

Depending on the mechanism and severity of the injury, patients with trauma-induced injuries may experience physiological disturbances. The most common cause of hypotension in trauma cases is either "hemorrhagic shock," or excessive blood loss, which is the primary cause of death for patients with severe injuries. When hypotension occurs in the context of trauma, additional causes of shock need to be taken into account after hemorrhagic shock sources have been examined. It is important to take into account relative hypovolemia from obstructed venous return in situations involving tension pneumothorax, cardiac tamponade, cardiogenic shock, and neurogenic shock.

When a trauma patient first presents, their arterial blood pressure readings might be deceiving if there is early bleeding. Compensatory reflexes through sympathetic, carotid sinus and aortic arch baroreceptors, and other low-pressure receptors can conceal the extent of bleeding. A later compensatory role is played by the pituitary's secretion of vasopressin and the renin-angiotensin system. These reactions permit an increase in heart rate, venous return, and total peripheral resistance through sympathetic vasoconstriction of the arterioles. The central nervous system additionally stimulates the sympathetic nervous system in cases of severe hypoxia and acidosis. Generally speaking, there are two phases to hemorrhagic shock: compensated and progressive. The features of each phase vary based on the amount of blood lost and acuity (Table 10.1).

Table 10.1. *Therapeutical Classification of Hemorrhagic Shock. NOM = non-operative management; PRC = packed red cells; OT = operating theatre; CA = cardiac; ARREST St-Y = sternotomy; TACC = thoracic aorta cross-clamping; HR = hypotensive resuscitation; ERT = emergency resuscitative thoracotomy; ALT = anterolateral thoracotomy; THR = titrated hypotensive resuscitation.*

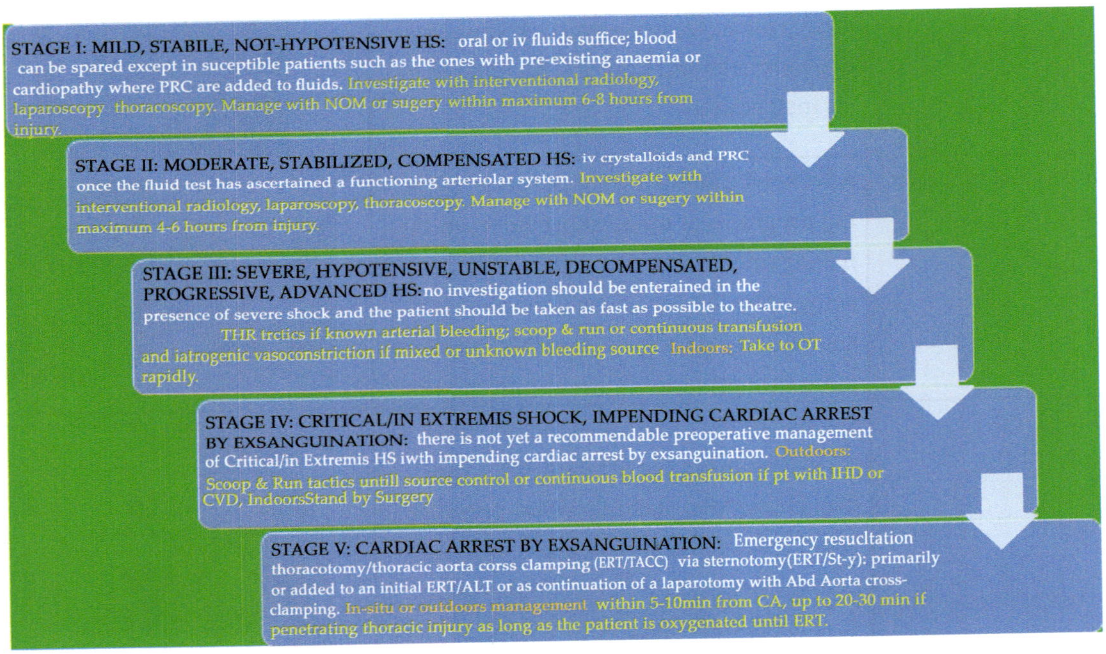

Source: Bonanno FG. Management of Hemorrhagic Shock: Physiology Approach, Timing and Strategies. Journal of Clinical Medicine. 2023; 12(1):260. https://doi.org/10.3390/jcm12010260.

When there is compensated hemorrhage, intact physiological compensatory mechanisms might be sufficient to maintain systemic perfusion without the need for medical assistance. Physiology alone may be able to replace between 10 and 15 percent of the blood lost. If resuscitation has been insufficient, hemorrhagic shock will worsen with more blood loss and eventually result in multiorgan failure. Heart failure, metabolic acidosis, and widespread tissue and cellular necrosis develop if insufficient perfusion continues (Figure 10.1).

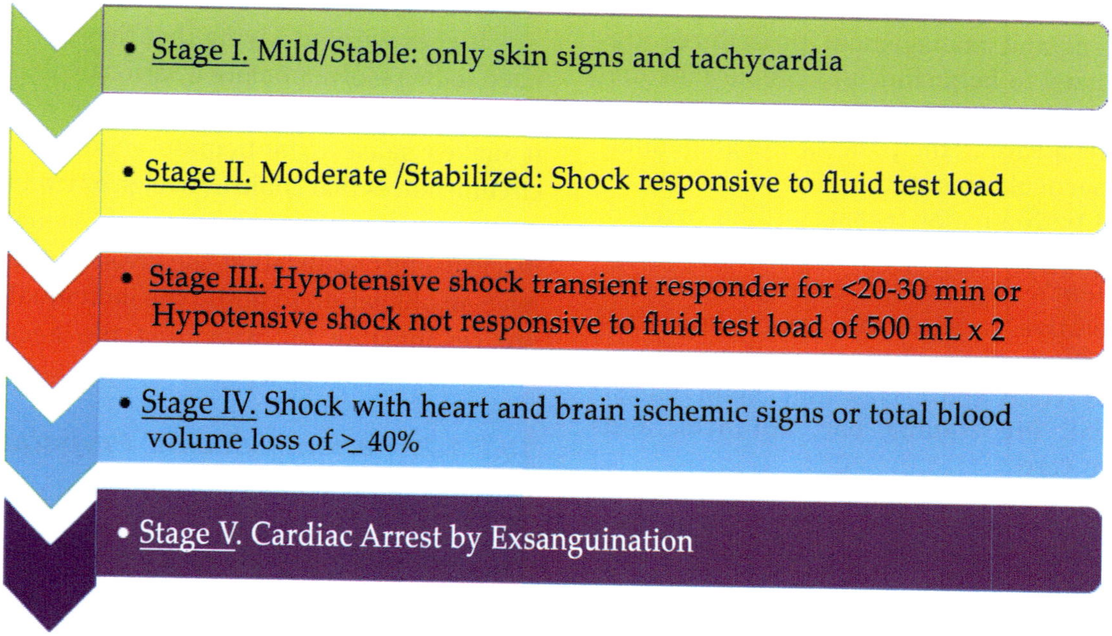

Figure 10.1. *Lethal triad.*

Source: Bonanno FG. Management of Hemorrhagic Shock: Physiology Approach, Timing and Strategies. Journal of Clinical Medicine. 2023; 12(1):260. https://doi.org/10.3390/jcm12010260.

Acute traumatic coagulopathy can result from injury caused by hemorrhagic shock and tissue hypoperfusion, which in turn trigger intricate interactions between intrinsic anticoagulants, inflammatory factors, and other cellular diseases. Factor shortage, hyperfibrinolysis, and platelet dysfunction are the causes of this coagulopathy. Additionally interfering with the coagulation process are iatrogenic factors of resuscitation. Acidosis, hypocalcemia, hypothermia, and hemodilution are some of these variables. The medical term for this is trauma-induced coagulopathy. A positive feedback loop that ultimately results in death is created by each of these processes. The triad of death, also known as the lethal triad, is widely understood to consist of hypothermia, coagulopathy, and acidosis. A threshold for severe, irreversible multiorgan failure may be crossed by hemorrhagic shock, making it irreversible even with blood transfusions and other treatments. (Brain Trauma Foundation, 2007; Centers for Disease Control and Prevention, 2015)

10.2. Initial Management

A coordinated, methodical approach to the history, examination, diagnosis, and treatment of a patient who has experienced a major trauma is necessary for successful patient management, and these procedures must be carried out concurrently. Frequently, initial treatment is started before a conclusive diagnosis is made. Every patient possesses a distinct set of injuries and mechanisms, which when paired with their premorbid condition, create an endless array of possible presentations. Many of the initial assessment and management procedures are standardized to help clinicians prepare for the unpredictable nature of trauma, and they also need to be aware of the policies and guidelines of their particular institution. The initial care of a patient with a major trauma will be covered in this section, with particular attention to the patient's stay in the emergency room. Intraoperative care can be greatly impacted by the initial management. A well-developed trauma system comprises four main parts: prearrival, the trauma bay, adjuncts, and definitive care.

10.2.1. Prearrival Preparation

A successful outcome depends on the trauma team's ability to provide quick, efficient care in advance of the arrival of a severely injured patient. This goes beyond simply making sure that the necessary equipment is there and working. While these assessments are crucial, there are additional organizational and patient-specific arrangements that must be taken into account.

10.2.1.1. Universal/Organization Preparation

- Designated trauma bay in the emergency department
- Who attends the trauma call?
- How are they notified?
- Policies and protocols regarding activation of
    - Emergency radiology
    - Emergency operating room (OR) use
    - Massive blood transfusion
    - Transport
    - Referral pathways to internal and external providers

It goes without saying that these problems need to be resolved before a seriously ill patient arrives. Trauma is an unpredictable event, so it makes sense to anticipate a unique set of circumstances that could outweigh or circumvent an organization's current readiness. As members of a learning organization, the involved clinicians have an obligation to notify the individuals who are responsible for providing the necessary resources in this case.

10.2.1.2. Patient-Specific Preparation

This needs to happen right before a patient with severe trauma arrives. To help with resource mobilization, the ambulance service should notify emergency department personnel about the patient's condition and injuries. A standardized handover tool is used by the majority of ambulance services worldwide to deliver critical information quickly and effectively. A mnemonic for identification of the patient, mechanism/medical complaint, injuries/information related to the complaint, signs (including vital signs and Glasgow Coma Scale [GCS] score), treatment and trends/ response to treatment is IMIST, which serves as an example of this tool. With this knowledge, the medical staff can start to make plans in advance for the patient's potential clinical needs.

10.2.1.3. Prearrival Briefing

The purpose of this briefing is to optimize team efficiency and performance. This enables all members of the team to introduce themselves, develop group situational awareness about the known condition of the patient, and to assign appropriate team roles.

10.2.2. Trauma Bay

10.2.2.1. Primary Survey

As soon as the patient arrives, the team's priority is to diagnose and treat life-threatening conditions quickly and simultaneously. Global adoption of the Advanced Trauma Life Support (ATLS) approach is widespread. Primary, secondary, and tertiary surveys make up its structure. The primary survey's goal is to locate and treat injuries that pose an immediate threat to life. It is arranged according to the ABCDE mnemonic (control of the airway and cervical spine, breathing and oxygenation, control of the circulation and bleeding, disability, and exposure). The ATLS course is a great way to start learning about trauma management. Most significantly, it offers a shared vocabulary and structure for organizing thought processes necessary for best individual and group performance.

10.2.2.2. Airway and Oxygenation

The establishment of a patent airway is of paramount importance to ensure a positive outcome for the patient. Rapid assessment is most easily achieved by asking the patient some simple questions. If the patient can speak, then the airway is usually patent. Intervention may still be required, but there is time to plan the safest treatment.

10.2.2.3. Management of the Airway and Trauma

There are numerous reasons why a patient might require an endotracheal tube to give them a permanent patent airway. First off, inducing anesthesia to perform an endotracheal intubation can be a risky and hazardous procedure. Ensuring proper tissue oxygenation is always the first priority. It is possible to optimize the patient's physiology and adequately prepare for an attempt at endotracheal intubation if a patent airway is maintained with basic airway maneuvers. In cases where the clinical circumstances permit, it is advisable to conduct a targeted neurologic evaluation before induction. In a patient who is sedated and has an endotracheal intubation, this can offer vital information that is very challenging to obtain. When it comes to intubating the trachea of a trauma patient in the emergency room versus an elective surgical patient in the operating room, there are various distinctions in technique.

10.2.2.4. Preoxygenation (Administration of Oxygen before Induction of Anesthesia)

It can be difficult to achieve preoxygenation in a patient with traumatic injuries. To provide a reservoir of oxygen in the patient's functional residual capacity (FRC) and prevent desaturation during the apneic phase of trachea intubation, preoxygenation aims to "denitrogenate" the lung. However, this process isn't as successful in trauma patients due to a lot of their injuries compared to a patient with less severe injuries. In particular, desaturation is more likely even with technically adequate preoxygenation if the injury lowers FRC or results in a shunt (lung units that are perfused but not ventilated). Such injuries include bleeding into the abdomen, diaphragmatic injury, tracheal aspiration of blood or gastric contents, hemothorax or pneumothorax, direct lung parenchymal injury, and rib fractures. The literature from emergency departments has addressed adding a backup oxygen source to provide apneic oxygenation during the peri-intubation period.

10.2.2.5. Fasting

All trauma patients should be assumed to have a "full stomach" even when many hours have elapsed since their last oral intake. As such, a rapid sequence induction (RSI) is considered standard practice. The use of cricoid pressure is common clinical practice but may worsen the view at laryngoscopy.

10.2.2.6. Altered Physiology

Those with major trauma who need emergency tracheal intubation are frequently the hospital's most critically sick patients. It is necessary to specify the rationale behind endotracheal intubation as well as how that physiologic insult affected the patient's reaction to laryngoscopy. For instance, even with optimal preoxygenation, rapid desaturation may still occur after apnea has been instituted if the cause of the endotracheal intubation was respiratory distress due to a major lung injury.

10.2.2.7. Hemodynamic Status

There are two main reasons why the hemodynamic response to anesthetics used to induce anesthesia is frequently overstated. First, despite the vasodilatory effects of anesthetic drugs, acute intravascular volume loss due to bleeding causes an inability to maintain cardiac output and arterial blood pressure. Second, the true intravascular volume state may be hidden by sympathetic overstimulation brought on by discomfort and pain; in such a case, inducing anesthesia may result in noticeable hemodynamic instability. Usually, this can be predicted by appropriately administering fluids intravenously, vasopressor availability and the availability of colloids, crystalloids, blood, etc.

10.2.2.8. Anesthetic Drug Choices

There is significant debate regarding the selection of medications to induce anesthesia in patients who are critically ill. Often used are propofol and, to a lesser extent, thiopental. When used to induce anesthesia, ketamine and etomidate might be more hemodynamically stable. The physician must have extensive knowledge and expertise with the anesthetic medications they intend to use, as opposed to utilizing a novel or unfamiliar medication. Because a very sick or hypovolemic patient has a relatively reduced volume of drug distribution, the dose of an anesthetic drug should generally be decreased. In these patients, there is preferential perfusion to vital organs like the heart, brain, and kidneys. Therefore, it is imperative to have a vasopressor on hand right away to treat any temporary hypotension brought on by the anesthetic medications.

10.2.2.9. Manual In-Line Stabilization

A laryngoscopy procedure may exert an excessive amount of force on the cervical spine. There should always be an effort to lessen this force. It is recommended that patients who have a suspected spinal injury be fitted with a hard collar. During laryngoscopy, the front of the collar should be released, and a second clinician should stabilize the patient's head and neck. Reducing cervical spine movement during laryngoscopy is the goal. Nonetheless, it's critical to adopt a realistic mindset because an unsuccessful endotracheal intubation attempt poses a far higher immediate risk (i.e., hypoxia) to the sufferer as opposed to slight neck movements. Before replacing the hard cervical collar, thought should be given to easing the manual in-line stabilization (MILS) to facilitate endotracheal intubation in the event of poor visualization of the glottic structures.

10.2.2.10. Choice of Laryngoscope

Video laryngoscopy has transformed how airways are managed in the emergency department and OR. The advantages of video laryngoscopy are numerous:

- Gives an adequate tracheal intubating view with reduced pressure and force
- Provides group situational awareness of the progress of laryngoscopy
- Improves visualization of larynx in more difficult patients without the need to change equipment

- Allows supervisors and trainers to provide dynamic feedback throughout the laryngoscopy

As stated before, clinicians must be familiar with the equipment they expect to use in the trauma bay.

10.2.2.11. Failed Endotracheal Intubation Drills

It is rare for endotracheal intubations to fail. Nevertheless, it is crucial to plan ahead and communicate clearly regarding the management of the unexpectedly difficult airway. In comparison to their elective counterparts, endotracheal intubation is probably going to be more challenging in traumatized patients. Spinal precautions, blood or foreign bodies in the airway, and the strain on the intubator are some of the factors that make the procedure more difficult. Plans for unsuccessful intubations must be clearly laid out, including what equipment will be required, where it will be located, and when staff members who are helping with intubation will be immediately available before anesthesia is administered. It is important to know in advance if staff members who work outside of an operating room are comfortable using equipment like surgical airway kits and laryngeal masks because they might not be familiar with them.

10.2.2.12. Posttracheal Intubation Care

Endotracheal intubation is not a therapeutic intervention in and of itself; rather, it is a means of delivering physiologic support. The transition of the patient to final care must continue to be the emergency department team's primary concern.

Several issues need to be managed immediately after intubation:

- Ongoing sedation—postintubation hypertension is common and should be avoided because of its effect on uncontrolled bleeding
- Ventilator and settings
- Disposition—where is the patient going next? To the computed tomography (CT) scanner, the OR, or intensive care unit (ICU)?
- Additional intravenous or arterial access, or both— these technical requirements should not delay movement to definitive care

10.2.2.13. Special Groups

Several special circumstances need to be considered when deciding on the management of the trauma patient's airway.

- **Airway burns:** Patients with airway burns require expedited management of their airway. Within a very short time, they can progress from minimal or no respiratory distress to a completely occluded airway due to edema. Warning signs of potential airway burns include facial burns, soot in the mouth/nose, carbonaceous sputum, explosive injuries to the upper body, and stridor.
- **Oral trauma:** Blood is often in the upper airway in trauma patients. Bleeding can range from a minor nuisance to a life-threatening hemorrhage. It is important to recognize this situation (i.e., blood in the airway) because induction of anesthesia can result in the rapid loss of a patent airway. Video laryngoscopes and fiberoptic scopes do not perform well when blood obscures the field of view. An additional suction source is

mandatory and a surgical airway team should be immediately available.

- **Direct airway injury:** Although uncommon, tracheal trauma should be suspected in any patient with direct penetrating or blunt trauma to the neck. Warning signs such as stridor and subcutaneous emphysema may be present. These airways should be managed only by experienced clinicians with early involvement of a head and neck surgeon

10.2.2.14. Circulation and Hemorrhage Control

Restoring adequate circulation and perfusion is necessary to guarantee that vital organs receive enough oxygen. First and foremost, we must halt any bleeding. A combination of the emergency department's procedures (direct pressure, suturing wounds), surgery, or angioembolization can be used to accomplish this. In addition, the anesthesiologist bears the responsibility of guaranteeing sufficient oxygenation of vital organs like the heart and brain. The term "damage control resuscitation" (DCR) refers to a resuscitative approach that avoids the risks of excessive resuscitation while offering circulatory support adequate to prevent irreversible end-organ damage. Other factors to take into account include acidosis, hypothermia, and calcium supplementation.

10.2.2.15. Disability

The neurologic system must be evaluated to detect potentially catastrophic injuries that need to be treated right away. Pupillary response, gross limb function, and the GCS score form the basis of this quick evaluation. Generally speaking, patients with a GCS score of less than eight need to be intubated.

10.2.2.16. Exposure

To avoid missing major injuries that are not visible, the patient needs to be exposed and inspected on all sides, including the back, for other injuries. Simultaneously, attention is required to avoid hypothermia in the patient as this affects coagulation, oxygen consumption, and mortality risk.

10.2.3. Adjuncts and Investigations

The diagnosis and management should be impacted by any ordered tests or investigations. Timely access to information can be a significant challenge in trauma patients, as clinical events can change drastically and quickly. Results with quick turnaround times, serial performance to track trends, and correlations with potential treatments that could enhance outcomes are particularly valuable.

10.2.4. Definitive Care and Transport

The process of treating the underlying physiologic issue is known as definitive care. Examples consist of removing the spleen, plating the fracture, and halting the bleeding. While some aspects of definitive care can wait until the patient's condition improves, others should be carried out immediately. Transferring the patient to a different medical facility for definitive care may be necessary, depending on the extent of their injuries and the capacities of each institution. In either case, the patient has to leave the emergency room.

10.2.4.1. Setting Priorities: What Is Next?

Determining the best place to treat the patient frequently leads to conflict. There may be disagreement regarding which injuries are the most clinically urgent and, therefore, where to treat them, depending on the severity of the injuries; alternatively, there may be logistical obstacles to treatment that make it impossible to treat the patient in one place for the entirety of their needs.

Serious injuries to the pelvis and brain are two examples. The operating room is the best setting for treating neurosurgical trauma; however, angioembolization is advised in the most recent guidelines for pelvic trauma. It can be challenging to decide which injury is more important, and the clinical specifics of each patient should be taken into consideration. These days, a lot of Level 1 trauma centers have hybrid operating rooms (ORs) where patients can receive both operative and angiographic interventions; in other words, the patient receives treatment instead of the other way around.

Conservative management during the acute phase is a reasonable alternative for many conditions. This gives time for the return of normal physiology, an explanation of the medical history, and a more thorough evaluation of the degree of injuries. Encouraging observation at the intensive care unit and conducting routine condition reviews is a very sensible and responsible course of action.

10.2.4.2. Local Care versus Transfer

When a patient's clinical requirements surpass the resources offered by the facility, the procedure for a prompt transfer starts. Knowing the local referral processes and getting assistance from the accepting hospital as soon as possible are crucial. It takes time to move a critically ill patient, and prompt communication with the accepting hospital makes it possible for the necessary resources to be prepared and mobilized. Regular review of the ATLS primary survey can optimize the patient's clinical status, regardless of the final destination. When transferring critically ill patients to a new facility, the standard of care they receive at the hospital should be maintained. Before beginning a transfer, specific equipment, staff skill mix, routes, and oxygen supplies should all be taken into account.

10.2.5. Decision-Making in Trauma

Multidisciplinary teams with complementary skill sets are needed in mature and complex systems like trauma and health care in order to achieve the best possible patient outcomes. To maximize team performance and restore some order to the potentially chaotic aftermath of a major trauma, a few basic strategies can be implemented.

10.2.5.1. Leadership and Followership

Conventional medical education emphasizes that a well-defined leader is necessary to guarantee the success of any resuscitation. A leader's primary responsibility is to serve as a hub for information and decision-making. On the other hand, people talk about good followership less frequently. Every team will always have a single leader, but there will also be multiple followers. The traits of a successful follower enable the leader to make the best choices possible at any given moment.

10.2.5.2. Graded Assertiveness

One method for voicing personal concerns to the team leader about priorities or decision-making in a way that preserves positive group performance is graded assertiveness. It is predicated on the idea that inadequate or inaccurate information forms the basis of bad decisions. Followers can voice their concerns and have a unique perspective on the situation. They can then constructively express their concerns by using the Probe, Alert, Challenge, Emergency Action (PACE) technique. Because of their importance and their typical access to information that followers may not have, team leader concerns may not always be given top priority.

10.3. Intraoperative Management

Due to trauma, a wide range of patients may require surgical or interventional procedures in the OR. It includes wounds to every organ and structure in the human body, regardless of severity. Some are very minor and straightforward, while others have clear implications and treatments related to particular organs. This section focuses on the latter group, which includes injuries to one or more organs that pose a life-threatening risk.

Table 10.2. *The Main Pain Ranking Scales in the Evaluation of Subjects with Trauma in Different Age Categories*

Age Category	Scale	Ranking	Interpretation
0 to 4 years	Faces, Arms, Legs, Cry, Consolability (FLACC) [**19,20**]	0 to 2 for each item Score from 0 to 10	0 relaxed-comfortable 1 to 3 mild discomforts 4 to 6 moderate 7 to 10 severe
0 to 4 years	Wong–Baker Faces®® [**21**]	Six different faces (6 scores)	
Over 4 years	Numerical Rating Scale (NRS) [**22**]	0: no pain 1 to 3 mild 4 to 6 moderate 7 to 10 severe	
Adults and Older	Visual Analogue Scale: (VAS) [**23**]	A 100 mm horizontal line with no pain written on the left and worst possible pain on the right side	
	Numerical Rating Scale (NRS) [**22**]	0: no pain 1 to 3 mild 4 to 6 moderate 7 to 10 severe	
Older	Pain Assessment in Advanced Dementia (PAINAD) [**24**]	Breathing, negative vocalization, facial expression, body language, consolability Score from 0 to 3 for each item 5 items considered	0 to 3 mild 4 to 6 moderate 7 to 10 severe

Source: Fabbri A, Voza A, Riccardi A, Serra S, Iaco FD on behalf of the Study and Research Center of the Italian Society of Emergency Medicine (SIMEU). The Pain Management of Trauma Patients in the Emergency Department. Journal of Clinical Medicine. 2023; 12(9):3289. https://doi.org/10.3390/jcm12093289.

To varied degrees, all current concepts that are recommended for patients who are bleeding profusely and have severe injuries can also be applied to those who are less injured. The patient who is heavily bleeding and has severe injuries typically presents in hemodynamic shock and requires life-saving measures. Massive bleeding, tension pneumothorax, cardiac tamponade, and severe cardiac contusion are among the differential diagnoses for a trauma patient in shock. The degree of shock may be exaggerated as a result of underlying medical conditions. There are three distinct stages to the care of seriously injured patients who are bleeding heavily. This distinction is predicated on disparate management principles, approaches, and physiologic features. During the initial stage, individuals experience uncontrollable bleeding. When the bleeding is at least partially under control, the second phase starts. When the patient's physiology begins to return to normal, the third and final phase is reached (e.g., arterial blood pressure). The division of the approach into these three phases accounts for the distinct treatment objectives for each phase as well as the variations in pace and pragmatism. It enables the supplier to understand the particular objectives for the assigned stage. These three stages are part of a continuum, with incredibly hazy boundaries (Table 10.2).

10.3.1. Phase 1: Uncontrolled Hemorrhage

When trauma patients experience significant bleeding that necessitates urgent surgery in the operating room, the medical team's only objective is to halt the bleeding as quickly as possible. Everyone participating makes every effort to achieve that goal.

Table 10.3. *The Main Phases of Trauma Care*

Stage of Care	**Element**	**Process**
Prevention	Analysing patients' data to establish the most valuable programs to prevent injury.	Road safety legislation such as alcohol screening, speed limit, and seatbelt, as well as good enforcement.
Prehospital	Dispatch and bystander's instructions, EMS care, triage, and transportation.	EMS Trauma protocol, fast and appropriate transportation to trauma care facility.
Hospital	Stabilisation and preparation for transfer to the higher-level trauma centre if needed. Definitive care (Trauma Centre or equivalent).	Activation of trauma team and preparation to receive patient.
Post-hospital	Rehabilitation services and home follow-up care.	Rehabilitation protocol and return to optimal activities.

Note: EMS = Emergency Medical Service. Adapted from "Indicators of the quality of trauma care and the performance of trauma systems" by Gruen, R., Gabbe, B., Stelfox, H., and Cameron, P., 2012, British Journal of Surgery, 99(1)v, pg 99

Source: Alharbi RJ, Lewis V, Miller C. International Perspectives of Prehospital and Hospital Trauma Services: A Literature Review. Trauma Care. 2022; 2(3):445-462. https://doi.org/10.3390/traumacare2030037.

There isn't time to wait for study results, to request more testing, or to speak with other experts. The anesthesia team's job is to make it easier to achieve hemostasis as soon as feasible. Anesthesia professionals face a demanding and ever-changing scenario when dealing with heavily bleeding patients who come to the operating room (OR) for resuscitation and hemostasis. Although additional staff can be very beneficial, they must be managed—ideally in a standard manner. An overly large team may find it difficult to work together and may experience difficulties. The patient needs to have their airway secured and be ventilated using only oxygen. By increasing the fraction of dissolved oxygen, the fraction of inspired oxygen (Fio_2) is maximized, which partially restores oxygen delivery by making up for hemoglobin lost. Implementing the massive transfusion protocol is another crucial institutional protocol (Table 10.3).

In the past, the anesthesia provider would aggressively restore the circulating volume and restore normal arterial blood pressure values by administering large volumes of crystalloids early on. This can cause the arterial and venous pressures to rise along with the cardiac output, which can then directly increase the rate of bleeding. This discontinued procedure would also cause hypothermia and coagulation factor dilution, which would increase bleeding. The idea of initial resuscitation has completely changed and been revolutionized over the last ten to fifteen years. Keeping the patient afloat as long as possible until the bleeding can be stopped is the primary objective of the initial resuscitation. The term "DCR" refers to the novel idea.

10.3.1.1. Damage Control Resuscitation

The cornerstones of DCR are permissive hypotension, restricted use of crystalloids and colloids, and early use of blood products. The goal of permissive hypotension is to take advantage of the body's natural reaction to bleeding. The driving force behind the bleeding is lessened as a result of the low venous and arterial blood pressures that follow and the reduction in cardiac output. The providers can also benefit from the body's natural response to blood loss, which is vasoconstriction in non-essential areas and rerouting blood flow to the most vital organs. To take advantage of this compensatory mechanism for as long as possible is the ultimate objective. Regretfully, it is impossible to determine with certainty when this mechanism is reaching its limits and the oxygenation of essential organs begins to suffer. Even though there is no consistent link between invasive or noninvasive systolic blood pressure (SBP) and organ microcirculation, SBP is nevertheless used as a very basic surrogate variable.

In contrast to normotensive resuscitation, animal models of shock show that resuscitation to 60% of the baseline mean arterial pressure (MAP) does not decrease regional organ perfusion; however, the less aggressive resuscitation does result in reduced blood loss. Brain perfusion did not differ between the two groups at the same time. Because of this, there is some expert consensus that patients who are actively bleeding should be able to tolerate SBP of 80 to 90 mm Hg until hemostasis is achieved, taking into account the patient's age, underlying medical conditions, and injury pattern. On one end of the spectrum, there is the young, healthy patient who has a significant abdominal bleed. Then, SBP in the range of 60 mm Hg may be tolerated for a brief period of time. Conversely, elderly patients who have multiple medical conditions and multisystem trauma involving the brain should have their SBP kept well above 100 mm Hg. These steps are taken in the interim until hemostasis is reached or the patient's condition worsens even more. The intravascular volume needs to be restored in the latter scenario. Crystalloids and colloids should be restricted in the early stages of the patient's treatment until further intravascular fluids are required. If not, the rate of bleeding will rise along with the cardiac output and intravascular pressures. The body will continuously use coagulation factors to try and stop the bleeding, which will cause their plasma levels to drop off quickly. A patient's chances of surviving a catastrophic bleeding episode are all adversely affected by these conditions. A brief period of improved physiology will result from returning vital signs to normal before the patient's coagulation capacity rapidly deteriorates and an increased bleeding rate disastrously exacerbates the whole situation. Large doses of crystalloids will also increase inflammatory response and exacerbate reperfusion injury. By reducing fibrinogen polymerization and platelet function, the administration of synthetic colloids will worsen coagulopathy.

As a result, the use of crystalloids and colloids has been reduced in the setting of severe hemorrhage. Instead, blood products are the fluids of choice for the resuscitation of massively bleeding patients. Packed red blood cells (PRBCs), fresh frozen plasma (FFP), and platelets are the mainstays for the initial resuscitation. Evidence is emerging that demonstrates the pragmatic and early use of these blood products in a fixed ratio (i.e., 1:1:1, PRBC: FFP: platelets). The benefit of using this approach is that the oxygen-carrying capacity is maintained or restored with the PRBCs, and the patient's ability to form clots is supported with the plasma factors in the FFP and platelet infusions. When transfusing large amounts of this combination of blood products, one should consider the additional supplementation of fibrinogen in the form of cryoprecipitate because fibrinogen is one of the key components of hemostasis.

Since the liver cannot resynthesize cryoprecipitate under such conditions, tranexamic acid, an antifibrinolytic, is administered to severely injured hypotensive patients to prevent coagulopathy early in the course of their illness. Vasopressors' function in providing hemodynamic support during this stage is still hotly debated. They should generally be avoided because additional vasoconstriction could jeopardize the blood supply to essential organs in a severely hypovolemic state.

10.3.1.2. Access to Intravascular Resuscitation

A patient who is bleeding excessively needs to have appropriate access to their vascular system to administer sufficient resuscitation. Two large-bore peripheral intravenous (PIV) lines should be inserted in any patient who has experienced significant trauma or trauma mechanism. They should ideally be placed in the upper extremities and should be 16 gauge or larger. Both the timeliness and integrity of meaningful venous access are crucial. Getting an 18-gauge PIV quickly is preferable to wasting time trying to find a difficult-to-find 14-gauge PIV.

Large-bore central access is usually beneficial for lengthy or substantial massive transfusions. Traditional large-bore (e.g., A catheter introducer sheath (8.5F) is inserted into the subclavian, internal jugular, or femoral veins. Ultrasound guidance is used to perform this if conditions allow. If PIV access is unreliable or delayed, intraosseous (IO) access can be used as a first-line solution. An IO line can be used to administer medication even though it cannot be used for rapid volume resuscitation. For an IO line in an adult, the humeral approach is the preferred location due to its close proximity to the heart and higher overall flow rates. Utilizing a contemporary rapid infusion system is crucial. The anesthesia team can swiftly and safely administer large volumes of warmed blood products thanks to the rapid infuser. Because rapid infuser systems are so powerful, it's important to keep a close eye on both the patient and the clinical situation to prevent over resuscitation (Table 10.4) (Figure 10.2).

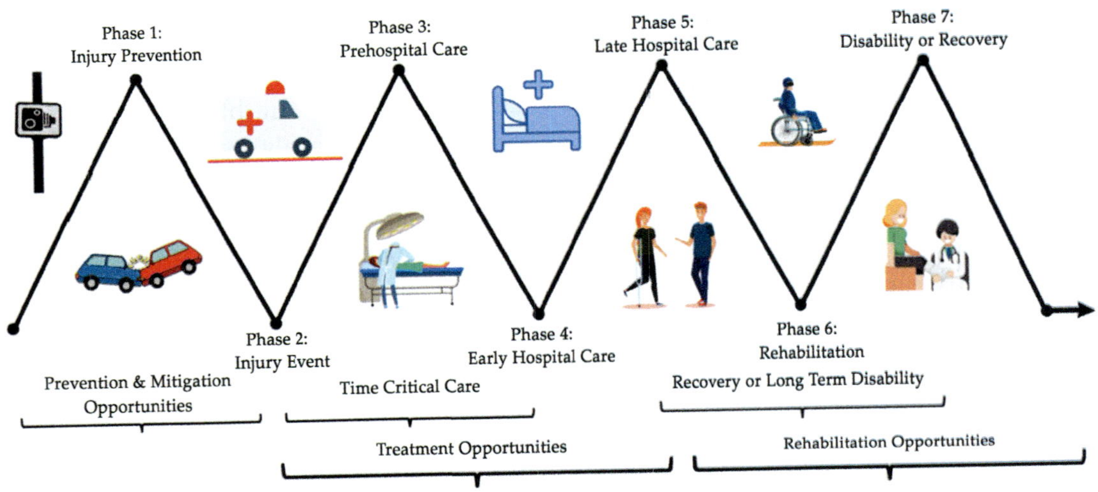

Figure 10.2. *Summary of a trauma patient's journey from injury to disability or recovery if death does not occur.*

Source: Alharbi RJ, Lewis V, Miller C. International Perspectives of Prehospital and Hospital Trauma Services: A Literature Review. Trauma Care. 2022; 2(3):445-462. https://doi.org/10.3390/traumacare2030037.

Table 10.4. *The ACS COT Trauma Centre Classification*

Level I	Lead hospital and tertiary care centre central to the system. Leads in all aspects of trauma care, from prevention to rehabilitation. Must admit at least 1200 trauma patients per year or have 240 patients with an Injury Severity Score (ISS) of greater than 15 or an average of 35 patients with an ISS of more than 15 for all general surgeons taking trauma calls. Either an attending surgeon or a resident at the postgraduate year 4 or 5 must be in-house 24 h a day. Resident may begin resuscitation but may not substitute for the surgeon. Expected that the attending surgeon will be in the emergency department within 15 min of patient arrival. Hospital must document the presence of the attending surgeon at least 80% of the time. While on call, surgeon must be dedicated only to that centre and can have no responsibilities at another centre. Backup call schedule must be available.

Level II	Must be 24-h in-house availability of the attending surgeon. Resident at the postgraduate 4 or 5 year or an attending emergency physician who is part of the trauma team may begin the resuscitation, but cannot substitute for the surgeon. Expected that the attending surgeon will be in the emergency department within 15 min of patient arrival. Hospital must document the presence of the attending surgeon at least 80% of the time. While on call, the surgeon must be dedicated only to that centre and can have no responsibilities at another centre. Backup call schedule must be available.
Level III	On-call surgeon must be available in the emergency department within 30 min of patient arrival. Must demonstrate a commitment to injury prevention, outreach activities to the local community, and education to all providers involved in the care of the injured patient.
Level IV	Located in a rural setting. Provides initial evaluation of injured patients. 24-h emergency coverage must be available by a physician.
Non-trauma centre	Delivers and regularly provides care to less severely injured patients Exists within the trauma system.

Source: Alharbi RJ, Lewis V, Miller C. International Perspectives of Prehospital and Hospital Trauma Services: A Literature Review. Trauma Care. 2022; 2(3):445-462. https://doi.org/10.3390/traumacare2030037.

The anesthesia team can give the patient and surgical team the crucial extra time they need until hemostasis is achieved when all of the previously mentioned procedures and methods are correctly used. Phase 2 of resuscitation starts when the bleeding is largely under control, at which point the approach's priorities and pace alter.

10.3.2. Phase 2: Controlled Hemorrhage

In phase 2, the anesthesia team should concentrate on a more customized, individualized approach once the major components of the bleeding source have been controlled. Phase 2 items may occur earlier and concurrently with phase 1 depending on the specifics of the case as well as the quantity and caliber of anesthesia providers available.

Invasive monitoring should begin at this point. The insertion should never delay or distract from the massive transfusion, the placement of intravenous lines, and the surgical hemostasis. Additionally, it is technically much easier to place an arterial line in a properly resuscitated patient.

Phase 2 involves a slowdown in the case dynamics, a reduction in blindness in the process, and a reevaluation of the patient's needs. The use of point-of-care testing (POCT) to direct resuscitation is a cornerstone during phase 2. To achieve this, one must consider the two primary physiological objectives of resuscitation: ensuring sufficient oxygen delivery and coagulation function. Normal intravascular filling and oxygen-carrying capacity are the primary determinants of oxygen delivery. The first is determined by looking at the patient's blood's hematocrit (Hct) or hemoglobin (Hb) concentration.

Targeted Hct values range from 18% to 28%, depending on the patient's age, comorbid conditions, and injuries. Numerous clinical indicators can be used to determine the intravascular volume status, including vital signs, urine output, and, if relevant, direct observation of the patient's heart and major vessels. In more challenging cases, a transesophageal echocardiogram (TEE) can measure the intravascular volume in more detail in cases of suspected cardiac comorbid conditions, cardiac contusions, and arrhythmias.

The patient's medical history, clinical presentation, standard laboratory coagulation tests, and point-of-care coagulation tests are the four main pillars of perioperative coagulation monitoring that the clinician must gather information from in order to determine the patient's coagulation status. The patient's medical history, if available, can provide details on prescription drugs and health issues that are connected to the coagulation system. A straightforward but essential diagnostic tool for coagulopathy existence and differential diagnosis is the clinical manifestation of the bleeding phenotype. It is necessary to correlate any abnormal coagulation test results with the clinical presentation. Procoagulant therapy should not be started in the absence of clinically significant diffuse bleeding since it raises the risk of thrombosis. The distinction between a surgical and nonsurgical source of bleeding can also be made with the aid of the clinical picture. Correction of the coagulation abnormalities is necessary to address the diffuse and more widespread pattern of nonsurgical bleeding. On the other hand, mechanical hemostasis must be used to control bleeding during surgery. Prothrombin is the main component of the typical laboratory coagulation tests.

10.3.2.1. Viscoelastic Testing

Viscoelastic point-of-care coagulation tests have established themselves as a standard for prompt evaluation of the circumstances previously mentioned during the last ten years. The thromboelastograph (TEG) and rotational thromboelastometry (ROTEM) are commonly used instruments for determining the type and extent of coagulation disruption and for directing therapeutic measures. A graphical output from both devices can direct the procoagulant interventions for the clinician. The three distinct phases of the TEG/ROTEM readout are the pre-clot formation phase, clot formation phase, and clot stability phase. Reagents are added to initiate the first phase, known as pre-clot formation, which activates the platelets and initiates the plasma coagulation cascade. In less than five minutes, this stage can provide the anesthesia provider with information regarding the coagulation cascade. If this phase is deficient, FFP and prothrombin complex concentrate (PCC) may be administered. The second stage lasts from the onset of clot formation until the maximum firmness of the clot is attained. The mass of functional platelets and the availability of fibrinogen are reflected in this phase. With the transfer, any flaws in the second phase can be fixed.

A goal-directed strategy and pre-established algorithms can be used to customize the treatment based on the data gathered from the four pillars of coagulation monitoring. This strategy also needs to consider the fact that procoagulant medication should always be used cautiously. Never correct a coagulopathy too much because doing so can raise the risk of major thromboembolic events.

Arterial blood gas analyses should be performed frequently after the bleeding has been controlled because they aid in directing PRBC transfusions and ventilation adjustments based on the patient's requirements. Furthermore, disruptions in the electrolyte (e.g., hyperkalemia and hypocalcemia) frequently arise and need to be treated.

Hypothermia should be avoided during resuscitation. By using forced air warmers, raising the room temperature, and only giving warmed fluids, this is accomplished. An esophageal temperature probe is inserted to help the clinician track the effectiveness of these interventions and to remind them to aim for normothermia (Table 10.5).

Table 10.5. *Transfusions in Injured Patients*

Authors	Statement	Conclusion
Malone et al. J Trauma 2006 [**38**]	The prevention of coagulopathy is superior to its treatment. Ratio 1:1:1 (red blood cells/plasma/platelet) is easy to use and the relatively higher plasma and platelet doses seems to be associated with improved outcome.	The fixed volume ratios might allow the number and rate of administered units of red blood cells to be used for primary treatment of bleeding.
Terence O'Keeffe et al. Arch Surg 2008 [**37**]	A massive transfusion protocol offers a number of benefits. Massive transfusion protocol was defined as receiving a 1:1:1 ratio of red blood cells, plasma, and platelets after at least 4 units of transfused red blood cells within 1 h of emergency department presentation or 10 units within 24 h of ED arrival.	Benefits: decreased blood product transfusions, improved time to transfusion, and reduced blood bank and hospital charges.
John B. Holcomb et al. Jama 2015 [**51**]	Plasma, platelets, and red blood cells in a 1:1:1 ratio vs. a 1:1:2 ratio	No significant differences in mortality at 24 h or at 30 days.
Guerado et al. Eur J Trauma Emerg Surg 2016 [**46**]	Massive bleeding is an acute life-threatening event. Massive transfusion is the transfusion of ≥10 red blood units within 24 h, the transfusion of >4 red blood units in 1 h, the replacement of >50% of the total blood volume by blood products within 3 h. Massive transfusion can provoke further complications and problems.	The early diagnosis of the source of bleeding is essential. The primary treatment is the surgical control of the source of bleeding in combination with resuscitation measures.
Michael S. Farrell et al. Emergency Medicine Clinics of North America 2020 [**53**]	In injured patients, crystalloid should be limited and blood transfusions should be initiated early. Blood products should be utilized in a balanced ratio and should be guided by viscoelastic assays and endpoints of resuscitation.	The main point is to address the cause of the hemodynamic instability or coagulopathy in injured patients to maximize the benefit of transfusions.

Rossaint et al. Critical care 2023 [**1**]	1. Rapid control of bleeding; 2. Coagulation support (fibrinogen concentrate or cryoprecipitate or red blood cells/fresh frozen plasma at a ratio of 1:1 or 2:1 as needed. A high platelet/red blood cells may be applied); 3. Fresh frozen plasma guided by PT and/or APTT > 1.5; 4. Fibrinogen supplementation if fibrinogen level < 1.5 g/L; 5. Factor concentrated based on laboratory coagulation parameters and viscoelastic evidence of factor deficiency; 6. Platelets to maintain platelets > 50 × 10^9/L in patients with ongoing bleeding and >100 × 10^9/L in patients with traumatic brain injury; 7. Management of antithrombotic agents.	Immediate detection and management of traumatic coagulopathy improves outcomes of severely injured patients.
Matthew R. Thau et al. Jama 2023 [**56**]	Endotypes derived from plasma biomarkers in injured patients were associated with a differential response to (plasma, platelets and packed red blood cells) 1:1:1 vs. 1:1:2 resuscitation strategies.	The molecular heterogeneity in injured patients has implications for a tailored therapy for patients at high risk for adverse outcomes.

Source: *Saviano A, Perotti C, Zanza C, Longhitano Y, Ojetti V, Franceschi F, Bellou A, Piccioni A, Jannelli E, Ceresa IF, et al., Blood Transfusion for Major Trauma in Emergency Department. Diagnostics. 2024; 14(7):708. https://doi.org/10.3390/diagnostics14070708.*

10.3.3. Phase 3: Restoration of Physiology

The patient's physiology is adjusted and restored during the third and last stage of resuscitation. This ought to happen after the resuscitation dynamic is under control and the surgical hemostasis is finished. The possibility of harm surpassing the benefits renders the DCR principles obsolete. In this phase, the intravascular volume is restored. Further cardiac output monitoring equipment can direct this procedure. The anesthetic should be gradually raised to a level close to 1 minimum alveolar concentration (MAC), if this level hasn't already been reached. At this point, it is possible to counteract anesthesia-induced vasodilation with low-dose vasoactive infusions. They shouldn't be utilized to make up for insufficient IVC resuscitation. Ongoing serial POCT helps assess how well the resuscitation went. Serum lactate and base deficit levels that are within normal limits are good markers of this accomplishment.

10.3.3.1. Anesthetics

As a general rule, arterial blood pressure values should be used as a guide when restoring adequate anesthetic levels, except the most severe bleeding. This idea is closely related to the quick intravascular space filling and enables the return of regular blood flow to all tissues.

In phase 2, gradual anesthetic administration ought to begin. Either incrementally increasing the concentration of inhaled anesthetic or administering repeated boluses of opioids can accomplish the stepwise deepening of the anesthetic.

10.4. Special Groups

10.4.1. Traumatic Brain Injury

A head injury that impairs normal brain function is referred to as a traumatic brain injury (TBI). Each year, over 15 million individuals seek treatment for traumatic brain injury (TBI) in emergency rooms, accounting for 30% of trauma-related fatalities in the US. TBI's long-term effects can include disability, a decline in overall quality of life, and impairment in cognitive and functional abilities.

Primary neurologic injury happens instantly upon injury and results in immediate neuronal damage. It is an irreversible injury. A major prognostic factor for traumatic brain injury (TBI) is the size of the initial injury. The brain injury that develops after the initial injury is known as a secondary injury. Intracerebral hypertension, hypotension, hypoxia, hyperthermia, coagulopathy, hyper- or hypoglycemia, and acidosis are common causes of secondary injury. Limiting secondary injury during the perioperative period is the anesthesia provider's main goal when managing traumatic brain injuries (TBIs) to enhance neurologic outcomes.

The process, degree, and kind of the injury all play a major role in the neurologic symptoms of traumatic brain injury. Skull fractures, hemorrhagic contusions, diffuse axonal injuries, and intracerebral, subdural, and epidural hematomas are among the various injury types. These wounds could be diffuse or focal. Although iatrogenic intoxication and other factors may occasionally result in misclassification, the GCS is frequently used to initially assess and classify TBI patients. The GCS scores for the visual, verbal, and motor domains should be reported individually. GCS components that cannot be tested ought to be documented. To determine the kind and extent of the injury, an early CT scan is essential. Similar to other trauma patients, ATLS is used for the first assessment. A TBI patient who is unable to maintain a patent airway due to reflex loss and is unable to ventilate or oxygenate themselves sufficiently should have an early definitive airway established. These variables are typically linked to additional concurrent injuries or a declining GCS score, which is typically 8 or lower. (Brain Trauma Foundation, 2007; Centers for Disease Control and Prevention, 2015) (Table 10.6).

Table 10.6. *Therapeutic Drugs with Anti-Inflammatory Action for TBI*

Drug	Route of Administration	**Preclinical Model**	**Inflammatory Events**
Dexamethasone	I.P.	WD	⇓ Microglia (CD68, MHC II) ⇓ Microglia (Endothelial-Monocyte Activating Polypeptide II, P2X4 Receptor, Iba-1)
Meloxicam	I.P.	M-WD	⇓ Lipid Peroxidation GSSH Nakatpase
Etazolate	I.P.	WD	⇓ IL-1β ⇓ Microglia (CD11b)
Carpofen	S.C.	WD	⇓ Microglia (Iba-1) ⇓ IL-1β, ⇓ IL-6 ⇔ IL-4, ⇔ IL-10
Indomethacin	I.P.	M-WD	⇓ IL-1β, ⇓ 6-Keto PGF1α
	I.P.	WD	
Nimesulide	I.P.	WD	⇓ 6-Keto PGF1a
Celecoxib	I.P.	WD	⇓ Il-1β, ⇔ IL-10
Meloxicam	I.P	WD	⇓ 6-Keto PGF1a
Etanercept	I.P.	FPI	⇓ TNF-α
Dexamethasone Melatonin	I.P.	CCI	⇓ MMP-2, ⇓ MMP-9, ⇓ Inos
Lipoxin A4	I.C.V.	WD	⇓ IL-1β, ⇓ IL-6, ⇓ TNFα, ⇓ GFAP ⇓ Microglia (CD11b)
Ibuprofen	I.P.	FPI	⇔ IL-4, ⇔ IL-10 ⇔ TNFα ⇔ IL-1α⇔ IL-6
Minocycline	I.P.	WD	⇓ microglia (CD11b)
	I.P.	WD	⇓ microglia, ⇓ IL-1β
Fenofibrate	P.O.	LFP	⇓ cerebral oedema ⇓ ICAM-1, ⇓ brain lesion
Pioglitazone and Rosiglitazone	I.P.	CCI	⇓ activated microglia (OX-42)
N-acetylcysteine	I.P.	WD	⇓ NF-kB, ⇓ IL-1β ⇓ IL-6, ⇓ TNF-α
Flavopiridol	I.P.	LFP	⇓ GFAP, ⇓ microglia
Roscovitine	I.C.V.	CCI	⇓ microglia (Iba-1)
Erythropoietin	I.P.	CCI	⇓ NF-kB, ⇓ ICAM-1, ⇓ IL-1β ⇓ TNF-α, ⇔ IL-6
	I.P.	WD	⇓ CCL-2 ⇓ microglia (CD-68)

Simvastatin	P.O.	CCI	⇓ TLR4, ⇓ NF-κB ⇓ IL-1β, ⇓ TNFα ⇓ Il-6, ⇓ ICAM-1
			⇓ Il-1β, ⇓ GFAP ⇓ IL-6, ⇓ TNF-α microglia (CD68)
Progesterone	I.P.	WD	COX-2, ⇓ PGE2, ⇓ NF-κB
	I.P./S.C.	CCI	⇓ IL-6, ⇓ COX-2, ⇓ NF-κB

⇑, increase; ⇓, decrease; ⇔, no change, I.P., intraperitoneal; S.C., subcutaneous; I.C.V., intracerebroventricular; P.O., oral; FPI, fluid percussion injury; CCI, controlled cortical impact; WD, weight drop; M-WD, Marmarou weight drop; MHC, major histocompatibility complex; CD68, cluster of differentiation protein 68; IL, interleukin; TNF, tumor necrosis factor; LFP, lateral fluid percussion; ICAM-1, intercellular adhesion molecule, MMP, metalloproteinase, COX-2, cyclooxygenase-2; NF-kB, nuclear factor-kB; GSSH, oxidized glutathione; CCL2, C–C motif chemokine ligand 2.

Source: Crupi R, Cordaro M, Cuzzocrea S, Impellizzeri D. Management of Traumatic Brain Injury: From Present to Future. Antioxidants. 2020; 9(4):297. https://doi.org/10.3390/antiox9040297.

The risk of intracranial insertion in TBI patients with facial or suspected skull base fractures should make nasal airways (and nasogastric tubes) as avoidable as possible. In cases of traumatic brain injury (TBI), additional indications for tracheal intubation include symptoms of intracranial hypertension or uncontrollably high blood pressure. When a patient's mental state and GCS score are getting worse, it is always advisable to secure their airway before transporting them.

When intubating a TBI patient, many of the same factors that apply to other trauma patients also need to be taken into account. These factors include hypoxia, inadequate fasting, unclear intravascular volume status, and the possibility of cervical spine injury in cases of blunt trauma. Patients with moderate to severe traumatic brain injury (TBI) account for 4–8% of cases of concurrent cervical spine injury, with a higher risk of high cervical injuries and mechanically unstable injuries. The cervical spine's integrity should be of special concern to the anesthesia provider. Rapid sequence induction of anesthesia and tracheal intubation should be carried out by skilled personnel, who should also open cervical collars and hold mechanical in-line stabilization. It's important to take into account extra variables like combativeness, concurrent airway injuries, elevated intracranial pressure (ICP) or impending herniation, and uncooperative patients. The question of whether video laryngoscopy (e.g., GlideScope) is better than traditional laryngoscopy when it comes to intubation. Video laryngoscopy (GlideScope) may result in a slightly longer time to endotracheal intubation but may also produce slightly less motion in the cervical spine and improve visualization of the glottis.

Hemodynamic stability should be the main goal when using anesthetics to preserve cerebral perfusion pressure (CPP). Because of their ability to lower cerebral blood flow (CBF) and subsequently lower the cerebral metabolic rate of oxygen (CMRO2) requirement, propofol and etomidate are frequently chosen. The use of ketamine in this population has not been associated with worse outcomes or increases in ICP, despite its controversial history. There is no discernible impact of nondepolarizing neuromuscular blocking medications on cerebral hemodynamics. ICP may theoretically rise in response to succinylcholine, but this effect has not been shown to be clinically significant and may be lessened by administering a defasciculating dose of a nondepolarizing medication.

Imaging may occasionally be followed by the need for emergency surgical care. Volatile anesthetics have the ability to "uncouple," or raise CBF while lowering CMRO2. Increased CBF doesn't happen until after 0 MAC in the case of sevoflurane and over 1 MAC in other cases. Less than one MAC should be used when using volatile anesthetics, with sevoflurane being the preferred option. Although total intravenous anesthesia (TIVA) is less titratable during abrupt, profound hypotension, which may happen during dural decompression, it may be preferred because it lowers ICP. There are data regarding the effects of TIVA and volatile anesthetics on cerebral hemodynamics, but no conclusive prospective outcome studies are available. When comparing the two anesthetic strategies, a retrospective study in combat-related traumatic brain injury did not find a significant difference in neurologic outcomes at discharge.

During the procedure, the patient is typically positioned in a reverse Trendelenburg position at an angle of approximately 30 degrees to aid in venous drainage. Fluid delivery intraoperatively requires a large-bore intravenous access. It is important to verify whether blood is available for transfusion. Surgery for complex depressed skull fractures close to venous sinuses carries an especially high risk of severe bleeding. Viscoelastometric testing or a conventional laboratory coagulation panel can be used to assess coagulopathy. For the purpose of continuously monitoring arterial blood pressure and drawing blood for multiple laboratory analyses, an arterial line should be implanted. The perioperative period should be spent adhering to the guidelines set forth by the Brain Trauma Foundation. Treating hypotension quickly is necessary to keep the CPP between 50 and 70 mm Hg. To reach euvolemia, intravascular fluid administration and resuscitation are typically necessary, particularly after mannitol administration. Typically, isotonic crystalloid is favored. When resuscitating ICU patients with brain injuries, the use of albumin may raise the risk of death in comparison to crystalloid. Avoiding hypoxemia is advised. To prevent blockage of cerebral venous drainage, attention should be given to peak inspiratory pressure and positive end-expiratory pressure. Hyperventilation is not recommended within the first 24 hours of injury unless treating impending herniation. Prophylactic administration of mannitol and antiseizure administration is recommended. Glucose should be monitored regularly. Hyperglycemia and hypoglycemia should be treated to avoid exacerbation of secondary injury. General recommendations are to treat blood glucose levels above 180 mg/dL. Most importantly, close communication with the operative team must be maintained prior to decompression and dural opening.

High ICP may, in turn, systemically cause heightened sympathetic activity in order to sustain CPP. We call this the Cushing reflex. Intravascular volume depletion may go unnoticed due to the release of catecholamines and an increase in systemic vascular resistance. After decompression and ICP normalization, sudden, profound hypotension can occasionally happen, especially in patients who are not receiving enough resuscitation. Prior to major decompression, anesthetic medication should be gradually tapered off, and vasopressors and inotropes should be on hand for administration. Blood should be on hand right away in case of an unexpected bleeding episode.

The surgeon should be consulted when deciding whether to extubate or keep the trachea intubated. Because there is a chance of hypoxia, postoperative hypoventilation, low consciousness, coexisting injuries, and the need for additional testing or treatment, many TBI patients continue to require tracheal intubation. It is important to transport these patients under close supervision. If the patient doesn't get better, sedation and a transport ventilator might be needed. To lessen bouts of agitation, bucking, or coughing, small-dose muscle relaxants may be taken into consideration when transporting TBI patients. Large-dose muscle relaxants should not be used for transport or at the conclusion of the procedure as they may cause a delay in the postoperative neurologic examination. Throughout the immediate postoperative phase, TBI variables should be maintained.

10.4.2. Spinal Cord Injury

When acute trauma impairs normal sensory, motor, or autonomic function, spinal cord injury (SCI) results. There are currently over 200,000 people living with SCI in the United States, where there are thought to be 12,500 new cases annually. The three most frequent causes of injury are assault, falls, and car accidents. The degree, scope, and severity of the injury all influence how SCI manifests itself. If the patient has no motor or sensory function below the level of injury, the injury can be considered "complete." Partial spinal cord injuries that leave some degree of residual sensory and motor function are referred to as incomplete spinal cord injuries. When describing the results of neurologic examinations, the American Spinal Injury Association (ASIA) classification is the recommended impairment scale.

When there is even the slightest suspicion of a spinal cord injury, patients should be transported or moved carefully, always wearing a cervical collar and taking strict precautions when rolling over. It is important to assess ventilation and oxygenation levels promptly. The diaphragmatic muscles can become weak and impaired after cervical spine injuries, particularly if the injuries are complete. Reduced vital capacity and the inability to cough up secretions are the results of this. The patient's capacity to breathe and take in oxygen may be made more difficult by concurrent lung injury brought on by trauma or long-term lung illness. Inadequate ventilation can manifest as paradoxical abdominal movement, increased work of breathing, and rapid, shallow breathing.

When intercostal and abdominal muscles are affected by thoracic and high lumbar injuries, these symptoms may manifest. An endotracheal tube should be inserted to secure the airway in the same way that it is for TBI patients. Up to 16 percent of SCI patients who are admitted also have a concurrent TBI diagnosis. The most common injury to this group of people with concurrent diagnoses was to the cervical spine. Within the first 24 hours following an injury, a patient with SCI may receive neuromuscular blockade with succinylcholine in a safe manner. It should be avoided, though, following 48 hours of injury due to the possibility of severe hyperkalemia upon administration. Patients with cervical or high thoracic injuries who undergo direct laryngoscopy and tracheal intubation have been observed to exhibit an exaggerated Bradycardic response and hypotension.

Due to disruption of sympathetic cardiac accelerator fibers, which results in unopposed parasympathetic innervation, high thoracic (typically T4 and above) and cervical SCIs may cause significant bradyarrhythmia and atrioventricular block (AV block) during the acute phase. Severe hypotension may also arise from sympathetic blockade and systemic vasodilation. This physiologic constellation, in addition to the motor and sensory findings below the level of injury, has been named "spinal shock." The use of inotropes, vasopressors, and isotonic fluid is part of the supportive treatment. After spinal shock has subsided, care should be taken to avoid giving the patient too much intravenous fluid replacement, as this could result in pulmonary edema.

MAP should be maintained, unless contraindicated by concurrent injuries, at 85 to 90 mm Hg for patients with SCI to maintain adequate spinal cord perfusion. Since there is evidence that high-dose steroids are primarily associated with adverse effects, including death, the American Association of Neurological Surgeons no longer recommends the administration of methylprednisolone.

10.4.3. Burns

Major burns can occur in isolation or in combination with other forms of traumatic injury. They can result in rapid deterioration. Organized and systematic advanced trauma management is paramount. In addition, there are some special considerations for patients with burns. This section will address some of the issues in the immediate management of a major acute burn patient. This section does not address issues that arise later in the management or intraoperative care.

10.4.3.1. Burn Severity

Burns are categorized based on their severity as superficial, partial-thickness, or full-thickness burns:

- **Superficial**—This burn affects the epidermis only (e.g., sunburn). It does not require any specific treatment other than first aid. Superficial burns are not included in the calculation of percentage body surface area (%BSA) affected.
- **Partial thickness**—This burn involves all of the epidermis and part of the dermis. It can further be divided into superficial dermal, mid-dermal, and deep dermal. These burns change in appearance as the burn destroys more of the dermis and vasculature; the pain ranges from minimal to extreme; color can be red to pale/white; and exudates can be high fluid to relatively dry. Blisters are often present. They may require surgical management.
- **Full thickness**—This burn involves complete destruction of all of the epidermis and dermis. It is white, insensate, and has a waxy or leathery appearance. This type of skin is called an eschar.

10.4.3.2. Estimating Burn Surface Area

The percentage of body surface area affected by burns determines how the patient will be managed going forward and whether they will need to be transferred to tertiary centers. The rule of nines is useful for localized burns to a specific body part, but it underestimates in the obese population because the patient's palmar surface is only thought to account for 1% of the total body surface area.

10.4.3.3. Types of Burns: Chemical, Electrical, and Thermal

Stopping the burning process is the first step in managing the burn. The best way to go about doing this will depend on what caused the burn. Take off anything that is easily removable from your body. Use flowing water to thoroughly irrigate the area. For certain chemical burns, this may require several hours.

Chemical Burns: Special Considerations

Make an effort to stop irrigation fluid from dripping onto unaffected skin. Continue rinsing until the pH of the skin or fluid (measured using litmus paper) is neutral. Use mineral oil instead of water to treat burns caused by elemental metals (such as sodium, potassium, magnesium, and lithium), as their reaction with water can exacerbate the burn.

Electrical Burns: Special Considerations

Because injuries have happened along that trajectory, look for entry and exit points. Rhabdomyolysis and compartment syndrome are possible consequences of underlying muscle damage. The amount of fluid needed has somewhat increased.

Thermal Burns: Special Considerations

As soon as you can, remove the heat source (e.g, setting fire to clothes). Keep up the long-term irrigation with cold water, but watch out for hypothermia. Keep an eye out for any related injuries (such as inhalational or other types of trauma).

10.4.3.4. Intravascular Fluid Management

Although there is still debate regarding the proper amount of fluid to administer and the end points to monitor, fluid management is a crucial component of contemporary burn care. Acute respiratory distress syndrome (ARDS) can occur three to five days after an injury, and there is growing awareness of the negative consequences of excessive intravenous fluid resuscitation (Figure 10.3).

There are several formulas used to estimate the amount of fluid required for resuscitation. About thirty to forty years ago, the majority were developed. Among the most popular is the Parkland formula, which has been modified to read 4 mL/kg/percent burn (adults) over the first 24 hours following burn injury.

During the first 24 hours, only crystalloid fluid is used because it is believed that the amount of protein leakage into the interstitial space is at its highest during this time, making colloids ineffective. A balanced salt solution, like lactated Ringer solution or Plasma-Lyte, is the most often used fluid.

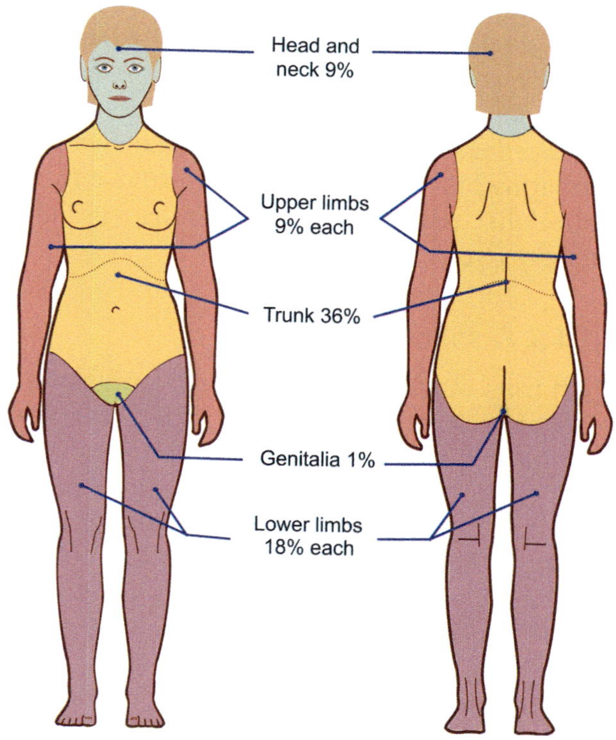

Figure 10.3. *The rule of nines—used to calculate %BSA (body surface area) burns.*

Source: By Jmarchn - Own work, CC BY-SA 3.0, https://commons.wikimedia.org/w/index.php?curid=107929836.

10.4.3.5. Airway

Erythema and the quick onset of edema in the damaged tissues are the hallmarks of burns. Swelling in the upper airway can cause complete obstruction of the airway and even death. Because of this, it's critical to keep a close eye out for burns that could impair breathing and to act quickly to begin intubation before swelling prevents it. To account for the anticipated swelling, think about inserting an endotracheal tube with an internal diameter of 0.5 to 1 mm less than would typically be used.

10.4.3.6. Pain

The degree of pain experienced can significantly impact one's quality of life. Every patient should receive analgesia as needed. For most patients, an opiate-based regimen with the addition of ketamine if needed usually offers adequate relief. These patients are extremely vulnerable to developing an opiate tolerance due to the prolonged nature and high level of pain involved in treating burns. It is best to seek advice from a specialist pain service as soon as possible after they start recovering.

10.4.3.7. Inhalation

Apart from the direct burn damage, combustion products can release harmful gases that are harmful to human health. Carbon monoxide is the most prevalent (CO). When compared to oxygen, CO has a substantially higher binding affinity for hemoglobin. Thus, the blood's ability to carry oxygen can be significantly reduced as a result of CO poisoning. The sole method for identifying CO poisoning is by using CO-oximetry on a sample of blood gas. Even in the presence of severe tissue hypoxemia, standard pulse oximetry monitors will read a normal value and are unable to identify CO poisoning. High concentration oxygen therapy dramatically lowers the half-life of carbon monoxide in the blood, and it is recommended that patients who may have inhaled CO be given high concentration oxygen as a precautionary measure.

10.4.3.8. Infection

One of the main reasons for delayed morbidity and death is infection. While empirical antibiotics targeting skin flora are adequate for the short term, sterile dressings must be applied to the burn site in order to restore the outer barrier against microorganisms. Additionally linked to an increased risk of infectious complications is over-resuscitation with fluids.

10.4.3.9. Eshcarotomies

The compliance of body tissues is greatly decreased by the escharring of full thickness burns. A compartmentlike syndrome may develop if there are eschars surrounding any portion of the body. This can impede ventilation around the torso, which is especially concerning. It might be necessary to perform eshcarotomies in this situation.

10.4.3.10. Transfer of Burn Patients

A burn center or unit that offers specialized treatment to burn victims is typically present in most places. For burn victims, such specialized care improves results. Consideration must be given to any additional related injuries and where they can be managed most effectively when it comes to the patient's transfer. There are situations when it makes sense to stabilize the severe visceral injuries at the trauma center and then later move the patient's care to the burn unit.

10.4.4. Extremes of Age

10.4.4.1. Pediatric Trauma

The most frequent cause of significant morbidity and mortality among children is trauma. For most clinicians, the sight of an injured child in the hospital usually causes anxiety. A better result can be achieved and the burden of the child's injury reduced by providing high-quality, cutting-edge trauma care. An overview of some of the problems that are particular to trauma in pediatric patients will be provided in this section. The fundamentals of ATLS serve as the cornerstone for managing pediatric patients.

10.4.4.2. Special Considerations

Nonaccidental injury

This differential diagnosis should always be

considered in pediatric injury. The majority of jurisdictions have mandatory reporting for child abuse. Warning signs include the following:

- Injury pattern inconsistent with developmental milestones (e.g., a 2-month-old rolling off the diaper changing table)
- Multiple injuries (especially if these appear to have been inflicted over a period of time)
- Frequent presentations - Inconsistent history of an incident

Pediatric physiology

Children's robust physiology allows them to conceal significant hemodynamic compromise. Confounders include pain, tachycardia, and a fear or stress response, among other symptoms. Once the compensatory threshold is reached, watch out for a sharp decline in quality.

Vascular access

Pediatric venous cannulation poses certain difficulties, even in patients who are well-hydrated. It may be nearly impossible when hemorrhagic shock is present. Early IO access is encouraged, and restoring a circulating volume should be the top priority. Some institutions operate on the tenet that you should try twice in two different places before using the IO approach.

Drug dosing

Accurate weight estimation of the child is crucial because most drug and fluid dosages are based on weight. The physician has two options for obtaining an estimate: asking a parent or caregiver, or using a tool like the Broselow Pediatric Emergency Tape. Pediatric patients still need to take certain medications into account when reducing their dosages.

Behavior

It is often difficult to get children to be compliant with treatment depending on their age. There should be consideration for the appropriateness of diagnostic tests such as CT and the requirement for the child to be still. Intubation may be required to facilitate the process.

Blood dosing

Little children have significantly less blood in their circulation, so even a tiny amount of blood loss can have a big impact. The estimated volume of blood in circulation in a 4-year-old child weighing 20 kg is merely 1600 mL. A 12-oz soft drink can's worth of loss, or 375 mL, represents more than 20% of the entire circulating volume. It's critical to look out for hidden bleeding sources and to act quickly. For every 10 mL/kg given, transfusion of red blood cells will result in an increase in hemoglobin of 2 to 2.5 g/dL.

10.4.4.3. Geriatric Trauma

The elderly trauma patient has special management needs, just like pediatric patients do. The elderly population does not have a high rate of morbidity or mortality due to trauma, but because of their advanced age, comorbid conditions, and use of medications, they are far more vulnerable to negative outcomes from subpar care. Once more, the cornerstone of all interventions is the advanced trauma management principles.

10.4.4.4. Special Considerations

Preexisting illness and physiologic reserve

An individual's capacity to withstand a significant trauma may be impacted by several medical conditions that are associated with aging. In addition, these patients have a significant chance of significant morbidity or death due to the physiologic reserve decline that comes with healthy aging.

Medications

Hemodynamic instability after trauma can be made worse by medications, such as antihypertensives, for relatively mild and well-managed conditions. Medicines that block β-adrenergic receptors can conceal the tachycardia brought on by blood loss.

Minimal impact trauma

Relatively minor mechanisms can result in significant injuries. Geriatric patients are more prone to fractures and head injuries. Subdural hematomas are particularly common.

Elder abuse

An increasingly recognized cause of injury to the geriatric population in long-term care facilities is abuse. This should be considered and explored especially in patients who are in care facilities and have reduced mobility or cognitive function.

End-of-life care

When implementing an intervention for a patient, it's critical to take appropriateness into account. Find out the patient's preferences and any prior restrictions on treatment orders, if at all possible. Keep your attention on interventions that can help the patient regain function at a level that they would find satisfying. Talk about this with the patient, their family, or both when you have the chance. You know it can be very tough in the midst of a major trauma.

10.4.5. Trauma in Pregnancy

Pregnant patients are fundamentally managed in the same way as any other trauma victim. The mother's and the fetus's outcomes will be maximized if advanced trauma management is the main focus. However, when treating a pregnant trauma patient, there are some particular issues to take into account. An overview of some of the factors and modifications to be aware of when treating a trauma patient who is pregnant will be provided in this section.

10.4.5.1. Causes of Trauma

Although they are more susceptible to harm, pregnant women experience the same kinds of trauma as non-pregnant women. There are a few unique circumstances to take into account. For instance, intimate partner violence rises in the course of pregnancy and must always be taken into account. Pregnant women also run the risk of not using seatbelts correctly, which can counteract the effectiveness of this countermeasure and cause an injury pattern that is different.

10.4.5.2. Anatomy of Injury

As the fetus develops during the pregnancy, the nature of maternal and fetal injury changes.

First Trimester: 0 to 13 Weeks Gestational Age

The uterus remains an intrapelvic organ; thus, it is well protected from blunt force trauma. There are the "usual" adult injuries to abdominal viscera. The embryo is nonviable; vaginal bleeding is a poor prognostic sign.

Second Trimester: 14 to 26 Weeks Gestational Age

The uterus moves into an extrapelvic position. There is a progressive, increased risk of direct fetal injury. The maternal organs gradually become more shielded.

Third Trimester: 27 to 40 Weeks Gestational Age

The maternal organs are relatively protected from injury by the uterus and fetus. Exception—the bladder is at increased risk. There is an increased likelihood of precipitating early labor.

10.4.5.3. Special Considerations

Maternal Physiology

Maternal physiology undergoes significant change to accommodate the growing fetus. Healthcare providers should be aware of specific changes that have a significant impact on treatment:

- Increased circulating blood volume that can mask significant blood loss
- Compensated respiratory alkalosis with the normal carbon dioxide partial pressure (Pco2) of about 30 mm Hg
- Increased clotting factors or hypercoagulable state toward the end of pregnancy; at term, a fibrinogen of 300 mg/dL would be abnormally low

Aortocaval Compression

In this phenomenon, the inferior vena cava and abdominal aorta may be compressed by the mass of the uterus and fetus, resulting in a 30% reduction in cardiac output. About 20 weeks is when the risk of aortocaval compression becomes clinically significant. A wedge of about 15 to 30 degrees is positioned under the right hip (left tilt) to stop this phenomenon, or the patient can be rotated with the help of a spine board. During a resuscitation, an alternate method is to have a helper manually move the uterus to the patient's left.

Maternal Airway

There is a higher likelihood of difficulty intubating a pregnant patient. This is due to several changes in anatomy and biomechanics:

- Increased generalized soft tissue edema that affects pharyngeal/laryngeal structures
- Increased breast size affecting chest compliance and positioning in the supine position
- Reduced FRC resulting in relatively rapid desaturation
- Lower esophageal sphincter incompetence resulting in higher risk of aspiration

To guarantee that there are no unavoidable negative events, the approach to the mother's airway needs to be done with extreme precision. Similar to patients who are not pregnant, spinal immobilization and adjuncts like video laryngoscopy should be taken into account.

Anti-D Immunoglobulin

Fetal Rh-positive antigen can cause isoimmunization in women with Rh (rhesus)-negative blood types. Patients who have experienced significant trauma during pregnancy, especially those with injuries to the abdomen, should be warned that there may be a chance of blood clots between the mother and the fetus. Anti-D immunoglobulin should be given to an Rh-negative mother to prevent long-term effects on subsequent pregnancies. This can be administered whenever the mother's blood type is established, but it should not be longer than 72 hours following the trauma.

Radiation Exposure

Pregnant women are naturally subjected to a great deal of radiation protection. Delays in diagnosing serious life-threatening conditions are the insult most likely to result in morbidity or death for both the patient and her fetus in the aftermath of a devastating trauma. Should an instantaneous, less radiation-intensive diagnostic modality be available (e.g., ultrasonography), then using it is suitable. Ionizing radiation use should be kept to a minimum while still making sure that the diagnosis is made as soon as possible.

Fetal Monitoring

Maternal stability should be attained before starting fetal monitoring. The people who monitor should be qualified and skilled enough to understand the data. For a fetus less than 24 weeks, continuous fetal monitoring is not advised unless full resuscitation and neonatal intensive care support are planned. Although the length of the monitoring is debatable, the majority of authorities advise starting with two to four hours. The uteroplacental unit's perfusion is not automatically controlled. Thus, even an asymptomatic decrease in the mother's cardiac output can show a marked decrease in the fetus's perfusion. A reevaluation of the mother's hemodynamics should occur upon any worsening of the fetal condition.

Delivery

To maximize either the mother's or the fetus's chances of survival, an early fetal delivery may be required. The only way to guarantee a successful resuscitation and control severe uterine or placental bleeding may be to deliver the fetus. Before performing any kind of surgical delivery, it is advisable to confer with colleagues who specialize in obstetrics and pediatrics. A perimortem cesarean section should be considered in the event of sustained cardiac arrest if spontaneous circulation has not returned after five minutes.

Specific Differential Diagnoses

The following diagnoses are unique to the pregnant patient and should always be considered in addition to standard differential diagnoses.

- An amniotic fluid embolus can cause potentially life-threatening hemodynamic collapse.
- Placental abruption is the process of inappropriate separation of the placenta from the uterine wall. The effect on the mother and fetus depends on the size and location of the disruption. Large disruptions can result in massive hemorrhage and fetal hypoxia.
- **Uterine rupture:** A major trauma can result in loss of containment of the fetus in the uterine cavity. This results in fetal parts being in the mother's abdominal cavity. It is a life-threatening obstetric emergency for both mother and fetus. Women who have had previous cesarean sections are at higher risk.
- **Eclampsia:** Although rare, eclampsia should be considered

in any pregnant woman with an altered conscious state. It is usually associated with hypertension (i.e., arterial blood pressure of more than 140/90 mm Hg) and proteinuria. (Steurer and Ganter, 2014)

10.4.6. Care for Trauma Patients in Non-OR Settings

Anesthesia providers are needed for many procedures performed on trauma patients outside of operating rooms. These processes take place at different resuscitation phases. Because of the unfamiliarity with the surroundings, equipment, and staff, providing care in these environments can present unique challenges. Before receiving additional triage, patients are frequently assessed in the CT scanner. The ICU or radiologic suites for interventional radiology (IR) or magnetic resonance imaging (MRI) are examples of additional locations. It is crucial to collect as much information as possible about the trauma mechanism, prior medical history, injuries, lab results, completed interventions, and the intended course of action. The patient's hemodynamic stability and airway patency should continue to be the anesthesia provider's primary concerns. It is imperative to maintain sufficient patient monitoring during both the procedure and the transport. Notifying trauma surgeons right away of any sudden or severe changes in the patient's condition is important. Respiratory therapists may be available to provide additional support if the patient needs any additional airway interventions or if they already have an established airway.

It is important to have emergency airway equipment and anesthetic induction and hemodynamic support medications on hand at all times. Every location should have access to suction as well, especially if thoracostomy tubes have been implanted. An anesthesia machine and a standard OR cart stocked with basic supplies and medication should be available for IR interventions that call for the presence of an anesthesia provider. The anesthesia provider must be prepared for active cardiopulmonary resuscitation if the patient is undergoing a procedure outside of the operating room and is still in the acute phase of care. This may mean having blood, fluid warmers, large-bore intravenous access, rapid transfusion machines, and invasive monitoring available. Maintaining normothermia and keeping an eye on the patient's temperature are important. Additional assistance from anesthesia technicians, nurses, and other ancillary staff members may be crucial due to the remote nature of certain locations. (World Health Organization, 2014).

A Closer Look

Geriatric Trauma

Geriatric trauma refers to physical injuries sustained by older adults, typically defined as those aged 65 and older, as a result of accidents, falls, or other traumatic incidents. As the global population continues to age, the incidence of geriatric trauma has risen, presenting unique challenges in both prevention and management within the healthcare system.

Older adults are more susceptible to trauma due to age-related changes in their bodies, such as decreased bone density, muscle mass, and sensory perception, which can increase the severity of injuries sustained from falls or accidents. Additionally, pre-existing medical conditions, such as osteoporosis, arthritis, and cognitive impairment, can further complicate the management of trauma in this population.

Falls are the leading cause of geriatric trauma, accounting for a significant proportion of injuries among older adults. Factors contributing to falls in the elderly include environmental hazards, medication side effects, gait and balance issues, and age-related decline in physical function. Fractures, particularly of the hip, spine, and wrist, are common consequences of falls in older adults and can have serious implications for mobility, independence, and overall quality of life.

Traumatic injuries in geriatric patients present unique clinical challenges due to age-related physiological changes, comorbidities, and polypharmacy. Older adults may have atypical presentations of trauma, with symptoms masked by pre-existing medical conditions or cognitive impairment, making timely diagnosis and intervention crucial for optimal outcomes. Additionally, the management of geriatric trauma requires a multidisciplinary approach involving emergency medicine, trauma surgery, geriatrics, rehabilitation, and social support services to address the complex needs of older patients.

Prevention plays a crucial role in reducing the burden of geriatric trauma, with interventions aimed at minimizing fall risk factors, promoting safe environments, and optimizing health and mobility in older adults. Strategies such as home modifications, exercise programs, medication reviews, and vision assessments can help mitigate the risk of falls and injuries among older individuals.

In conclusion, geriatric trauma represents a significant public health concern with implications for healthcare systems, caregivers, and society as a whole. By understanding the unique needs and challenges associated with trauma in older adults, healthcare providers can implement targeted interventions to prevent injuries, improve outcomes, and enhance the overall well-being of this vulnerable population. World Health Organization, 2014.

Summary

- Physiologic derangements in patients who have suffered trauma-induced injuries depend on the mechanism and severity of the injury. Most commonly, hypotension in trauma is the result of severe blood loss or "hemorrhagic shock," which is the main cause of fatality in critically injured patients.
- Hemorrhagic shock and tissue hypoperfusion subsequently lead to complex interactions between inflammatory factors, intrinsic anticoagulants, and other cellular dysfunctions that can cause acute traumatic coagulopathy after injury.
- Mature and complex systems such as health care and trauma require multiple individuals with different and complementary skill sets to work together toward the common goal of achieving the best patient outcomes.
- Graded assertiveness is one technique for communicating personal concerns about decision-making or priorities to the team leader in a way that maintains constructive group performance.
- The spectrum of patients who need to go to the OR for surgical or interventional procedures as a result of trauma is vast. It encompasses injuries of all levels of magnitude in all organs and structures of the human body.
- Permissive hypotension aims to utilize the body's physiologic response to hemorrhage. The resulting low venous and arterial blood pressures and the decrease in cardiac output lead to a reduction in the driving force behind the bleeding.
- Traumatic brain injury (TBI) is defined as an injury to the head that disrupts normal brain function. Over 15 million people are seen in emergency departments for TBI each year and it contributes to 30% of trauma deaths in the United States.
- The patient is usually placed in a reverse Trendelenburg position of approximately 30 degrees during the procedure to facilitate venous drainage.
- Spinal cord precautions should be immediately undertaken when suspecting an injury, including a cervical collar and strict roll precautions whenever transporting or moving patients.
- Fluid management is an important cornerstone of modern burns management; however, controversy still exists about the correct amount of fluid to give and the appropriate endpoints to be monitored.
- Burns are characterized by erythema and the rapid onset of edema in affected tissues. When this happens in the upper airway the swelling can result in total airway obstruction and death.
- Infection is a major cause of delayed morbidity and death. Although empiric antibiotics addressing skin flora are sufficient for the immediate management, coverage of the burn surface with sterile dressings is essential to reestablish the external barrier to organisms.

References

1. Brain Trauma Foundation, American Association of Neurological Surgeons, & Congress of Neurological Surgeons. (2007). Guidelines for the management of severe traumatic brain injury. *Journal of Neurotrauma, 24*(Suppl 1), S1–106.
2. Centers for Disease Control and Prevention. (2015). Injury prevention & control: Data & statistics (WISQARS). Atlanta, GA: Centers for Disease Control and Prevention.
3. Dawson, S., King, L., & Grantham, H. (2013). Improving the hospital clinical handover between paramedics and emergency department staff in the deteriorating patient. *Emergency Medicine Australasia, 25*, 393–405.
4. Duchesne, J. C., McSwain, N. E., Cotton, B. A., et al. (2010). Damage control resuscitation: The new face of damage control. *Journal of Trauma, 69*(4), 976–990.
5. Dutton, R. (2012). Haemostatic resuscitation. *British Journal of Anaesthesia, 109*(Suppl 1), i39–i46.
6. Enlav, S., Sela, H., & Weiniger, C. (2013). Management and outcomes of trauma during pregnancy. *Anesthesiology Clinics, 31*(1), 141–156.
7. Feinman, M., Cotton, B., & Haut, E. (2014). Optimal fluid resuscitation in trauma: Type, timing, and total. *Current Opinion in Critical Care, 20*(4), 366–372.
8. Frieden, T., Houry, D., & Baldwin, G. (2014). Report to Congress on traumatic brain injury in the United States: Epidemiology and rehabilitation. Atlanta, GA: National Center for Injury Prevention and Control, Division of Unintentional Injury Prevention.
9. Ghobrial, G., Amenta, P., & Maltenfort, M. (2014). Longitudinal incidence and concurrence rates for traumatic brain injury and spine injury—A twenty-year analysis. *Clinical Neurology and Neurosurgery, 123*, 174–180.
10. Grathwohl, K., Black, I., & Spinella, P. (2008). Total intravenous anesthesia including ketamine versus volatile gas anesthesia for combat-related operative traumatic brain injury. *Anesthesiology, 109*, 44.
11. Heron, M. (2015). Deaths: Leading causes for 2011. *National Vital Statistics Reports, 64*(7), 1–96.
12. Holly, L. T., Kelly, D. F., Counelis, G. J., et al. (2002). Cervical spine trauma associated with moderate and severe head injury: Incidence, risk factors, and injury characteristics. *Journal of Neurosurgery, 96*(3 Suppl), 285–291.
13. Lancman, B., & Jorm, C. (2015). Taking the heat in critical situations: Being aware, assertive and heard. In R. Iedema, D. Piper, & M. Manidis (Eds.), *Communicating Quality and Safety in Healthcare* (pp. xx–xx). Cambridge, England: Cambridge University Press.
14. MacKenzie, E., Rivara, F., & Jurkovich, G. (2006). A national evaluation of the effect of trauma-center care on mortality. *New England Journal of Medicine, 354*, 366–378.
15. Morrison, J., Dubose, J. J., Rasmussen, T. E., et al. (2012). Military application of tranexamic acid in trauma emergency resuscitation (MATTERs) study. *Archives of Surgery, 147*(2), 113–119.
16. National Spinal Cord Injury Statistical Center. (2013). Facts and figures at a glance. Birmingham, AL: University of Alabama.

17. Roberts, I., Shakur, H., Coats, T., et al. (2013). The CRASH-2 trial: A randomized controlled trial and economic evaluation of the effects of tranexamic acid on death, vascular occlusive events and transfusion requirement in bleeding trauma patients. *Health Technology Assessment, 17*(10), 1–79.

18. Robitaille, A., Williams, S. R., Tremblay, M. H., et al. (2008). Cervical spine motion during tracheal intubation with manual in-line stabilization: Direct laryngoscopy versus Glide Scope video laryngoscopy. *Anesthesia & Analgesia, 106*(3), 935–941.

19. Spahn, D. (2013). Management of bleeding and coagulopathy following major trauma: An updated European guideline. *Critical Care, 17*(2), R76.

20. Steurer, M., & Ganter, M. (2014). Trauma and massive blood transfusions. *Current Anesthesiology Reports, 4*, 200–208.

21. Study Group PROPPR, Holcomb, J. B., Tilley, B. C., Baraniuk, S., et al. (2015). Transfusion of plasma, platelets, and red blood cells in a 1:1:1 vs a 1:1:2 ratio and mortality in patients with severe trauma: The PROPPR randomized clinical trial. *JAMA, 313*(5), 471–482.

22. The SAFE Study Investigators, Australian and New Zealand Intensive Care Society Clinical Trials Group, Australian Red Cross Blood Service, George Institute for International Health, Myburgh, J., Cooper, D. J., Finfer, S., et al. (2007). Saline or albumin for fluid resuscitation in patients with traumatic brain injury. *New England Journal of Medicine, 357*(9), 874–884.

23. Turkstra, T., Craen, R. A., Pelz, D. M., & Gelb, A. W. (2005). Cervical spine motion: A fluoroscopic comparison during intubation with lighted stylet, Glide Scope, and Macintosh laryngoscope. *Anesthesia & Analgesia, 101*(3), 910–915.

24. Vourch, M., Asfar, P., & Volteau, C. (2015). High-flow nasal cannula oxygen during endotracheal intubation in hypoxemic patients: A randomized controlled clinical trial. *Intensive Care Medicine, 41*(9), 1538–1548.

25. Walters, B., Hadley, M., & Hurlbert, R. (2013). Guidelines for the management of acute cervical spine and spinal cord injuries: 2013 update. *Neurosurgery, 60*(Suppl 1), 82–91.

26. Weingart, S., & Levitan, R. (2012). Preoxygenation and prevention of desaturation during emergency airway management. *Annals of Emergency Medicine, 59*(3), 165–175.

27. World Health Organization. (2014). Injuries and violence: The facts 2014. Geneva: World Health Organization.

28. Zeiler, F., Teitelbaum, J., West, M., & Gillman, L. M. (2014). *Neurocritical Care, 21*(1), 163–173.

INDEX

Z

Printed and bound by CPI Group (UK) Ltd, Croydon, CR0 4YY
18/09/2026
14965065-0001